P9-DMB-731

THE FEED ZONE COOKBOOK

THE FEED ZONE COOKBOOK

Fast and Flavorful Food for Athletes

BIJU THOMAS & ALLEN LIM

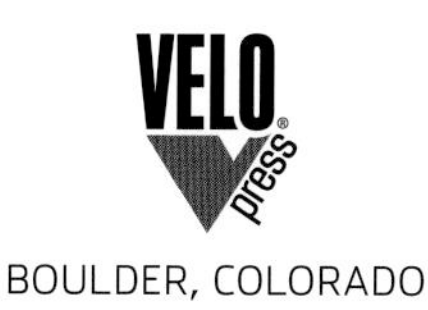

BOULDER, COLORADO

velopress®

3002 Sterling Circle, Suite 100
Boulder, Colorado 80301-2338 USA
(303) 440-0601 ⋆ Fax (303) 444-6788 ⋆ E-mail velopress@competitorgroup.com

Distributed in the United States and Canada by Ingram Publisher Services

Library of Congress Cataloging-in-Publication Data
Thomas, Biju.
The feed zone cookbook: fast and flavorful food for athletes / Biju Thomas and Allen Lim.
p. cm.
Includes index.
ISBN 978-1-934030-76-9 (hardcover: alk. paper)
1. Athletes—Nutrition. 2. Cooking. I. Lim, Allen. II. Title.
TX361.A8T56 2011
613.2024796—dc23
2011028918

For information on purchasing VeloPress books,
please call (800) 811-4210 ext. 2138 or visit www.velopress.com.

★

Text set in Stainless and Caecilia.

12 13 / 10 9 8 7 6 5

CONTENTS

In the Feed Zone Lab

In the Feed Zone Kitchen

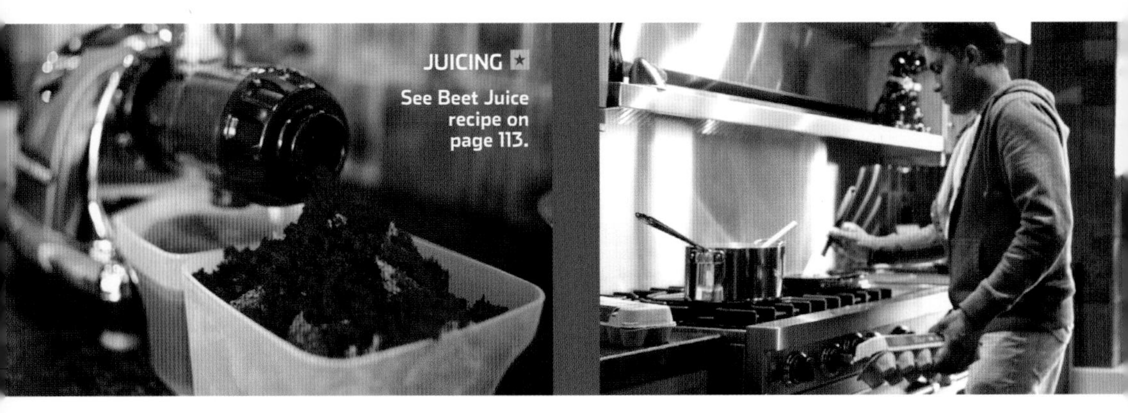
JUICING ★
See Beet Juice recipe on page 113.

"BIJU'S RECIPES ARE MIND-BLOWINGLY SIMPLE, BUT THEIR FLAVORS AND QUALITY ARE AS GOOD AS A FIVE-STAR RESTAURANT. . . . BIJU WILL INSPIRE YOU TO WANT TO COOK." *—Matthew Busche, RadioShack pro cycling team*

Recipes Not to Miss

Portable Foods

At the Back

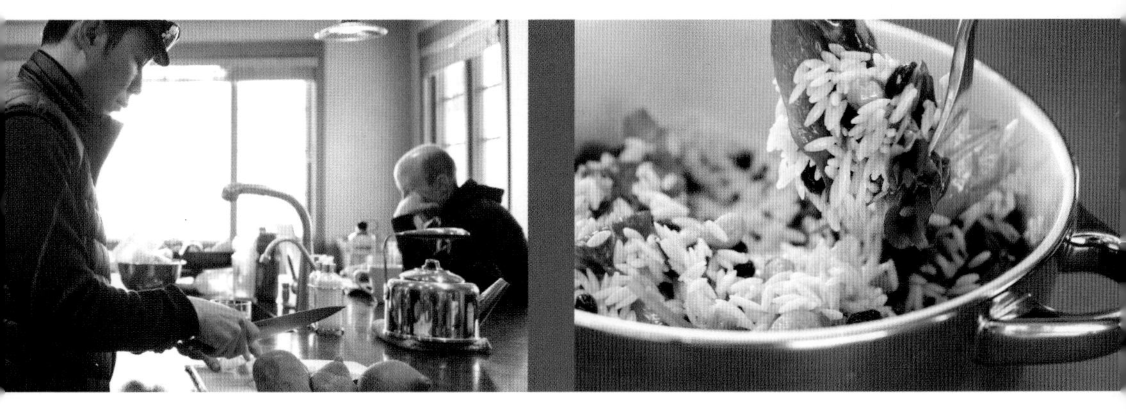

"ALLEN LIM HAS ALWAYS PREACHED EATING REAL, NATURAL FOODS AS THEY PROVIDE FAR MORE OF WHAT WE NEED FOR ENERGY AND RECOVERY THAN ANY SUPPLEMENT. . . ."

—*Lucas Euser, Team SpiderTech*

Foreword

OVER THE COURSE OF MY LAST 15 YEARS AS A PROFESSIONAL CYCLIST, diet and nutrition have played a significant role in my performance, but getting the right food at races hasn't always been possible and didn't become a serious problem for me until the 2011 season. I ended up hospitalized at the Tour of Catalunya in March due to complications that stemmed from an old stomach injury and the poor quality of food at the race.

These health problems came in the midst of early season preparation and I was concerned that I would not be at my best by the Tour of California, which was the most important race of the year for me next to the Tour de France. So I returned to the States to get some rest and to try and get my diet and training back on track. I needed some real help so I asked Allen and Biju if they would be willing to support me during a two-week training camp in Park City, Utah. They agreed and as soon as they arrived they got to work. Not knowing what might cause problems for my stomach, they took a back-to-basics approach: simple meals with minimal ingredients so I could begin to relearn what worked and what didn't.

My mornings started with a big bowl of oatmeal with Biju's toasted nut mix, poached eggs, and a glass of beet juice. For long training rides, I ate primarily chicken sausage rice cakes. After the ride, gluten-free pasta salad, chicken fried rice, or a hot soup. For dinner we had everything from pan-seared steak to pasta with smoked salmon, and Biju's chicken tikka masala, followed by a beautiful salad. For dessert, a big bowl of fruit with honey and yogurt. I felt myself getting stronger every day. I was also learning new recipes and picking up some skills in the kitchen as I watched Biju and Allen cook each day.

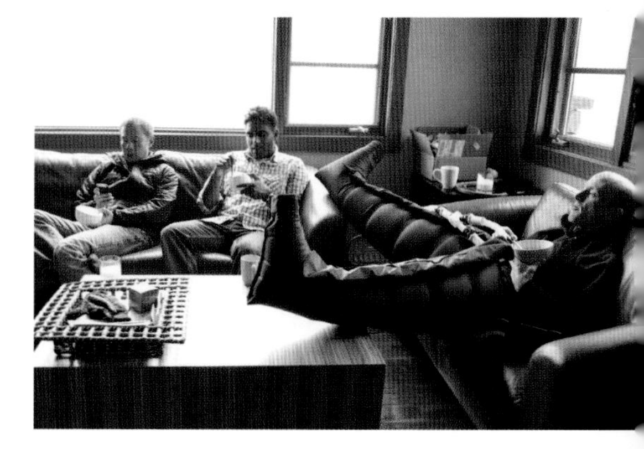

I FELT MYSELF GETTING STRONGER EVERY DAY. ★

AFTER THE BIGGEST WIN OF MY CAREER, **I FOUND MYSELF MAKING BIJU'S RECIPES.**

By the time we were done with the training camp, I was confident that I would have decent form at the Tour of California, but I also knew that it wasn't going to happen unless Biju and Allen came to cook for the team. The night before the start of the race, Biju and Allen showed up in a beat-up "Cruise America" RV. Using two butane burners, one propane stove, and a handful of pots and pans they began cooking the best race food our team has ever eaten. The European riders were totally unaccustomed to eating food this good at a race. They were amazed by how great their legs felt and lamented the fact that they didn't have this advantage earlier in their career.

Best of all, when we sat down at the dinner table for a great meal it took our minds off of the race and brought us together as a team. As we dined on park benches under a borrowed tent, riders who had been on the same team for years were talking, laughing, and telling stories we'd never heard before. We had escaped the typical drudgery of eating for the sake of eating. We felt great and by the end of the race we had won the two hardest stages and finished with Chris Horner winning the overall and me in second.

Right after the Tour of California, I went on to win the Tour of Switzerland, erasing a 2-minute deficit in the final time trial to win by 4 seconds. It was the biggest win of my career and something I could have hardly imagined sitting in the hospital in Spain only 2 months before. Equally surprising was the fact that after that win, I found myself making Biju's recipes. I even made Allen dinner one evening. It wasn't quite as good as Biju's cooking but it was still one of the best pre-Tour meals I've ever cooked. So not only did Biju and Allen help salvage a disastrous start to my 2011 season and turn it into one of my best, they actually got me into the kitchen, cooking these recipes.

LEVI LEIPHEIMER
RADIOSHACK PRO CYCLING TEAM

Foreword

THE FOOD THAT FUELS ME AS AN ATHLETE is incredibly important. On any given day I will only feel as good as the food I have eaten before, during, and after my ride. Garbage in, garbage out.

Nowhere is this more evident than in the middle of a multi-day stage race. Not only is bad food poor athletic fuel, but the last thing I want to see or eat after riding hard for 5 hours for the fourth day in a row is some white bread, pasta, and flavorless boiled chicken. Putting that food into my tired body doesn't do much good, but even more so, it just cracks me mentally.

I know that there are good, healthy, and easily accessible ingredients and dishes out there that would be much better for me in a race. But in a race a cyclist is usually limited to what the team or race organization provides, which is almost always cost-cutting, nutrient-starved dishes. So when the opportunity presented itself at a few races during the 2011 season, Allen and Biju would sneak me some real food—the good stuff—at dinnertime. I would walk past the buffet to a corner in the hallway where they would dish me up some quinoa salad, fresh beets, and a proper piece of meat. Healthy and delicious, those morsels made my day and gave me confidence that I had what I needed to recover properly for the next day of racing.

Immediately following some of the stages at the Tour of California I would sneak out of my team bus to find the little motor home that was Biju's test kitchen. Coconut water and rice cakes were the perfect choices for refueling right after a hard effort. Tasty and effective.

There are so many foods out there that are packed with nutrients, easy to find, and easy to make. *The Feed Zone Cookbook* is full of recipes from Allen and Biju that epitomize the athlete's two greatest purposes in sitting down for a meal: to optimize performance and to maximize the pleasure that comes from eating.

After all, sport is too hard to not enjoy the food that fuels you!

TIMMY DUGGAN
LIQUIGAS-CANNONDALE PRO CYCLING TEAM

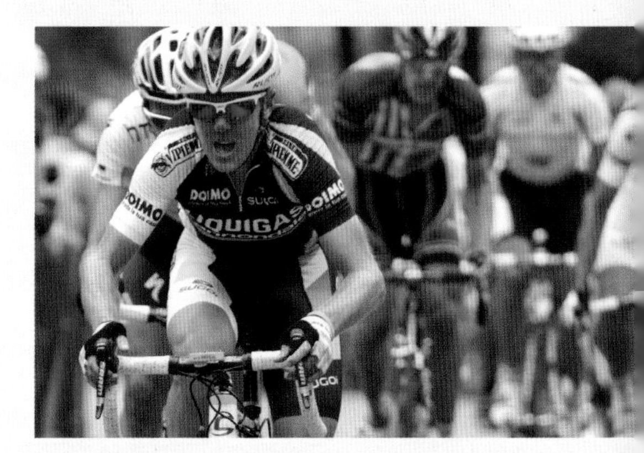

INTRODUCTION

By Allen Lim, Ph.D.

Science and Practice

I started working on the Pro Cycling Tour just a few months after finishing my doctorate in integrative physiology at the University of Colorado at Boulder. I was extremely confident in the quality of my education and the work that I had put into it. I had established an intimate knowledge of energy metabolism, taught courses in exercise physiology and nutrition, and performed research on the physical and metabolic demands of professional cycling in both the lab and the field. When it came to discussing topics like bioenergetics and nutrition, I could talk carbohydrates, fats, and proteins in a kind of caloric cacophony, reciting the precise script of biochemical pathways that controlled them. I knew the science, I was proud of it, and I felt ready to put it into practice.

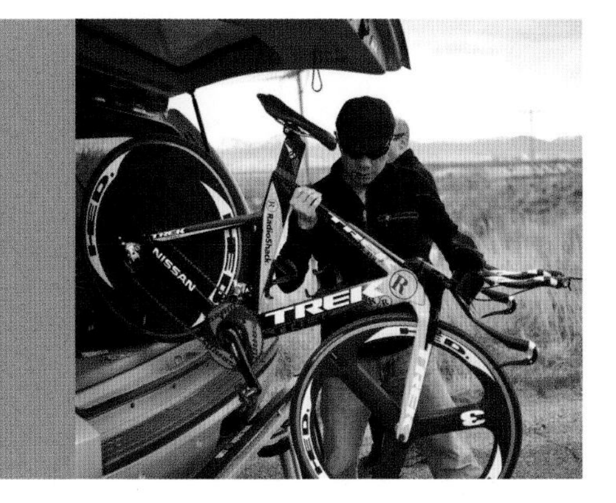

Given my education, it wasn't a surprise that I was constantly being asked questions about what to eat, how much to eat, and when to eat it. However, it became immediately clear that my scientific vocabulary was of little use in helping the athletes I worked with to optimize their diets. Teaching professional athletes the chemistry behind ATP synthesis or the array of steps necessary to store muscle glycogen just didn't matter if I couldn't help them plan the meals they needed throughout their day. I was speaking the wrong language. I wasn't a chef or a dietician. In fact, I wasn't doing much better with my own diet. I'd spent most of the previous decade eating my meals over the kitchen sink, in front of my computer, or while walking across campus—behavior that was perfectly normal for a "starving" graduate student. But on my first night in Europe I watched one of the athletes I was coaching pour a bowl of cereal for dinner, and I knew we all had to do better.

WHILE THERE IS SOMETIMES A LARGE CHASM BETWEEN SCIENCE AND PRACTICE, SUCCESS IN EITHER IS A LOT MORE ABOUT THE PROCESS OF DISCOVERY THAN THE REGURGITATION OF FACTS OR TECHNIQUES. ★

I needed to teach the athletes simple, practical recipes. In some cases I needed to teach them how to shop for food, how to chop vegetables, or how to literally fry an egg. Even for the riders who did have skills in the kitchen, I was continually looking for ways to translate my scientific knowledge into practical meals.

So, like any good scientist, I called my mom. Pen and paper in hand, I bombarded her with questions. What was that thing wrapped in bamboo leaves that we used to eat when I was a kid? What ingredients do I need for that noodle dish? How did you make that amazing curry? And what were those rice cake desserts we use to pick up at the bakery in China Town? When I couldn't find all the answers in science, my instinct was to look for answers in my heritage and upbringing. Michael Pollan summed it up well: "Culture is what your mom fed you."

Fortunately or unfortunately, as a Chinese American immigrant by then living in Europe, the answers I came up with were at times totally incongruous with the old-school European cycling culture I encountered. With little reverence for the conventions that surrounded me, one day I decided to put a rice cooker in the team bus to replace the crusty baguette sandwiches the riders were normally given after the races with fresh rice. I did this not because of something I had read in a scientific journal but because it was easy and because it was what I knew. But for many *soigneurs*, cooks, and especially the team bus driver, this was blasphemy. I was subjected to a load of racial slurs for my disruptive ways, but it was well worth it. The riders appreciated and thrived on the change. The feedback from the riders—their stomachs and their performance—became an essential part of what's guided me in the years since that day.

The rice cooker and all of those recipes from my mom initiated a valuable dialog with the athletes. I started asking them as many questions as they asked me. We began teaching each other. Why do you like eating rice and scrambled eggs for breakfast? Do you think oatmeal with poached eggs works as well? Is a boiled

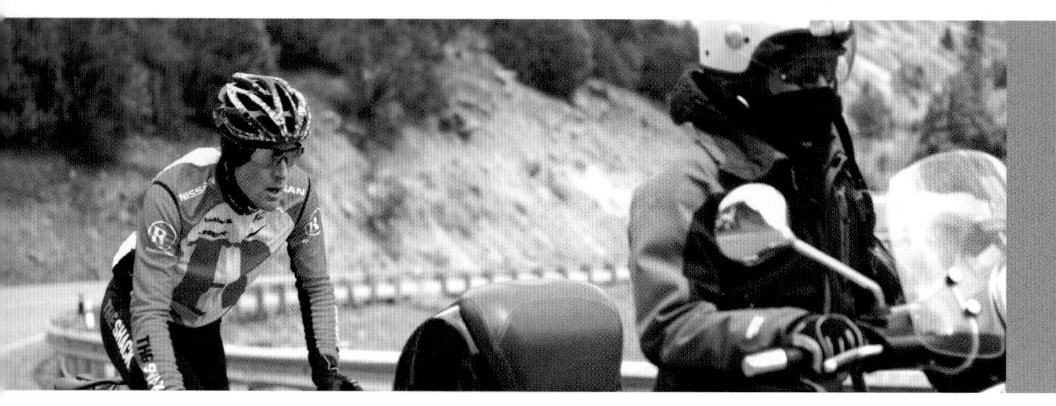

potato with salt and parmesan better or worse than an energy bar? Is it easier on your stomach when you eat the salad before or after the main course? How much fiber can you handle? Do you like Chinese food? For me, this process of question and answer was a natural and exciting one. While there is sometimes a large chasm between science and practice, success in either is a lot more about the process of discovery than the regurgitation of facts or techniques.

A Real-World Study of One

Coming full circle, I've come to lean heavily not on scientific knowledge per se but on the scientific process—on constantly creating and testing questions and possible answers. But unlike research in the lab, practicing science, especially when it comes to diet and nutrition at home or on the road, means embracing individual variability as significant. Everyone is different. Instead of trying to prove that something works for a group, it's often better to recognize when something does or doesn't work for an individual. Rather than shunning science as the wrong language, I started encouraging athletes to become keen observers of their own bodies—to pay careful attention to the relationship between what they eat and how they perform. In science there is a principle called Occam's Razor, which essentially states that all things being equal, the simplest solution or the solution derived from the fewest number of assumptions is the right one. On a very basic level, if something you eat makes you feel like crap, then, all things being equal, stop eating it.

Unfortunately, reality isn't so simple. We make many assumptions based on limited information. Nutrition and nutrition science are complex and ever-changing fields. Every year new knowledge is created that can both inform and confuse the process. Add to this the incredible number of food products and supplements claiming to make us champions. From energy bars to gels and shakes, the sheer hype and volume of information can easily conflict and overwhelm.

Beyond these products and supplements, there are also far too many diet trends being pushed to athletes that cover the spectrum from veganism to paleoism, from gluten-free to gluten-rich. While some diets are based on blood type and others on body type, what they all have in common are bold claims and fervent believers.

However, the real problem, the real complication, is the fact that we are all human. Our diets are easily influenced not only by trends but by personal preference and the ease or availability of certain food products. We all have our guilty pleasures, foods we love to eat even though we know they don't always make us feel good or perform well. But what we eat is fundamentally an opportunity for and a reflection of personal responsibility.

It's true that the human body is extremely adaptable. I have seen athletes survive some of the biggest races in the world on diet plans, foods, and products as varied as their individual personalities and cultures. But our goal here is to do more than survive. Our goal is to optimize and

REGARDLESS OF DIET, PREFERENCE, OR THEME, WHAT SEPARATES A GOOD DIET FROM A GREAT DIET ARE THE INGREDIENTS ONE STARTS WITH. › BEGIN WITH FRESH, WHOLE FOODS THAT COME IN THEIR OWN WRAPPER WITH AS MANY OF THEIR PARTS INTACT AS POSSIBLE. ★

thrive—to use real food as a real weapon. What you call your diet or how you label it is far less important than the ingredients you use to build it. Like proper training, the inherent quality and diversity of what we choose to eat is key to optimal health and performance.

A Better Way to Eat

This idea about quality and diversity is essential to how I've come to see nutrition. Regardless of diet, preference, or theme, what separates a good diet from a great diet are the ingredients one starts with. Begin with fresh, whole foods that come in their own wrapper with as many of their parts intact as possible—foods that are minimally processed, grown locally and preferably organically by real farmers, not by multinational corporations.

With respect to variety, we are quick to deconstruct our foods as carbohydrates, fats, proteins, and calories or by their fiber, mineral, vitamin, sodium, or antioxidant content. But this classification does little to inform us about the incredible number of vegetables, fruits, grains, and life that exists on the planet that we use as food sources. More important, our current reductionist thinking barely addresses all of the unique and distinct effects that whole foods can have on the complex array of systems controlling our mind and body. As an example, quercitin, a powerful antioxidant commonly found in foods like apples and onions, has been heavily marketed in recent years as a potent nutritional supplement. But quercitin is only one of hundreds of flavonoids or polyphenols found in fruits and vegetables. While it may be purported as an "all-star" compound, there's controversy as to whether it works as well on its own compared to when it's supported by its entire team, as is the case when it's part of a whole food. In fact, most natural systems exhibit a phenomenon called emergence, which describes properties or attributes that can't be explained by the individual parts that make them up. The joy we get from a home-cooked dinner with friends and family is a simple example of emergence and the

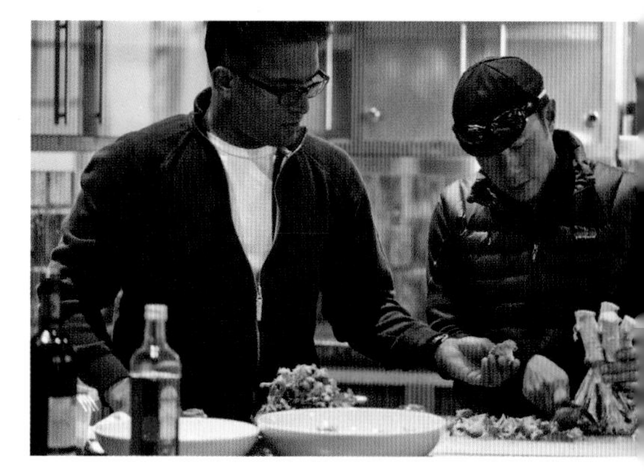

benefit of adopting a holistic approach to food even as an athlete.

Regardless of your athletic talent or aspirations, the meals that fuel you are best when made, as much as possible, from scratch and with real intent and care. However, making meals from scratch and taking the time out of our already busy schedules is hard. This fact has spawned many of the processed and pre-packaged products we commonly think of as sports food or accept as part of the American diet. Though these products are convenient and can play an important role in supplementing an athlete's diet, this convenience belies a simple truism about athletics: Being an athlete is hard. And if you want to reach your potential, it's unlikely that the best way will be easier or more convenient.

Perhaps this is why the hardest job at the Tour de France, aside from riding in it, is the work taken on by the team chef. The inherent difficulty, importance, and emergence associated with preparing fresh, wholesome dishes make the team chef one of the most important staff members on a professional cycling team.

Over the past several years, I've had the great privilege of working with a number of incredible chefs at some of the world's biggest cycling events, including the Tour de France. Some, like Americans Barbara Grealish and Sean Fowler, who cook domestically and in Europe, respectively, for the Garmin professional cycling team, have been incredibly influential in helping me understand how to better feed and nourish the athletes I work with. They had the skills that were a critical bridge between theory and execution. I've also spent a great deal of time fighting with the "old-school Euro" chefs on the Tour—a fact that further highlights the cultural biases we all, including myself, literally bring to the table.

Chef Biju

Regardless of perspective, however, having someone cook for you or fighting over what someone cooks for you is very different than having the know-how and motivation to

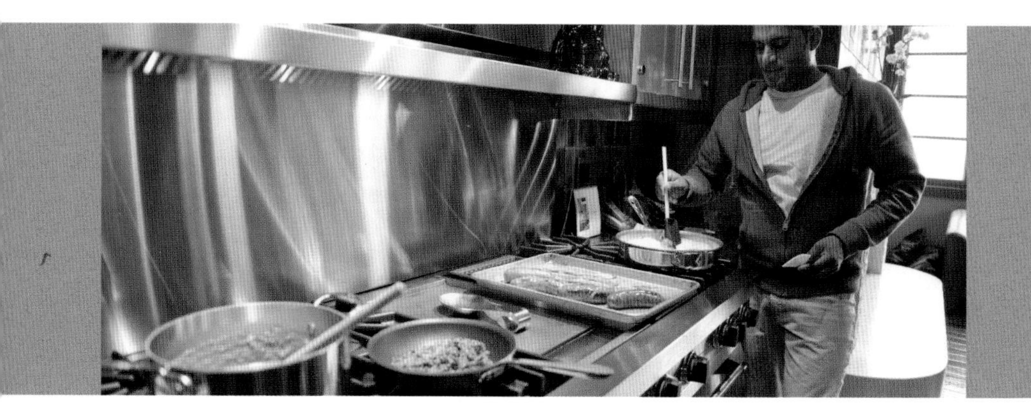

cook for yourself. For me, this knowledge and motivation really came together after I met Chef Biju Thomas. Biju was catering a dinner party for Jonathan Vaughters, the founder of the Garmin professional cycling team, whom I had been working for at the time. His meal was incredible—not just delicious but profoundly simple and nourishing. I immediately began talking to Biju about his cooking style, about food, and about helping me make great nutrition through great meals more accessible for the athletes I coached.

Biju and I quickly became friends through the process. Not only did we share a common love of food and cycling, we had similar upbringings. We both immigrated to and were raised in the United States, we both grew up riding and racing bikes, and we were both caught between incredibly diverse food cultures that ran the gamut from ethnic street food to over-the-top family gatherings that featured recipes from India, where Biju is from, or from China and the Philippines, where my family is from. Through our shared experiences and especially through Biju's passion and talent, we took our conversations about diet and nutrition a step further; instead of talking with athletes about food theory, we began actually cooking with them, not just cooking for them.

This book is a manifestation of countless conversations, endless days on the road in hotel kitchens, race meals made in cramped motor homes, and the often comical times cooking with our very close friends, many of whom just happen to be some of the best professional cyclists in the world. We put this book together not as a bible or manifesto on diet and nutrition but as a reference for athletes looking for no-nonsense, race-proven ideas, who are also willing to take the time and energy to cook the recipes that we know just work.

These recipes and the format they are laid out in also reflect a dichotomy we all experience in both sport and life—the balance between sitting down for a home-cooked meal versus having to eat on the run or, more aptly, on the bike. Some meals are handheld or portable to accommodate eating in the middle of a race or on the way to the office after a hard morning of training.

WE BELIEVE THAT BY SHOWING YOU RECIPES WE USE AND LOVE, INSTEAD OF ARGUING OVER THIS VERSUS THAT, WE CAN BETTER HELP YOU REACH YOUR GOALS. ★

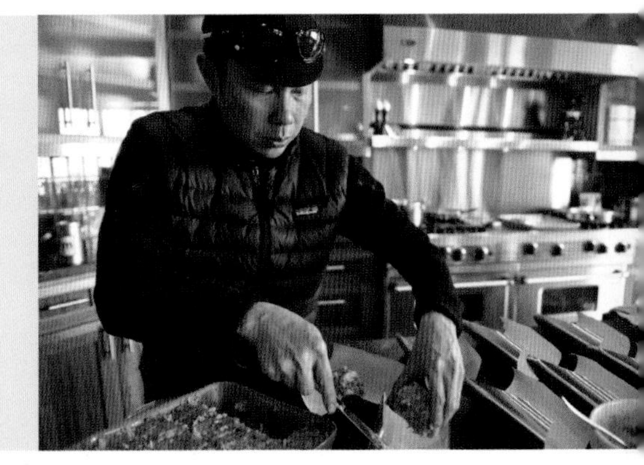

AS NIETZSCHE PUT IT, "YOU HAVE YOUR WAY. I HAVE MY WAY. AS FOR THE RIGHT WAY, THE CORRECT WAY, AND THE ONLY WAY, IT DOES NOT EXIST." ★

What all these recipes have in common are fresh, wholesome ingredients that stand up to the demands of performance and fit into our busy schedules.

Because these meals are designed to feed athletes who are committed to maximizing their potential, they are clearly not designed for losing weight or to treat disease or to promote a particular diet agenda. Harold and Kumar may have gone to White Castle, but Biju and I went to a whole lot of bike races. As a result, many of these meals are carbohydrate-heavy, do have a lot of fat, and do have more salt than many nutritionists or doctors would consider healthy. Yes, we use a lot of cholesterol-laden eggs and a lot of white rice in our recipes as well as real sugar instead of artificial sweeteners, butter instead of margarine, and the occasional bar of chocolate. Moreover, we realize and make no apologies for the fact that no matter how hard we try, these recipes are not without our own cultural and life biases because, right or wrong, they are born from actual experiences with real athletes as well as some pretty good ideas from our moms.

We believe that by showing you recipes we use and love, instead of arguing over this versus that, we can better help you reach your goals. We know that cooking real food is much better than tearing open packages for dinner because a scientist in a laboratory claims that the globs of deconstructed food bits inside of them will increase your maximal oxygen consumption. So we hope you enjoy and we encourage you to experiment, to play and tinker with our recipes, to figure out what works for you, and to realize that at the end of the day, you alone are responsible for your health, well-being, and performance.

★★★ **This book is a manifestation of** countless conversations, endless days on the road in hotel kitchens, **race meals made in cramped motor homes**, and the often comical times cooking with our very close friends, many of whom just happen to be some of the best professional cyclists in the world. › We put this book together not as a bible or manifesto on diet and nutrition but as a **reference for athletes looking for no-nonsense, race-proven ideas**, who are also willing to take the time and energy to cook the delicious recipes that we know just work.

In the Feed Zone Lab

Food Timing

When it comes to meals for athletes, it's rare for a day to be made up of a traditional breakfast, lunch, and dinner. Our focus is on timing our food with training or racing: pre-workout, workout, and post-workout. Because most of our riders still eat breakfast and dinner at a normal hour relative to the rest of the world, we've kept the breakfast and dinner categories. However, the approach to these meals will still be somewhat unconventional for endurance athletes. We have also added "Portables" and "Après" menus to bring attention to what you eat during training and immediately afterward.

PRE-WORKOUT

In general, most athletes find that eating about 3 hours before competition or about 2 hours before training works very well. When competing, it's important to give yourself ample time to digest your food and to be very satiated by your pre-competition meal. Sometimes athletes will have a little snack (typically a rice cake) or energy drink about 30 minutes before competition to keep their blood sugar normal.

In training, there can be more flexibility, depending upon its nature. A lot of the pros tend to spend their first hour on the bike going easy or warming up, so they can afford to eat a little closer to training.

One thing to realize, however, is that eating about 1 to 1½ hours before training or competition can lead to a really rough first hour. This is because insulin levels spike at about 1 to 1½ hours after eating. This can cause a short-term dip in blood glucose levels as insulin works to clear glucose from the blood stream—a situation that can be exacerbated by exercising muscles that can take up glucose without the need for insulin. As a result, some athletes often feel a little hypoglycemic, or "bonky," during the first part of their ride. I've seen some riders wait until they start exercising to eat if they are running late for a training ride. It's not an optimal approach, but sometimes it works better than crashing during the 1- to 1½-hour window. I also recommend foods with a little more fat and protein prior to long workouts. A lower glycemic index can help prevent the big blood-sugar spikes.

WORKOUT

When exercising, especially if the activity is very hard, I recommend that athletes replace about half of the calories they burn per hour with calories from solid food and a 4 percent sports drink (4 grams per 100 ml, or about 80 kcals per 500 ml water bottle). For a pro cyclist in a typical race this formula may work out to about 100 grams of carbohydrate, or 400 kcals per hour.

POST-WORKOUT

After racing or training more than 4 hours, it's critical that you eat at least 4 grams of carbohydrate per kilogram of body weight within 30 minutes of finishing. For exercise lasting less than 2 hours, the goal is 2 grams of carbohydrate per kilogram of body weight. This amounts to about 500 to 1,000 kcals for a 150-pound athlete, depending on the duration of training. Generally speaking, this means that you will eat as much as possible right after getting off the bike if it has been a hard day of training. After an easy day of training, you will eat enough to take the edge off. We need to eat immediately after exercise because our muscles are extremely sensitive to insulin during this time. Insulin brings carbohydrate into the muscle, where it can be stored as glycogen. Consequently, eating right after exercise helps to better restore muscle glycogen.

For some athletes, just changing the timing of when they eat can be the difference between adequate and inadequate muscle glycogen stores, even if the total calories ingested are the same. When you eat foods with a very high glycemic index immediately after exercise, you increase the speed at which calories are replaced. In fact, post-exercise is one of the few times that you can indulge in sweets and desserts with fewer negative consequences.

DINNER

For most athletes, dinner will be eaten between 6 p.m. and 8 p.m., depending on the training day. When athletes have a calorically adequate and nutritious meal immediately after exercise, dinner is usually the one meal where I caution them against overindulging and encourage them to eat the bulk of their daily greens, fruits, and vegetables. Of course, every training day and situation may be different, but in training it normally works best if you don't stuff yourself at dinner. In contrast, the opposite tends to be true in stage races. That is, make sure you're satiated and full in the middle of a competition.

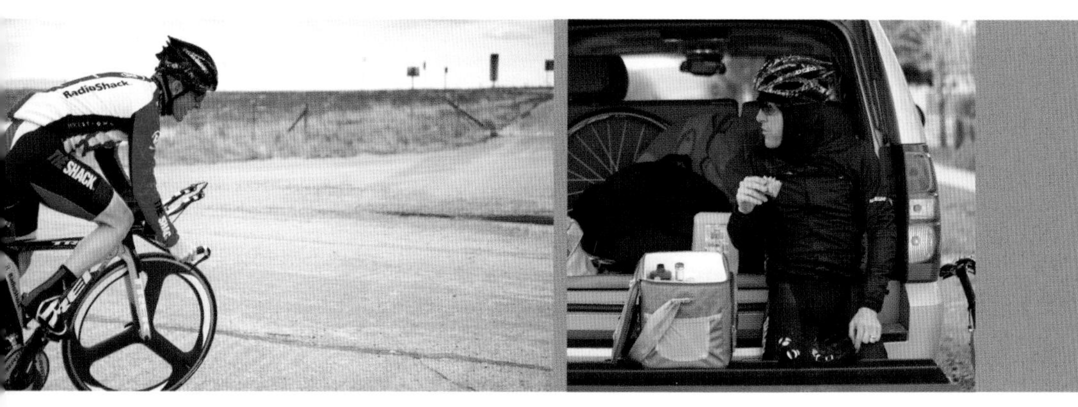

THERE'S NO DOUBT THAT THE EFFORT OF COUNTING CALORIES AND BEING EDUCATED ABOUT THE FOODS YOU EAT CAN GO A LONG WAY TO HELPING YOU MAINTAIN OR REACH AN OPTIMAL BODY WEIGHT. ★

How Hungry Are You?

I've spent much of my professional career thinking about, measuring, and researching energy balance. So when portable power meters like the CycleOps PowerTap became readily available and it became possible to directly measure how much energy a cyclist transferred to the bike, I knew we had reached a landmark in training technology (see "How a Power Meter Measures Calories"). There's no doubt that power meters have transformed the sport of cycling. And unlike other sports, it's now possible to directly measure how many calories you're burning on the bicycle, giving you an exact figure to gauge how much you need to refuel.

While this technology helps us to know how many calories we've burned in training, it doesn't tell you how much you need to eat to stay in energy balance over the course of the day. There are still the calories you need to fuel your activity outside of training, which can be very difficult to measure. You still need to read food labels or look up calorie estimates for whole foods. And finally, you still need to keep track of the actual food you eat as well as portion sizes. It may be a lot of work, but there's no doubt that the effort of counting calories and being educated about the foods you eat can go a long way to helping you maintain or reach an optimal body weight. This is one of the reasons why we've included the nutritional information for each recipe in the book. To keep things easier, the nutritional information at the bottom of the recipe covers just the recipe in its simplest form. Nutrition facts for optional ingredients can be found in Appendix A.

HOW A POWER METER MEASURES CALORIES

A power meter measures energy mechanically using units of measure called joules. One thousand joules is equal to 1 kilojoule, also written as a kjoule or a kj.

Energy in food, however, is measured as the amount of heat given off when that food is burned using units of measure called calories. One thousand calories is equal to 1 kilocalorie, also written as a kcal or as a Calorie with a capital "C" on nutrition labels in the United States.

One kcal or Calorie is roughly equivalent to 4 kjoules (1 kcal = 4.126 kjoule). So, if you burn 100 Calories of food on the bike, that would be equivalent to 400 kjoules of energy released by your body. But the human body is only about 20 to 25 percent mechanically efficient, meaning only about a quarter of the

This is all good information, but there are even easier methods for determining how much to eat. The bottom line is that most of us know when we've had too much to eat. Most of us know when we're hungry. On the Pro Cycling Tour, just like in real life, the riders don't eat their meals with a scale on the table to measure their portions. We don't follow our riders around with face masks or make them sleep in hermetically sealed rooms with temperature sensors to measure metabolic rate. Like you and me, cyclists look at themselves in the mirror, twist and turn, and maybe even jump up and down a bit to see what jiggles and then wait for the narcissism or self-loathing to begin (as if it weren't already in full bloom).

At the end of the day, your gut is the best barometer for how much to eat. As a general rule of thumb, when you're in a period when you're not training or are training very little, it's okay to be hungry. When you are training, be a little hungry. And when you're getting close to a major competition or event and when you are competing, make sure that you aren't hungry.

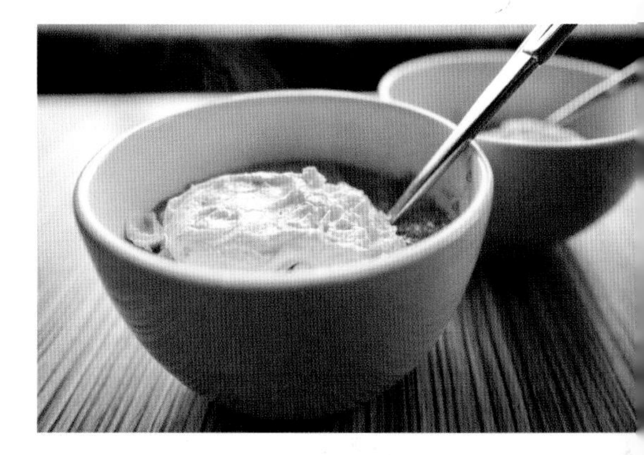

When you are racing in any endurance sport, one of the last things you want to happen is to bonk, to hit that point where you're out of muscle glycogen, chewing at your own flesh, totally disoriented as your blood sugar drops like the stock market in the middle of a Bernie Madoff–induced crash.

This possibility scares me so much that while driving support behind Ben King during his solo breakaway at the US Pro Championships, I drove right next to him

energy we burn actually gets transferred to the bicycle to turn the pedals. As a result, a power meter measures only 20 to 25 percent of the energy we burn. The rest is wasted as heat. If you burn 100 Calories of food on the bike, which is equivalent to 400 kjoules, your power meter will read 100 to 120 kjoules of work.

To clarify, if you have a power meter and it reads 1,000 kj (i.e., kilojoules, or kjoules) at the end of a ride, by a quirk of nature, this is equivalent to 1,000 to 1,200 kcals of energy that your body has burned. And since we substitute the word Calorie with a capital "C" in the United States to denote a kcal, a 1,000-kj ride is equivalent to what we normally think of as 1,000 to 1,200 food Calories (on nutrition labels in the United States) or 1,000 to 1,200 kcals (on nutrition labels in most other countries).

when he slowed a bit just before the final hour of the race and started yelling at him to eat and drink as much as possible. He asked me, "How much?" and I screamed back at him in a frantic rage, "Until you start to throw up on yourself!" He pounded a Coke, drank a bottle of water, and gorged on whatever was in his pockets. He then went on to make history by being the youngest rider to ever win the US Pro Championships. Despite my advice, he never puked on himself.

While sometimes you want to eat as much as possible, other times you need to figure out ways to eat less. Just before the Tour de France, Levi Leipheimer was impressed by how satiated he felt after eating watermelon, excited that he had just found a low-calorie food that could help him take the edge off his final push to make race weight for the Tour. Reclining in satisfaction for a moment in his La-Z-Boy after just putting down four watermelon wedges, he suddenly freaked out, wondering if the reason he felt full had nothing to do with the water and bulk of the watermelon but its caloric content. Jumping out of his chair, he yelled, "How many calories are there in watermelon?" I yelled back, "I have no clue." He rushed to his computer and started searching and returned 85 Calories per 250-gram wedge, or about 340 Calories for the four wedges he'd just eaten. Not knowing if that was good or bad, I pointed out that the 1,000 grams of melon he'd eaten would be equivalent to 4,000 Calories if it were pasta or 9,000 Calories if it were a stick of butter. Satisfied, he returned to his chair, his melon belly well calibrated and content. Less than an hour later, he was hungry again.

Hunger's Reality Check

To make sure that your hunger barometer is on track, it's also a good idea to get a body weight scale and track changes in your weight over the long haul. A scale offers consistent and objective feedback, which can help us to better understand how our training, rest, and diet affect our performance and our body.

GOING TO BED HUNGRY

I've seen a number of athletes gauge hunger in relation to how they sleep. This seems to work well because most of the riders I work with know that they still need to eat enough to be able to train productively. Much of the caloric monitoring and potential hunger tends to happen in the evenings, and this can have a direct bearing on how they feel before falling asleep. If they eat too little and are really hungry, they might have difficulty falling asleep. If they eat just enough, they might be a little hungry when they go to bed, or at least hungry enough that they could have a glass of almond or rice milk (I don't know a lot of riders who drink real milk) and a cookie (I know a lot of riders who like eating cookies). Although they are aware of this level of hunger, it isn't enough to disturb their sleep. If they overeat, they tend to fall asleep easily, resting peacefully in their

Another good reason for a scale and frequent weighing is to understand the natural fluctuations that occur throughout the day and season. Depending upon our hydration status, there can be big peaks and valleys in our body weight. The extra power that you gain from an increase in body water always improves your power-to-weight ratio. In contrast, a drop in power caused by dehydration is not offset by the drop in weight, leading to a decrease in your power-to-weight ratio. Getting used to these daily fluctuations in your body weight allows you to gain perspective on your actual race weight rather than getting fixated on what might otherwise be a lot of noise.

Divergent Ideas on Diet

TO CARB OR NOT TO CARB

There is an overwhelming amount of scientific and real-world evidence that demonstrates that a diet rich in carbohydrates is critical to success in endurance

MAKING WEIGHT

If you are interested in **losing weight**, I recommend that you make it your goal to lose **one pound per week**. One pound of fat is equivalent to 3,500 Calories. This amounts to a 500-Calorie deficit each day, which means you will be going to bed a little hungry.

In the meantime, some additional things that might help the process of controlling body weight include **getting more sleep, exercising before breakfast, watching fat intake, eating smaller meals more frequently** throughout the day to take the hunger edge off, and **drinking lots of fluids** or **eating more bulky, high-fiber foods**, which can help you feel satiated on fewer calories.

little food coma. But if they really overeat, especially on kilos of raw scampi in Italy, the thermic effect of food or energy needed just to digest turns them into hot furnaces, and they have real problems all night. Understand that this is completely anecdotal and I have no idea if there is a causal relationship between daily fluctuations in energy balance and sleep. It's just another observation made from where I stand in the carbon-spandex jungle.

*** As a general rule of thumb, when you're in a period **when you're not training or are training very little, it's okay to be hungry.** When you are training, be a little hungry. And when you're getting close to a major competition or event and **when you are competing, make sure that you aren't hungry.**

THERE IS AN OVERWHELMING AMOUNT OF SCIENTIFIC AND REAL-WORLD EVIDENCE THAT DEMONSTRATES THAT A DIET RICH IN CARBOHYDRATES IS CRITICAL TO SUCCESS IN ENDURANCE SPORTS. ★

sports. Carbohydrates are stored in the body as liver and muscle glycogen. Without it, an athlete's ability to perform at high intensity is severely diminished, and when it is depleted the dreaded bonk is a distinct possibility.

Fear of glycogen shortfalls has spawned carbohydrate-loading strategies among endurance athletes, especially in the week or days leading up to an event. Many athletes eat as much as 10 grams of carbohydrate per kilogram of body weight per day before an event. For an average male rider weighing 154 pounds, or 70 kg (2.2 lbs, per kg), that's 700 grams of carbohydrate per day. At 4 Calories per gram of carbohydrate, that's 2,800 Calories. Eating lots of carbohydrate is a logical and straightforward idea.

There is also research that calls this strategy into question. By severely limiting carbohydrate intake while training, athletes deplete glycogen stores. The theory is that while athletes are training in a glycogen-depleted state, significant adaptations are made in their ability to utilize fat as a fuel source, hopefully helping to spare glycogen sometime in the future. As the glycogen-depleted athlete gets close to competition, there is a shift back to a high-carbohydrate diet. Having been severely depleted, the body super-compensates, allowing more glycogen to be stored. By competition time, the athlete will theoretically enjoy the best of both worlds—an enhanced fat-burning ability that spares glycogen and more glycogen on board for the critical high-intensity efforts that can make or break races.

As interesting as this train–low glycogen, race–high glycogen idea is, it does come with risk. I tried this strategy with Blake Caldwell in 2008, the year that he placed second at the US Pro Championships by about 1 pixel. Earlier that summer, enthusiastic to try the new strategy, Blake significantly reduced his carbohydrate intake during an incredibly difficult training block that had him setting out from Girona, Spain, on long rides to the Pyrenees. Unfortunately, the added stress was too much, and the scales tipped. Blake became very sick and lost about a week of training. Blake is the most even-tempered rider I've ever known, but I've never seen anyone as angry with anyone as he was with me for suggesting the change in diet (and rightfully so).

Blake doesn't race professionally anymore, so we can joke about that time when I told him not to eat carbs and then sent him off to ride in the Pyrenees. Ever since that experience, I've been extremely careful about watching an athlete's carbohydrate intake. I still believe the idea of short-term depletion has merit, but it needs to be done, if at all, with real care and caution.

GLUTEN

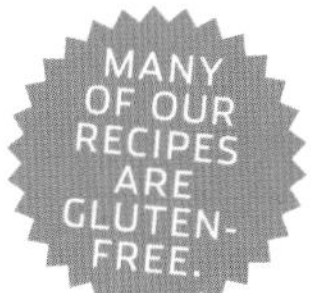
MANY OF OUR RECIPES ARE GLUTEN-FREE.

In the 2008 Tour de France, the Garmin cycling team did something that no other team had done before—the team went almost entirely gluten-free, or, more correctly, wheat-free. The idea came about when some of our doctors hypothesized that going wheat-free would help reduce the inflammatory load on our riders over the course of the race. A few of our athletes knew they were sensitive to wheat and had already successfully changed their diet. This made it easier to entertain the idea of putting the entire team on a similar diet.

But to shun pasta at the Tour de France? That's like going to China and not eating rice. Actually, it's exactly like going to France and not eating bread—a bit loony and seemingly impossible. Even though there wasn't much if any evidence supporting the notion that athletes without celiac disease would fare better on a gluten-free diet, I was eager to see what would happen. Moreover, because my own diet had never relied heavily on wheat for obvious cultural reasons, I thought it was an idea worth exploring.

So we did it. While David Millar and Danny Pate totally cracked by the end of the Tour, the rest of the riders all felt that the change really helped them. Most typically, they noted that they didn't feel as bloated or heavy, were mentally sharper, and had fewer stomach problems. Whether this was due to the removal of gluten or just due to our chef Sean Fowler's amazing cooking, we will never know. We didn't draw blood and look for any inflammatory markers—we only had experience to guide us.

Since then, I've had other athletes try a wheat-free diet, and the reviews are mixed and highly individual. After Biju spent a week cooking gluten-free for Lance Armstrong, Lance gave the definitive thumbs-down on the project, while his close friend, John "College" Korioth (who was on the same diet and training with Lance), had one of his best weeks ever on the bike.

Some riders have listened to their bodies to craft their own strategy. Levi Leipheimer and Christian Vande Velde occasionally

TO DATE, I'M NOT AN ADVOCATE OF EITHER A GLUTEN-FREE OR A GLUTEN-RICH DIET. BUT IF ATHLETES TELL ME THEY ARE DOING BETTER WITHOUT WHEAT, REGARDLESS OF THE PRESENCE OR ABSENCE OF CELIAC DISEASE, I AM LIKELY TO BELIEVE THEM. ★

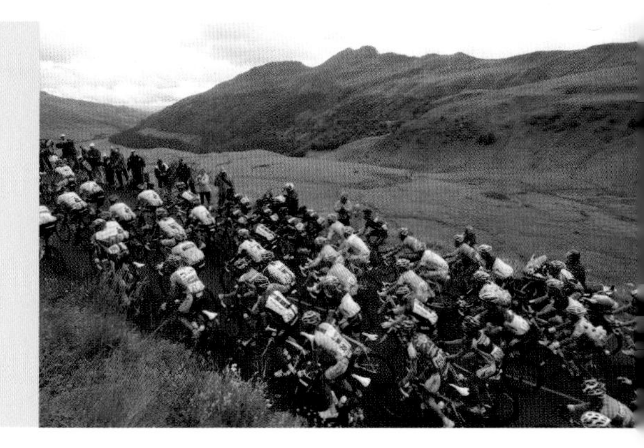

adopt a gluten-free diet while making weight or racing, and eat a more traditional diet in the off-season or during periods demanding more calories and glycogen. This mixed approach seems to work well for them. Like most ideas in this book, you need to carefully experiment and decide what's right for you.

To date, I'm not an advocate of either a gluten-free or a gluten-rich diet. But if athletes tell me they are doing better without wheat, regardless of the presence or absence of celiac disease, I am likely to believe them. For this reason, many of our recipes are gluten-free.

Whether the recipes contain gluten or not, we worked hard to make sure that each dish is nutritious and tastes great. In fact, at the 2011 Tour of California, Biju and I tested most of these wheat-free recipes on the RadioShack professional cycling team without telling them. One evening we brought a huge bowl of gluten-free quinoa-based pasta to the dinner table. On first bite, some of our European riders, Markel Irizar, Dmitriy Muravyev, and Haimar Zubeldia—riders who would not be caught dead at a bike race without pasta—began raving. I let Levi Leipheimer break the news that this was not their mom's pasta. By the end of the race, the entire team had one of its strongest performances to date, with Chris Horner and Levi Leipheimer finishing first and second, respectively.

WHERE'S THE MEAT?

At the 2011 Tour de France, David Zabriskie started the race intending to do something few other athletes have been known to do at the Tour—rely on a vegan diet (with the occasional piece of fish) to get him around France. Whether a vegan diet works for an athlete competing at one of the hardest sporting events in the world is debatable. If you believe the rest of the 197 Tour riders not on this diet, the answer would be no.

Today's Tour de France athlete may need anywhere from 1.5 to 2 grams of protein per kilogram of body weight per day. This is due to the long duration and intensity of the Tour, which makes it difficult to take in

GET IN ON THE SECRET

It's difficult to find a sports drink that is not full of artificial colors, artificial sweeteners, and synthetic flavoring agents. When I worked with the Garmin team, our athletes often complained of stomach problems after a few hours—the notorious sugar "gut rot." Like most athletes, their solution was to dilute their sports drink, but this in turn dilutes valuable sodium intake.

To solve this problem and create a more natural product, I began working with Dr. Stacy Sims from Stanford University, and in 2009 we started to make a custom sports drink from scratch that does not contain any excess ingredients. If you are looking for a wholesome sports drink alternative, ours may be ordered online at www.secretdrinkmix.com.

enough carbohydrate. When this happens, the body turns to protein as a fuel source. But at 1.5 to 2 g per kg of protein, a 70-kg (154-lb.) Tour rider would need 115 to 140 grams of protein per day—the equivalent of 19 to 23 eggs, which is a tough mark to hit. However, if an athlete eats enough carbohydrate during a race, protein will be spared as a fuel source.

Given that David has been a professional cyclist for 12 years, I really believe he knows his body best. After all, he began having one of the best seasons of his entire career when he started eating vegan. If anyone could finish the Tour on a vegan diet, it would be David, and I, for one, was rooting for him. Unfortunately, David was forced to abandon the Tour on stage 9 after breaking his wrist in a high-speed crash. That's a situation that diet couldn't prevent.

We've included vegetarian dishes in this cookbook because when you are not competing at the professional level it's more feasible to maintain a vegetarian or vegan diet, as most people require only 0.5 to 1.0 grams of protein per kilogram of body weight per day. In addition, most of the breakfast, portable, and après dishes in this book can be made with or without meat depending upon your own preference.

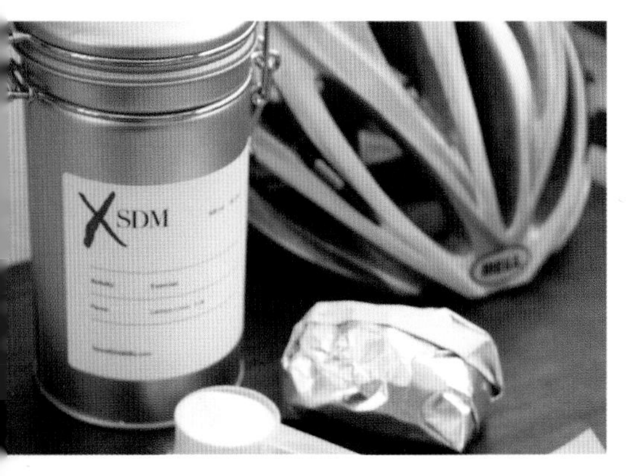

Hydration

With all of this talk about food, we would be remiss if we didn't also talk about one of my personal obsessions—proper hydration. While we can live for weeks without food, we can only live for a few days without water. This same concept applies to performance. We have enough glycogen and fat stored in our bodies to allow us to perform at a wide range of intensities and durations without eating, but we would not be able to sustain these same performances without drinking.

Similar to our philosophy on food, we believe that starting out with the best ingredients and not having a bunch of artificial or superfluous ingredients is key when thinking about hydration. But this doesn't mean that we recommend drinking strictly water during exercise. On the contrary, when exercising, especially in the heat or when sweat rates are high, there is no situation when water alone is superior to a sports drink with about a 4 percent carbohydrate solution (4 grams per 100 ml, or 80 kcals per standard small 500-ml cycling bottle) and some sodium (300 to 400 mg per 500-ml bottle).

Over the course of training or competition you'll want to hydrate enough to limit your losses to no more than 3 percent of your body weight. The best and easiest way to track your hydration status is to simply weigh yourself before and after exercise.

In the Feed Zone Kitchen

How We Use Macronutrients

CARBOHYDRATES

We are generous with carbohydrates because this is a book for endurance athletes who burn lots of calories in training. Endurance athletes need energy, especially carbohydrate energy stored as muscle and liver glycogen. In many ways, one of the most performance-enhancing substrates available to us is glycogen. For all the controversy over performance-enhancing drugs and all of the ignorant belief that athletes can't win without them, it angers me when athletes don't eat enough and bonk. In fact, many times when an athlete complains about being fatigued or riding like crap on the bicycle, the problem is depleted muscle glycogen—something that can be easily remedied by increasing carbohydrate intake through eating foods like pasta, rice, potatoes, bread, couscous, and other whole grains.

PROTEIN

With respect to eating meat, most of our recipes call for chicken or beef, with pork and fish specified on occasion. Of course, we use a lot of eggs, and small amounts of bacon are included to add flavor to dishes. We tend to stick with proteins like chicken, beef, and eggs because most of our athletes are comfortable eating and cooking these foods, and they are readily available when traveling. In addition, dark meats like beef are high in iron and can help prevent athletes from becoming anemic. We avoid shellfish due to concerns over food safety, especially at races when we have limited space and store our food in coolers.

FAT

Use olive oil or butter, not margarine. And if your stomach allows, try going for whole-fat instead of low-fat. There are several reasons to get over your fear of fat:

- **Fat is a vital nutrient and plays a critical role in a wide number of bodily functions.**
- **Fat aids in the absorption of vitamins.**
- **Fat provides padding and protection to our vital organs.**
- **Fat can make a meal more satiating, resulting in more reasonable portions.**
- **A "whole-fat" product can contain fewer calories than the nonfat or low-fat version.**

Let's face it—fat makes almost any meal taste better, and enjoyment is part of living a balanced life.

Building Your Plate

There are plenty of nutrition books out there that specify the percentage and type of food you need to be eating. Although it's sometimes necessary and nice to boil it down to these figures and just tell someone to consume a meal with 60 percent carbohydrate, 25 percent fat, and 15 percent protein, it's not always practical to achieve those numbers. Keeping a careful food diary can help you intuitively know how to meet your dietary goals, but most of the athletes I work with don't keep detailed food diaries. They generally rely on what they see on the plate to build a complete meal. It's like getting a workout prescribed to you by duration, intensity zones, and power values versus planning a ride on a map and figuring out how hard to go over particular sections. With that in mind, we're going to use the map here and give a little bit of advice about how we go about building a plate.

Although most of the recipes in this book are shown as actual dishes, we recommend setting a table family-style because everyone can build their plate as needed. We always start with an ample amount of carbohydrate as a base—rice, oats, potatoes, cereal, pasta, or other grains. The bulk of your calories will come from that base, and the portion size will depend upon how hungry you are.

Instead of thinking of foods like rice or potatoes as the side dish, think of meats or other protein sources as the side dish that flavors and complements the base. In countries like India and China, where protein is often scarce for the majority of the population, this is a common way of serving meat because it makes a little go a long way. This same idea works for endurance athletes. Many of our protein dishes are designed as sauces or stews that you can use to dress and add flavor to your carbohydrates.

After you add some flavor to your plate, make sure that you always have a big salad and lots of greens on hand. While the carbohydrates form the bulk of our energy needs, the plants we eat are vital to maintaining a high nutrient density and are a real key to great nutrition. Much of the time, we roast, grill, sauté, or stir-fry our vegetables to shrink them down and allow more to be eaten. At races, I normally recommend having the riders eat their fruits and vegetables after they eat the main dish so that we fill them up first on the essential carbohydrates they'll need for the next day. In training, however, we often do the opposite so that the riders can watch their calories and maintain an ideal body weight.

Finally, we do have a few dessert items. As part of a well-rounded diet, planning

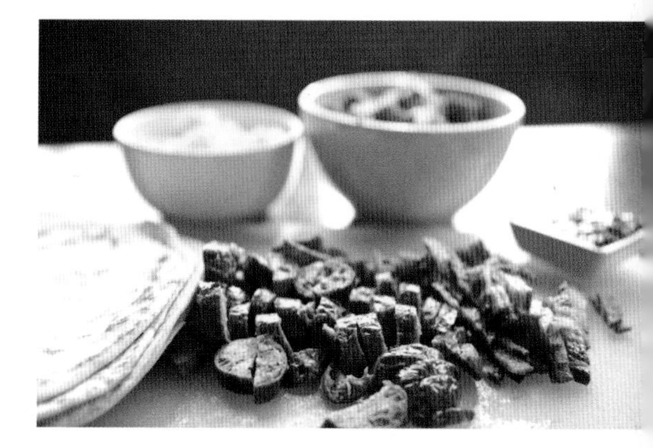

a dessert is better than feeling restricted and then bingeing. At the races, a very common and simple dessert is simply a plain or flavored yogurt with a bowl of fresh fruit with honey and **Toasted Nut Mix, page 276.** ★

Feed Zone Cooking Guidelines

Before you begin cooking, there are a couple of things you need to know to use this cookbook effectively.

We encourage you to substitute ingredients. You might be inclined to substitute ingredients for any number of reasons: to save time, to use things you have on hand, or simply for personal preference. All we ask is that you not trade quality ingredients for highly processed ingredients with no nutritional merit.

Substitutions endorsed›

- Tofu or soy protein for meat
- Brown rice for white
- Gluten-free replacements
- One vegetable for another
- Parsley for basil, etc.

Unacceptable substitutions›

- Artificial sweeteners
- Instant foods (especially rice or oatmeal)
- Fake fats (margarine)

Also, if you do substitute and the recipe doesn't work, then try it again with the original ingredient. Many of our recipes are quite malleable; others, especially items on the Portables menu, are not.

Take shortcuts—especially if it helps to cure your takeout habit. We recognize that the kitchen presents a real learning curve for some athletes. Whenever possible buy the real deal, not pre-packaged, pre-cooked substitutes. Try to fill your shopping cart with food that is in its own wrapper. Naturally, there will be occasions when you need to pick up a rotisserie chicken for a quick dinner, and we are well aware that most athletes don't make their own salsa or cook their own beans (though the nutritional value is usually better when you do).

Shortcuts endorsed›

- Canned beans (for dry beans)
- Prepared salsa
- Store-bought pizza dough
- Frozen vegetables (for fresh vegetables)

Make room for some indulgences in moderation. You may find that we cook with what some people consider "blacklisted" foods. At times, we'll use certain ingredients not typically considered healthy because they taste better, they're less processed, and it's saner to not fixate on avoiding particular ingredients. Any food can be bad in excess, but when we eat these foods in moderation, there is potential for great benefit and nutritional value.

Indulgences endorsed (in moderation)›

- Pork, bacon, red meat, chicken thighs
- Cheese
- Dessert

Have staple ingredients cooked and ready. One way to save a lot of time with our recipes is to pre-cook or prep the ingredients that you use most often: pasta, rice, potatoes, grains, vegetables, and selected meats. When we have spare time when traveling with the team, we will pre-cook pasta and rice, chop and cook meats that will be used in stews or burritos, and pre-cut lots of vegetables for either cooking or juicing. When hunger strikes, we can quickly boil some water or heat up a pan to bring life back into the food.

When you look over the breakfast and après recipes, you'll notice that many times ingredients are listed as "cooked." Having a container of rice or pasta in the fridge ready to go means 10–15 minutes saved, whether you are making rice and eggs before a big ride or throwing together a honey chicken wrap after you return home starving. You'll find a special section in Basics that explains how to prepare your favorite carbs and proteins, aptly named "Cooked and Ready."

⚠ WARNING!

THE RECIPES IN THIS BOOK CONTAIN KNOWN ALLERGENS SUCH AS BACON, DAIRY PRODUCTS, SOY, EGGS WITH YOLKS, NUTS, FLOUR, AND SUGAR.

Remember many of our dishes freeze well, so take the time when you have it to prepare for when you know you'll be on the move.

Our food is meant to be recycled. One of the great skills that I've learned from Biju is the art of recycling or re-purposing leftover food. Not only does this skill stretch your food budget and reduce waste, it's the key to making homemade meals with minimal prep time. Many of the dinner dishes can be used as a base for portable foods or for quick dishes immediately after a ride. For example, we often take leftover meats, rice, and potatoes and use them as a base for

LIVING ON MEATBALLS

One season Christian Vande Velde was staying at my place in Boulder, Colorado, for a two-week training camp. His stay coincided with the untimely demise of the cooling pump in my freezer. Further complicating things, my freezer was packed with one-quarter of a free-range, grass-fed cow. I had a lot of meat that needed to be cooked right away. That evening Christian, Biju, Mike Friedman (aka "Meatball"), and I made enough meatballs to feed a small army. In celebration of our effort, we had a classic dish of spaghetti and meatballs. Those meatballs were so good and so abundant that the next day after training, Christian had meatballs over rice. Later that evening I had some meatball sliders. Eventually, we cooked up more pasta . . . you get the idea. Christian and I took a small hiatus from meatballs following that experience. ★ Be sure to try Biju's meatballs, page 234.

burritos. With the addition of a little salsa and cheese, these burritos are a hit on the team bus, whether for a snack or immediately after the race.

Common Ingredients

With these principles in mind, we want to expound on some of the common ingredients in our recipes that you might have preconceived ideas about or might not be familiar with.

RICE

We often use white rice with our athletes because it cooks faster, has a higher glycemic index (which can be good immediately after training), and is culturally what we're accustomed to. Brown rice is a fine substitute in most of the recipes (rice cakes being the exception).

Be careful about substituting. Calrose and jasmine rice are recommended in many cases and are always recommended for rice cakes. We also use basmati rice sometimes, but never for the rice cakes, as the rice won't stick together. Just don't try to use microwavable or instant rice for any recipe in this book. Why? Because the dishes won't taste very good, if they actually turn out, and because Biju and I will take it as a personal offense.

EGGS

We use the entire egg, and lots of them. Eggs do contain quite a bit of cholesterol, and for the average American the conventional wisdom is that this may lead to an increase in blood cholesterol and thereby increase the risk of heart and peripheral vascular disease. A number of factors can affect the relationship between dietary and blood cholesterol—namely, physical activity and genetics. If you're not physically active, you might want to restrict yourself to 1 to 2 eggs a day on average over the course of a week. If you have a family history of high cholesterol or know that you have high cholesterol, you might already know that you need to restrict the amount of eggs in your diet.

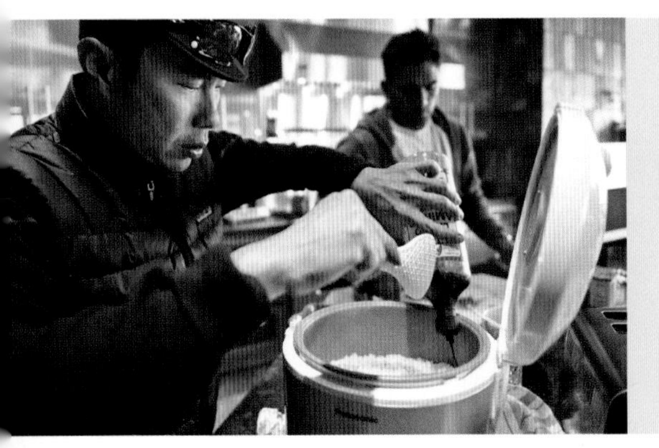

IT'S ALL ABOUT THE RICE COOKER

I once spent an entire season scouring obscure Asian markets in Europe for the best rice cookers available on the continent, securing a few of them for the team I was working with, and converting the riders to a predominantly rice-based diet. My triumph was short-lived. The guys returned to the bus following their first race of the next season only to learn that

The truth is, eggs are a very easy and convenient source of very high quality protein. Protein quality is graded on a scale, with a 1.0 being the highest grade of protein. The egg white is the only protein that scores a 1.0, and it is what all other proteins are effectively graded against. In addition, cholesterol is an essential backbone for all anabolic hormones in the body and is a vital nutrient. In the end, just as sugar alone is not going to give you diabetes, having cholesterol in your diet isn't going to give you a heart attack. If you have concerns, talk to your doctor; in addition, get regular checkups and know your own body. The fact that we use eggs in our cookbook doesn't remove your responsibility, nor does it spell doomsday.

SUGAR

Sugar is a vital energy source, especially for competitive cyclists. For example, in the Tour de France, simple sugars, especially in sports drinks, can make up the majority of the calories consumed. Imagine if one

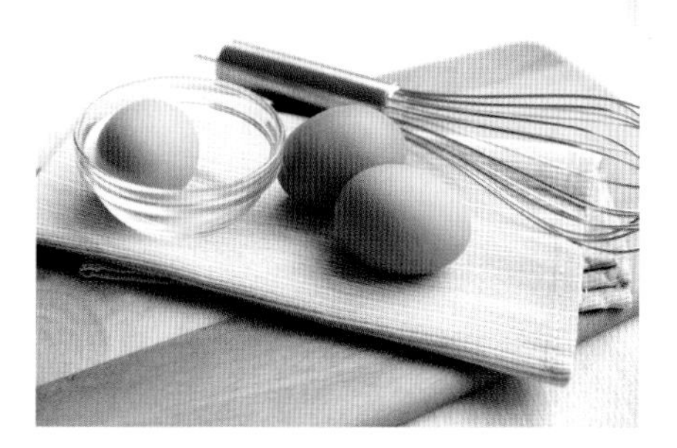

of those athletes tried eating all of those calories in solid form. He would produce so much fecal matter that he literally would be sitting on the toilet for 5 hours the next day, rather than in his saddle. And while I concede most of us are not riding in the Tour, just because sugar is normally associated with nutritionally poor processed foods doesn't mean that it doesn't have a role in wholesome meals made from scratch or in sports drinks during exercise.

You can use the following sugars interchangeably in most of our recipes: brown sugar, honey, maple syrup, agave nectar. Brown sugar is the most affordable and accessible option. All of these are real sugars.

my precious equipment had deliberately been left at the *service course*. As consolation, they were offered microwavable rice that came conveniently packaged in plastic bags. The ensuing series of confrontations between hungry riders and team personnel are a little too gruesome to recount here. By the next race, one of the riders (a seasoned pro with Grand Tour podium finishes to his name) took it upon himself to bring his own rice cooker onto the bus. Sadly, even that rice cooker was later confiscated as rogue non-sponsor-issued contraband, after which crusty baguettes began to reappear.

One moral to this story is that as much as we may try, it's difficult to change old, foolish habits. Buy a rice cooker while you are feeling inspired, and you'll grow so attached to it that if someone steals it as they did mine, it will feel like somebody stole your bike.

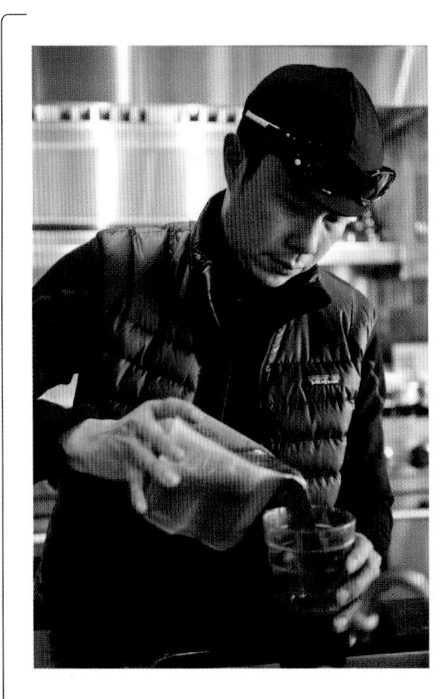

JUICING

Juicing improves the nutrient density of athletes' diets by significantly increasing the quantity of fruits and vegetables they can handle without the worry of an unbearable amount of fiber load in their GI tract. Drinking juice is especially beneficial before and after training.

Beet juice, in particular, is high in dietary nitrates. Recent studies have shown that it can actually improve economy, or gross mechanical efficiency, meaning more power is being produced for a given amount of oxygen consumed or energy burned. The ability to produce more power without using more energy can have huge ramifications over a day of hard racing or several hard days of racing. And for this to occur with a simple glass of beet juice a day is pretty amazing.

Bailey, S. J., P. G. Winyard, A. Vanhatalo, J. R. Blackwell, F. J. Dimenna, D. P. Wilkerson, et al. 2009. Dietary nitrate supplementation reduces the O_2 cost of low-intensity exercise and enhances tolerance to high-intensity exercise in humans. *Journal of Applied Physiology* 107(4): 1144–1155. › Lansley, K. E., P. G. Winyard, J. Fulford, A. Vanhatalo, S. J. Bailey, J. R. Blackwell, et al. 2011. Dietary nitrate supplementation reduces the O_2 cost of walking and running: A placebo-controlled study. *Journal of Applied Physiology*, 110(3): 591–600. › Larsen, F. J., E. Weitzberg, J. O. Lundberg, and B. Ekblom, 2010. Dietary nitrate reduces maximal oxygen consumption while maintaining work performance in maximal exercise. *Free Radical Biology and Medicine*, 48(2): 342–347.

ARTIFICIAL SWEETENERS

The issue of artificial sweetener in our foods is political and dirty. In 1958 Congress passed the Delaney Clause, which prohibited any ingredient, at any dose, known to cause cancer in animals or humans from being used in the U.S. food system. In 1977 a Canadian study found that rats exposed to high doses of the artificial sweetener saccharin developed cancer; as a result the Food and Drug Administration proposed banning saccharin (Arnold et al., 1977, Long-term toxicity study with orthotoluene-sulfonamide and saccharin, *Toxicology and Applied Pharmacology* 41(164), Abstract no. 78). But the public wanted its diet soda, so Congress overruled the FDA and delayed the ban for two years until more research could be done. That moratorium is still in place, and other

SALT

Sodium is one of the most important electrolytes in the human body. It controls the function of every cell in our body, propagating electrical signals through our nervous system and playing a vital role in fluid balance. We lose a lot of salt and electrolytes when we exercise—between 700 mg and 1,000 mg of sodium per liter of sweat, or about 350 to 500 mg of sodium per standard 500-ml bottle of sports drink. Most sports drinks don't contain enough sodium, and if we don't get enough sodium in our diets, then when we exercise, our function can deteriorate. In fact, we can become paradoxically more dehydrated by drinking water alone because the body increases urine output to maintain the concentration of sodium. Of course, some individuals are salt-sensitive and can experience a dangerous rise in their blood pressure when they consume too much salt. If you know you feel really bloated and your blood pressure skyrockets when you add a lot of salt to your food, then do the rational thing and put the shaker down.

artificial sweeteners have been introduced since. Even though lab animals have been shown to develop cancer when exposed to some artificial sweeteners, they remain the only exception to the Delaney Clause and are generally recognized as safe (GRAS) by the powers that be. That's like saying something is "kind of" safe.

There are many sources of sodium in our meals. Most of the recipes in this book call for sea salt, liquid amino acids, or low-sodium soy sauce. The latter two can be used interchangeably. If you are watching your sodium intake, try a spray version of the liquid amino acids or salt and add textured salt only after you finish cooking. This will allow the salt taste to be more pronounced despite using less salt.

Tools and Appliances

We did our best to make sure that you could make these recipes with the basic pots, pans, and mixing bowls that most people have in their kitchen. However, there are some kitchen appliances that we find invaluable and that you might not have:

Rice Cooker› You can buy a really simple automatic rice cooker at your local department store. But for the same price (around $30 to $80), you can likely find a much nicer rice cooker with a locking lid at an Asian supermarket. If you're single or cooking for two, a 5-cup rice cooker will work great. If you're cooking for a team or a large family, a 10-cup rice cooker is a better choice.

Slow Cooker› Our Après menu includes several one-pot recipes that are designed to be made in a slow cooker (also called a crockpot) and then served on rice or pasta. Some of the bowls on the Dinner menu can be prepared in the same way. The nice thing about a slow cooker is that you can pile in all of the ingredients and head out for a long ride, and food will be ready to eat when you return. A heavy cast-iron pot is

The Athlete's Kitchen

There are a handful of staples that athletes should always have on hand›

IN THE FRIDGE

- Seasonal fruits & vegetables
- Eggs
- Protein (chicken, beef, or plant protein)
- Tortillas (whole wheat, corn)
- Yogurt
- Milk (almond, rice, dairy)
- Parmesan
- Fruit & vegetable juice
- Nut butter (peanut, almond, Nutella)
- Fresh citrus (lemons, limes)
- Fresh herbs (parsley, basil)

IN THE PANTRY

- Rice (calrose, jasmine)
- Pasta (couscous, orzo, angel hair)
- Grain (quinoa)
- Potatoes (russet, sweet)
- Flour (all-purpose, gluten-free)
- Beans, canned or dried
- Fish, canned albacore
- Stock (chicken or vegetable)
- Oils (olive, grapeseed, canola)
- Vinegars (balsamic, red wine, apple cider)
- Sea salt & pepper grinders
- Spices (cinnamon, chili powder, cumin, curry powder, nutmeg)
- Soy sauce, low-sodium
- Spicy (Sriracha, sambal, tobasco)
- Sweet (brown sugar, raw sugar, honey, maple syrup, agave, jam, molasses)

Naturally, there are a few appliances and tools that you'll need as well›

APPLIANCES

- Rice cooker
- Food processor (small, inexpensive)
- Blender
- Slow cooker

Optional

- Dutch oven
- Juicer
- Heavy stock pot

You don't need a well-stocked kitchen to make good food. We cook in motor homes.

OTHER TOOLS

For cooking

- 10-inch sauté pan
- 4.5–6 quart large pot
- Baking sheet
- 8- or 9-inch square pan
- Muffin tin

For prep

- Cutting board, synthetic
- Knives of assorted sizes
- Measuring cups
- 8–10" steel mixing bowl
- Spatula and spoon set
- Strainer

TIP Discount retailers like T.J.Maxx and Ross often have kitchen supplies at a good price.

an alternative to the slow cooker, though you might prepare an après dish the night before to avoid leaving it unattended. (And even then, you wouldn't want to cook it more than two hours.)

Small food processor› Rather than spend 30 minutes chopping vegetables for these recipes, get a small food processor. You will have more time to eat and relax.

Juicer› A masticating juicer is much easier to set up and clean than the cheaper alternatives. Also, it grinds the produce, yielding more juice with an overall better taste. Having used multiple juicers, we think the masticating juicer is well worth the investment.

To put all of this into some perspective, at the Tour of California in 2011, we prepared all of our meals out of a rented motor home cooking on two butane stoves and the single propane stove in the camper using only two pots, two sauté pans, two rice cookers, two mixing bowls, a food processor, a big brownie pan, the miscellaneous knives and utensils we brought from home, and Levi Leipheimer's masticating juicer. Much of this was actually borrowed from Andy Barr, owner of the Drunken Monkey sushi restaurant in Truckee, California, and from the Truckee Police Department (special thanks to Chief of Police Nicholas Sensley and Andy for getting us through the week).

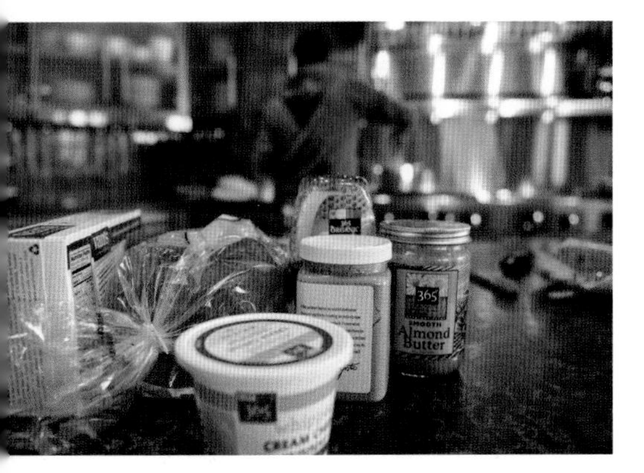

* * *

Finally, realize that these recipes are a foundation for a strong diet, but they aren't the only foods that we feed our athletes. For example, we buy lots of boxes of cereals for the guys to eat for breakfast, though I still discourage relying solely on a bowl of cereal for dinner. Depending upon the race and the availability of our chef or rice cookers, we still give athletes protein drinks or high-calorie energy drinks immediately after a race to help restore muscle glycogen and fluids. And despite trying to meet most of our riders' nutritional needs through diet alone, there are many instances where we supplement with things like a multivitamin, iron, fish oil, vitamin C, and calcium. Ultimately, this book is not a full treatise on diet and nutrition. What follows is a small sample of what we eat and what we've fed athletes in the past. We hope these recipes give you ideas, get you in the kitchen cooking your own meals, and show you the fundamental principles that shape our approach to everyday eating. Most importantly, we want to showcase wholesome meals as a critical advantage in sport and life.

★★★

Conventional wisdom says **breakfast is the most important meal of the day** because it's the first meal of the day. In our world, it's the most important meal of the day **because it's typically the first meal before training or racing.**

Consequently, our Breakfast menu includes many recipes that are quick to make and easy to digest. But you don't need to confine these recipes to morning. You can have them anytime or prepare them in advance to have as snacks so your blood sugar doesn't dip before you head out to the race.

Our bowls are the smallest and simplest recipes—items like oatmeal or sweet rice porridge. The handhelds can be wrapped and eaten on the go, and our potato cakes and burritos work well on the bike too. The big plates are intended for the times when you need a lot of calories and have plenty of time to digest your food. **At the races, our breakfast table is set with dishes from each of these sections.**

BREAKFAST

BOWLS

HANDHELDS

BIG PLATES

V **VEGETARIAN**
G **GLUTEN-FREE**

SERVING SIZES

Beware serving sizes in this book that are typically larger than normal. If you are not training, reduce your portion or cut some calories by using less sugar. If you do work out in the morning the extra calories will fuel your training or help you recover.

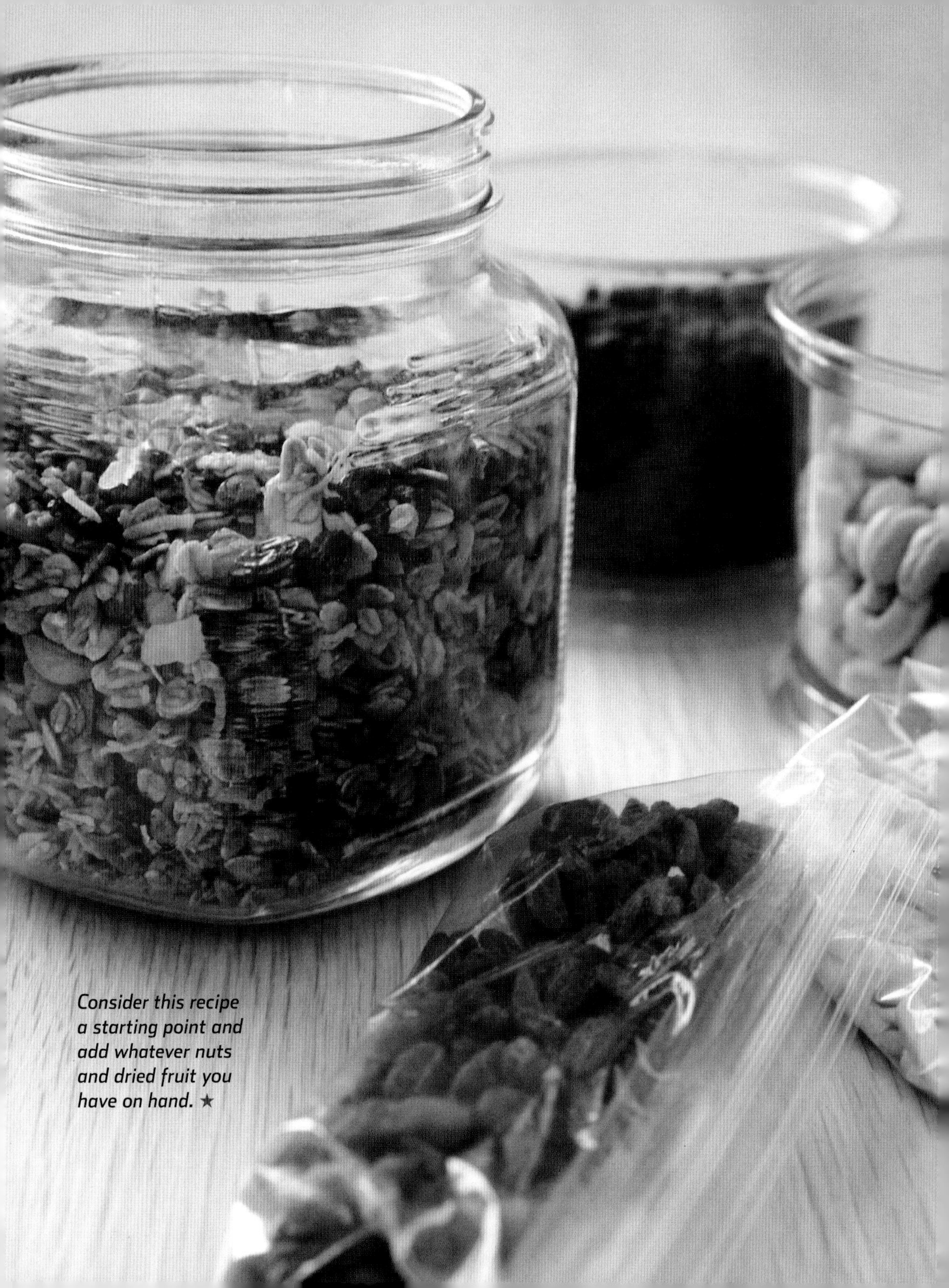

Consider this recipe a starting point and add whatever nuts and dried fruit you have on hand. ★

SERVINGS› 8
TIME› 5 minutes prep,
bake 1 hour

Granola

Most granola contains some sort of oil, but we use fruit juice and syrup or agave nectar to give our oats moisture before baking. There are countless ways to enjoy granola throughout the week: as a cold breakfast cereal, combined with steamed milk for a quick and healthy "oatmeal," or mixed in with yogurt for a midafternoon snack.

4 cups "old-fashioned" rolled oats

½ cup brown sugar

1 cup unsweetened shredded coconut

½ cup maple syrup or agave nectar

¼ cup unfiltered apple juice

1 ripe banana

OPTIONAL ADDITIONS
(use up to ½ cup of each)

slivered almonds

chopped cashews

pine nuts

golden raisins

dried goji berries

currants

1. Heat oven to 300 degrees.
2. In a large bowl, combine oats, brown sugar, and coconut.
3. In a blender, combine maple syrup, apple juice, and banana. Process until smooth.
4. Add the contents of the blender to the bowl and stir. You may have to add another splash of apple juice if the granola seems too dry.
5. Spread mixture evenly onto a cookie sheet lined with parchment or waxed paper. Bake 45 minutes.
6. Add any combo of the optional ingredients, if desired. Stir granola, and bake for an additional 10–15 minutes or until granola is desired shade of brown. Allow granola to cool completely.

Makes about 6 cups. Transfer to airtight jar or container and store in the fridge for up to one week.

PER SERVING (¾ cup)› Energy 453 cal • Fat 12 g • Sodium 6 mg • Carbs 83 g • Fiber 10 g • Protein 13 g
Nutrition for optional additions can be found in Appendix A.

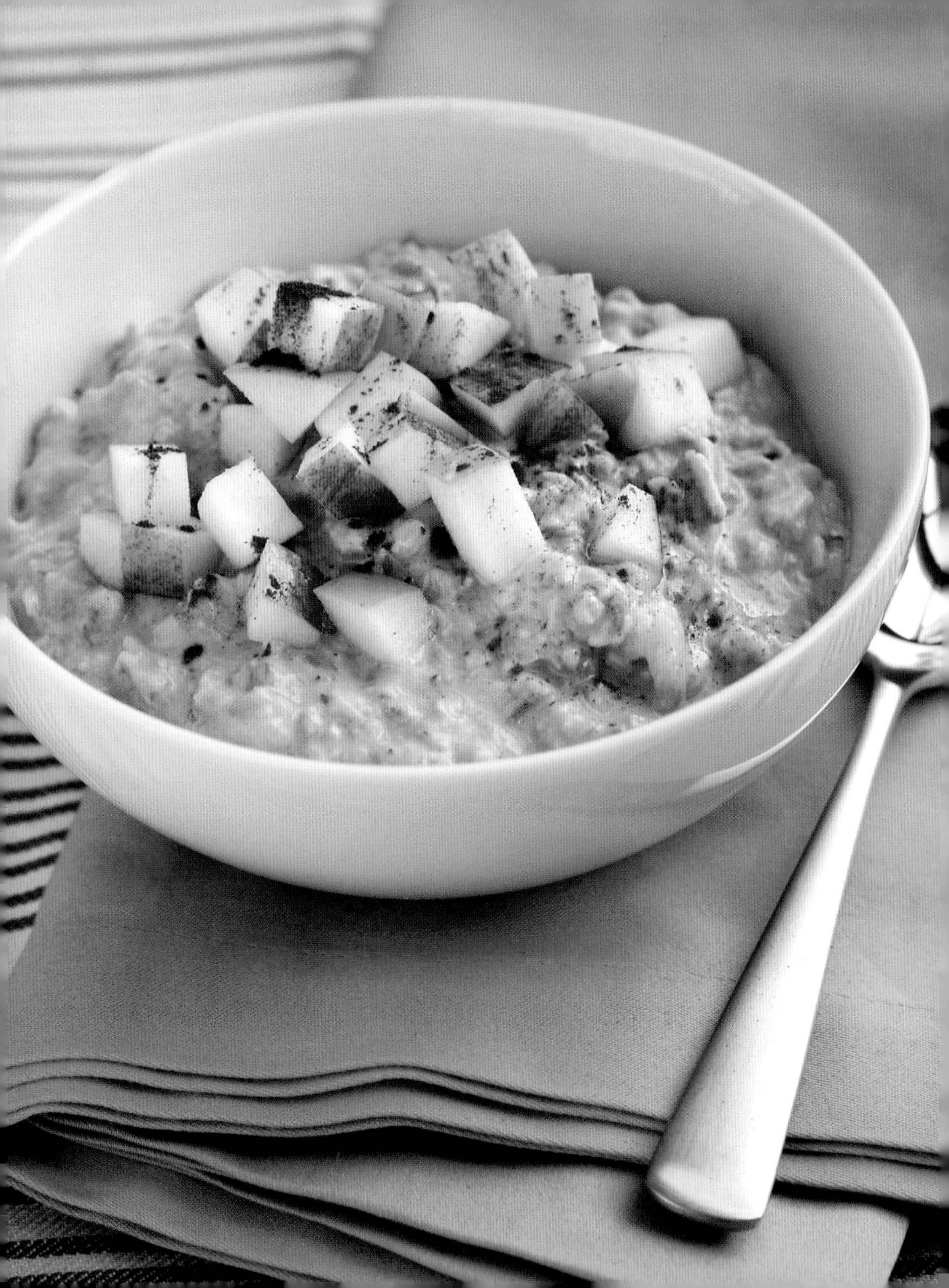

SERVINGS› 2
TIME› 10 minutes,
store overnight

Muesli

If you've traveled around Europe racing bikes or as a tourist, you know how common muesli is at hotels and little inns. It turns out to be an incredibly simple dish for any athlete who does not want to spend much time thinking about breakfast. Make a fresh batch each night and set in the fridge; enjoy what's leftover for a post-ride snack.

1 cup "old-fashioned" rolled oats

1 cup milk

¼ cup yogurt

1 small apple, diced

¼ cup chopped pecans or walnuts

sprinkle of ground cinnamon

OPTIONAL ADDITIONS

2 tablespoons honey or maple syrup

1 mashed ripe banana

¼ cup applesauce

fresh fruit

1. Combine all ingredients (including any optional additions) in a medium bowl. Mix thoroughly.

Cover the bowl, and store in the fridge overnight.

PER SERVING› **Energy** 479 cal • **Fat** 15 g • **Sodium** 79 mg • **Carbs** 76 g • **Fiber** 10 g • **Protein** 19 g

Nutrition for optional additions can be found in Appendix A.

SERVINGS› 2
TIME› 10–15 minutes

Biju's Oatmeal

Rice or pasta are common pre-race breakfast staples for professional cyclists, but at the 2011 Tour of California Chris Horner and the RadioShack team proved that oatmeal can be the breakfast of champions. Levi Leipheimer has mastered our recipe, and we hope it will become your favorite standby food too.

- 1 cup water
- dash of salt
- 1 cup "old-fashioned" rolled oats
- 1–2 cups milk, depending on desired thickness
- 1 tablespoon brown sugar
- 1 tablespoon molasses
- 1 banana, chopped
- ¼ cup raisins

OPTIONAL ADDITION

Toasted Nut Mix (page 276)

1. In a medium saucepan, bring the water and salt to a low boil. Add oats and cook, stirring frequently, about 5 minutes.
2. Add milk and brown sugar, and return the mixture to a low boil. Add molasses, banana, and raisins, continuing to stir until oatmeal reaches desired thickness. Remove pan from heat. Let rest for 10–15 minutes if you have the time.

Finish with a sprinkle of ground cinnamon and a splash of milk.

TIP Use any kind of milk—dairy, soy, almond. Start with 1 cup and add more to achieve your desired consistency.

PER SERVING› **Energy** 490 cal • **Fat** 6 g • **Sodium** 181 mg • **Carbs** 102 g • **Fiber** 10 g • **Protein** 19 g

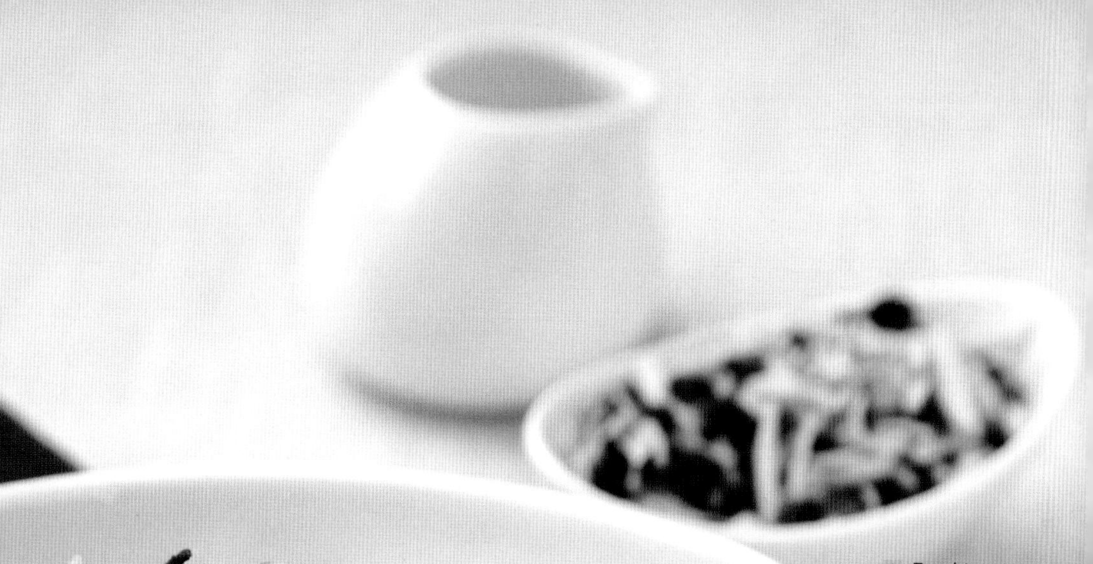

★ For this easy Toasted Nut Mix, see page 276.

SERVINGS› 2
TIME› 10 minutes

Quinoa and Berries

Quinoa is a great gluten-free alternative to traditional breakfast cereals. We serve it warm, typically with our favorite berries and nuts. It's also delicious topped with poached eggs or piled with yogurt.

1 cup quinoa, rinsed and drained

1 cup water

1 cup milk

dash of salt

1–2 tablespoons honey

½ cup fresh blueberries

chopped walnuts or pecans (optional)

1. In a medium saucepan, combine the quinoa, water, milk, and salt and bring to a gentle boil, watching to prevent the milk from boiling over. Turn the heat down and let simmer until most of the moisture has evaporated.
2. Add honey; stir. Cover and let sit for a few minutes.

Top with fresh berries, along with any other desired garnishes—such as chopped nuts, yogurt, or a sprinkle of brown sugar.

PER SERVING› **Energy** 426 cal • **Fat** 6 g • **Sodium** 356 mg • **Carbs** 78 g • **Fiber** 7 g • **Protein** 18 g
Nutrition for optional additions can be found in Appendix A.

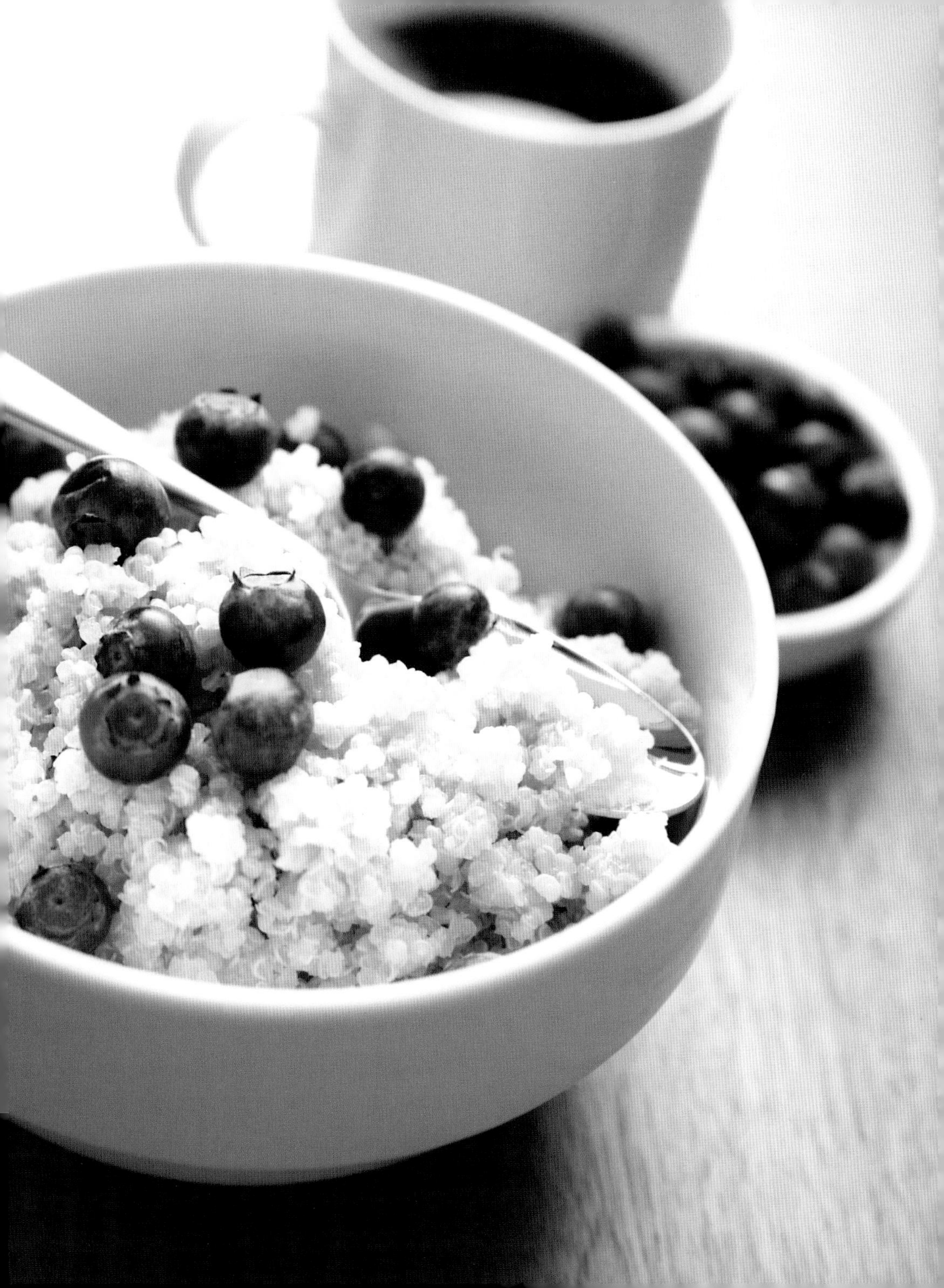

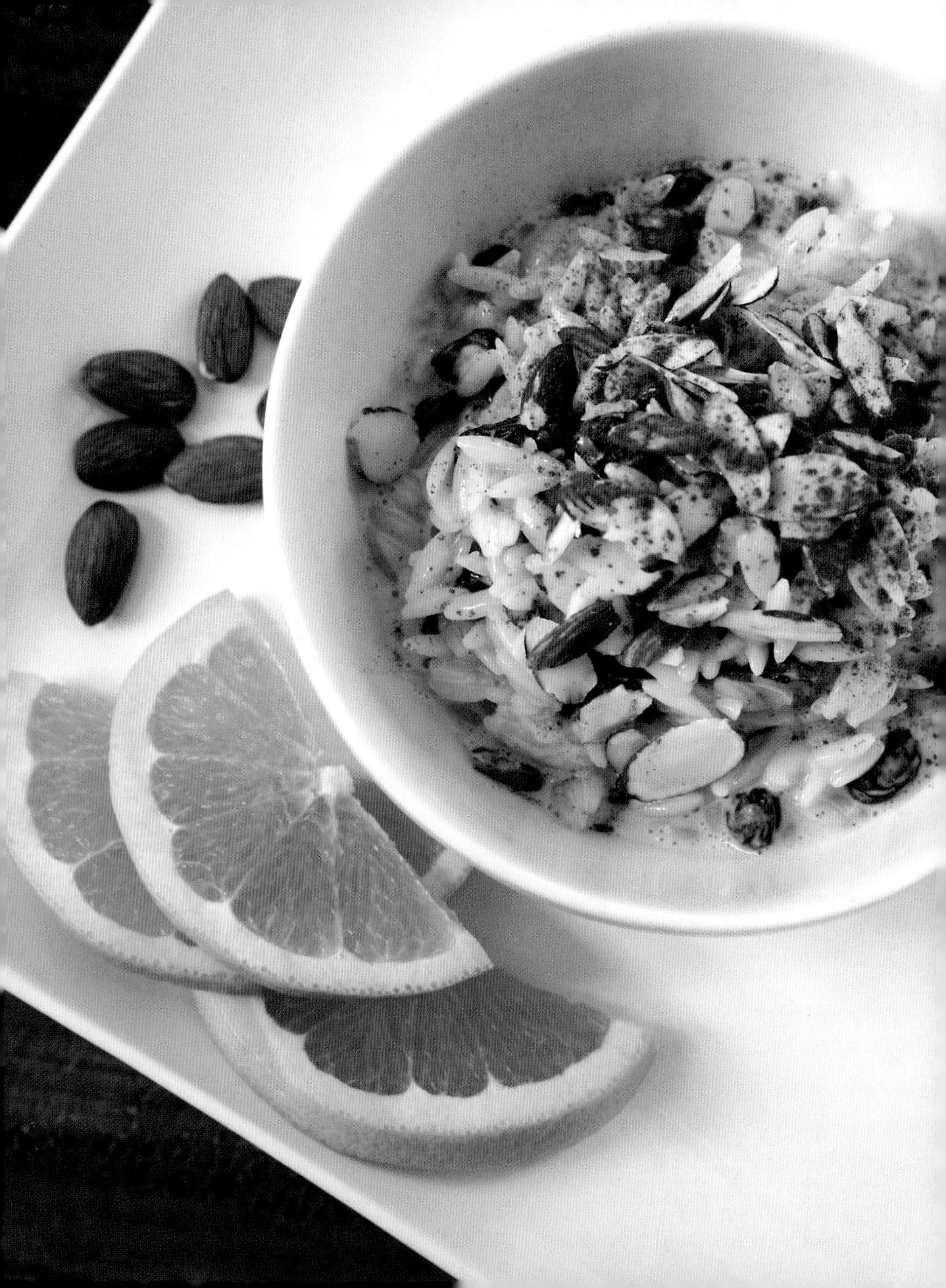

SERVINGS› 2
TIME› 5 minutes

Orzo with Dried Fruit

This is an easy last-minute breakfast if you have cooked orzo on hand. Almond milk is the perfect pairing for the texture and flavor of orzo, but other types of milk may be substituted. If you've already finished your workout, double up on the dried fruit for more fiber.

2 cups almond milk

COOKED **1 cup cooked orzo**

¼ cup raisins, currants, or chopped dates

2 tablespoons brown sugar

1. In a saucepan over medium-high heat, bring almond milk to a gentle simmer.
2. Add orzo, dried fruit, and brown sugar; stir. Cook until warm, approximately 3–5 minutes.

Divide orzo into two bowls. Top with slivered almonds, ground cinnamon or nutmeg, and more brown sugar, if desired.

TIP For an everyday low-calorie bowl, add just half of the brown sugar, which amounts to 40 calories saved.

PER SERVING› **Energy** 242 cal • **Fat** 5 g • **Sodium** 182 mg • **Carbs** 88 g • **Fiber** 3 g • **Protein** 12 g

Nutrition for alternatives can be found in Appendix A.

SERVINGS› 2
TIME› 5 minutes

Sweet Rice Porridge

Leftover rice makes a fast, filling breakfast. With the help of the egg yolk and the banana, you'll get just enough protein and sugars. This recipe is not too different from our Leftover Rice Pudding (page 259), which is served as a dessert. We made it a bit lighter here so you can start your day with a treat.

- 1½ cups milk
- 1 egg yolk
- COOKED 1 cup cooked rice
- 1 ripe banana, sliced
- 1 teaspoon vanilla extract
- 2 tablespoons brown sugar
- dash each of salt and ground cinnamon
- fresh berries (optional)

1. Whisk together milk and egg yolk in a medium pot and heat gently.
2. Add the cooked rice, banana, vanilla, brown sugar, salt, and cinnamon. Cook and stir for 5–10 minutes or until mixture comes to a gentle boil.

Transfer to a bowl or plate and top with fresh berries, if desired.

PER SERVING› **Energy** 405 cal • **Fat** 7 g • **Sodium** 173 mg • **Carbs** 71 g • **Fiber** 3 g • **Protein** 16 g
Nutrition for optional additions can be found in Appendix A.

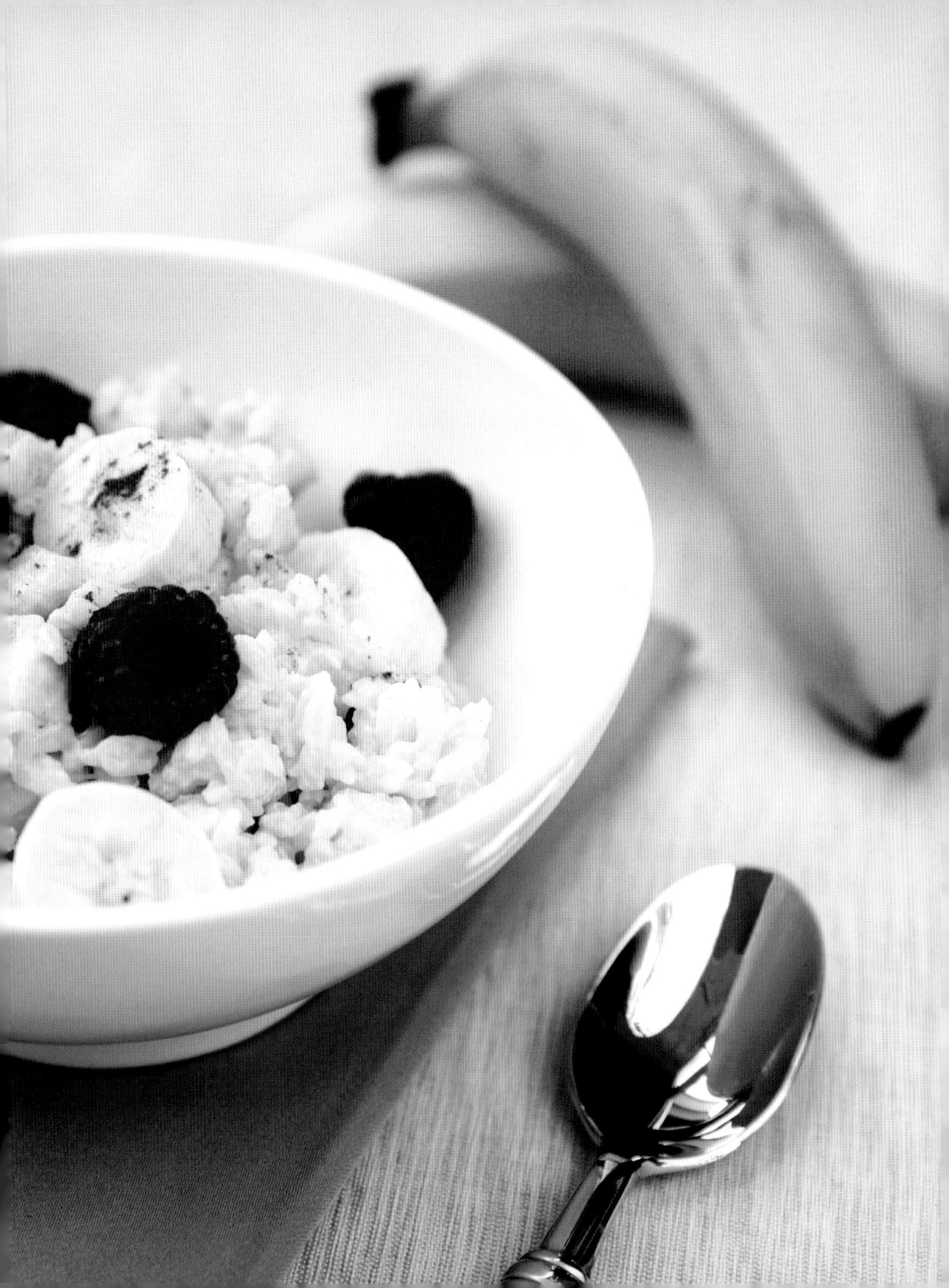

SERVINGS› 1
TIME› 15 minutes

Ham and Swiss Sandwich

This is an indulgent breakfast sandwich that will trump any take-out sandwich around. Our instructions include homemade mayonnaise, but to save time you can substitute purchased mayo.

- 2 slices of rustic bread
- olive oil
- handful of salad greens
- freshly squeezed lemon juice and salt
- 1 egg
- 1 thick slice Swiss cheese
- 2 ounces shaved ham
- Red Pepper Mayonnaise (page 292)

1. Brush one side of the bread slices with olive oil, and toast oil-side down in a sauté pan.
2. Meanwhile, toss the salad greens with a bit of olive oil, lemon juice, and salt.
3. In a small pan, cook the egg over easy. Turn off the heat.

Place toasted bread on a plate with the untoasted side face-up. Top one slice with cheese, ham, and the cooked egg. Add greens, drizzle with mayo, and place the second slice of bread on top.

PER SERVING› **Energy** 525 cal • **Fat** 19 g • **Sodium** 915 mg • **Carbs** 63 g • **Fiber** 5 g • **Protein** 24 g

★ For tasty Red Pepper Mayonnaise, see page 292.

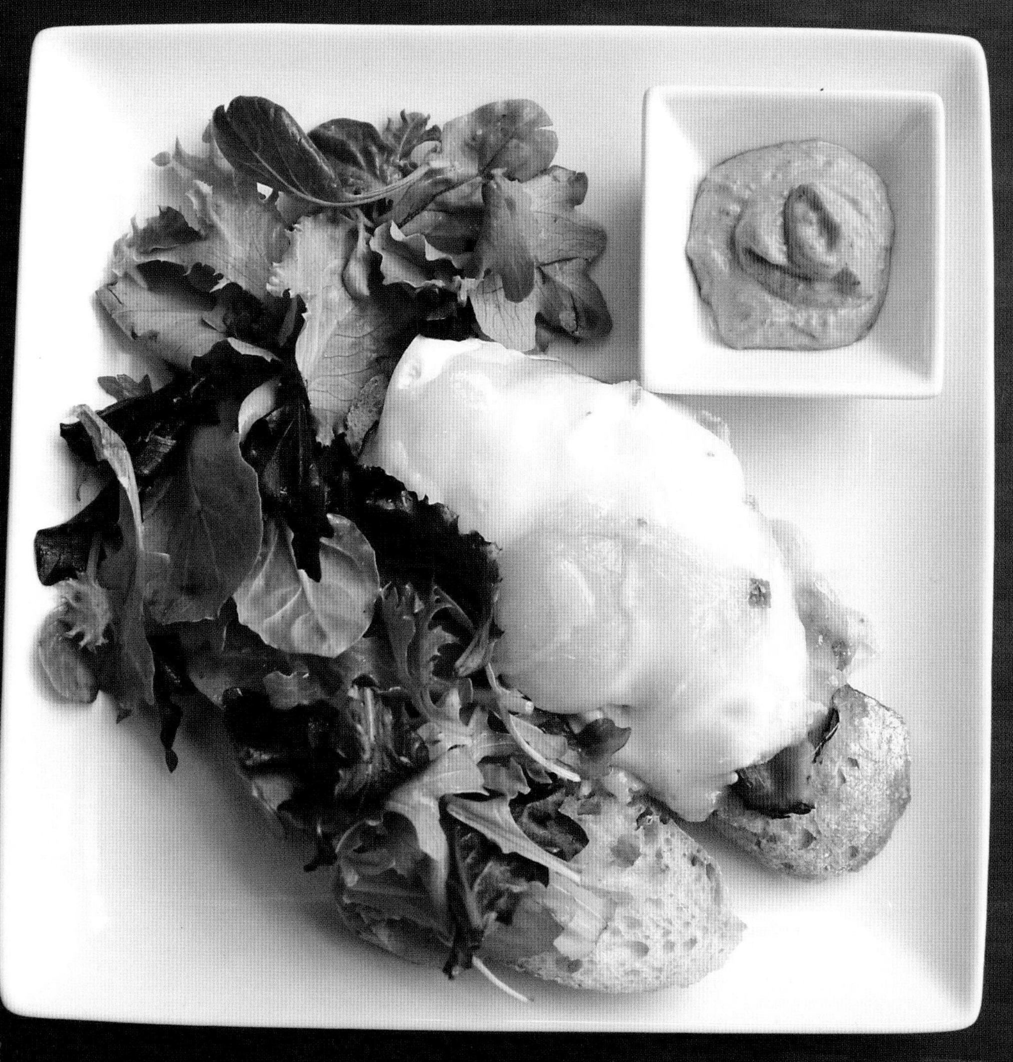

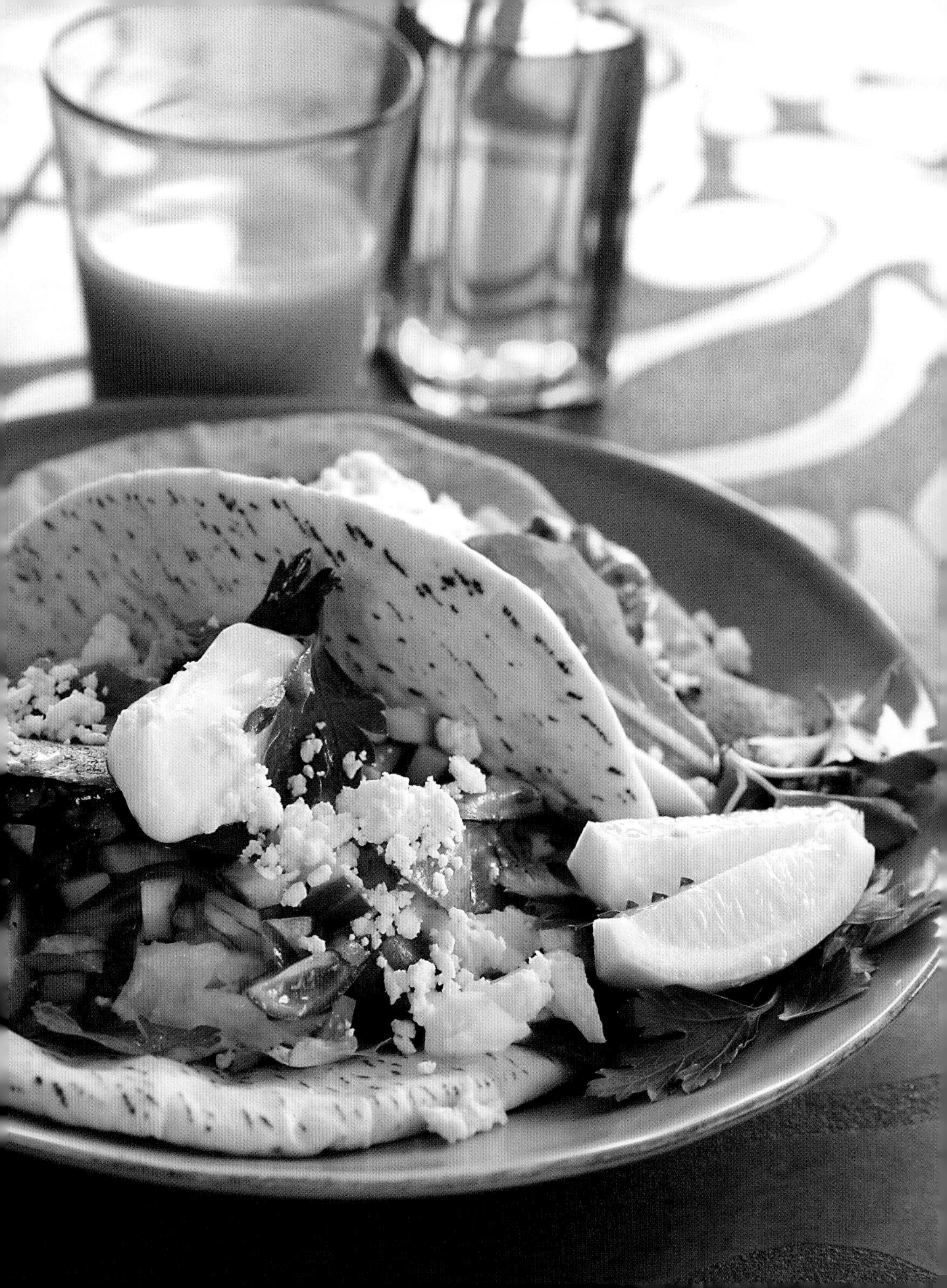

SERVINGS› 2
TIME› 15–20 minutes

Mediterranean Pita

This pita is best with lots of veggies, so it's an ideal post-ride or recovery-day meal. As with all of our recipes, you can use meat you have on hand, but should you try gyro meat (lamb), it will not disappoint. If you'll be enjoying it before you ride, load it up with steamed white rice or potatoes in place of the veggies.

VEGGIES

1 cup mixed greens

½ cucumber, chopped

½ tomato, chopped

¼ onion, chopped

1 tablespoon parsley, coarsely chopped

DRESSING

¼ cup plain yogurt

1 tablespoon olive oil

juice of 1 lemon

2 pitas

olive oil

2 eggs

¼ cup lean gyro meat

¼ cup crumbled feta cheese

1. Combine veggies in a large bowl.
2. To make the dressing: Blend all ingredients together in a small bowl. Add a splash of water if using Greek yogurt. Season to taste with salt and pepper.
3. Brush the pitas with olive oil and warm them in a pan. While they are warming, scramble the eggs in another pan. Once the eggs are cooked through, sauté the gyro meat. Remove both pans from heat.

Top or stuff the pitas with the veggies (or rice or potatoes), then scrambled eggs, meat, and feta. Top with yogurt dressing. A fresh squeeze of lemon finishes it perfectly!

PER SERVING› **Energy** 450 cal • **Fat** 25 g • **Sodium** 771 mg • **Carbs** 39 g • **Fiber** 2 g • **Protein** 17 g

SERVINGS> 1
TIME> 10 minutes

Egg and Greens Sandwich

Dark wilted greens with the flavors of olive oil and lemon juice are the star of this sandwich. Use the darkest, most bitter greens you can find for a nice contrast and added nutrient boost after your workout. Mustard, beet, or collard greens; kale; or spinach will do nicely.

- 1 cup fresh greens, tough spines removed
- 2 thick slices of rustic bread
- olive oil
- 2 eggs, lightly beaten
- lemon wedge
- grated parmesan

OPTIONAL ADDITIONS

- tomatoes
- salsa

1. In a shallow pan heat about 1 inch of water and a dash of salt; bring to a boil. Add greens and cook until wilted, about 3–5 minutes. Drain in a colander. Set greens on paper towels to dry.
2. Brush both sides of bread with olive oil and toast in a hot pan or under broiler for just a few minutes. Keep a close eye so as not to burn the bread.
3. In a sauté pan, cook eggs to your liking.

Pile the greens and then the eggs onto the toasted bread. Add a squeeze of lemon juice, a bit of shaved parmesan, and salt and pepper to taste.

TIP There's no need to be precise with your greens. One cup translates to a big handful, and add more if you want an extra dose of this superfood.

PER SERVING> **Energy** 537 cal • **Fat** 16 g • **Sodium** 700 mg • **Carbs** 71 g • **Fiber** 6 g • **Protein** 28 g
Nutrition for optional additions can be found in Appendix A.

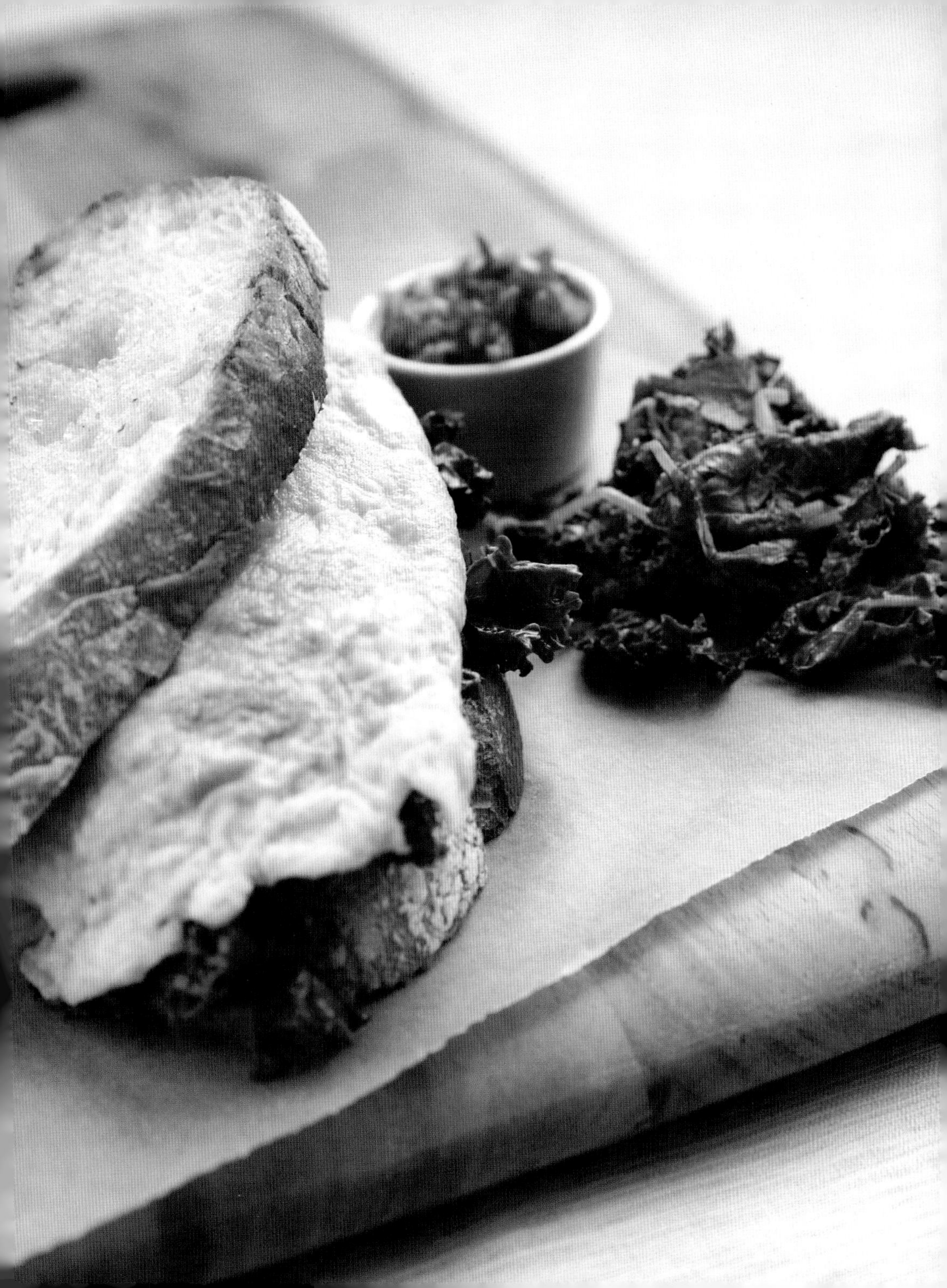

SERVINGS› 1
TIME› 15–20 minutes

Egg and Chorizo Sandwich

Chorizo is a highly seasoned ground pork sausage that's popular in Spain and Mexico. If you can't find it at your local grocery, substitute any other kind of link sausage. Flavor this good isn't exactly low-fat, so rather than frying the egg, try poaching it.

2–3 ounces chorizo
¼ cup sliced onions
white vinegar
1 egg
2 slices of rustic bread
olive oil

OPTIONAL ADDITIONS
grated parmesan
fresh basil

1. Bring a sauté pan to medium-high heat. Add chorizo and onions. Cook, stirring occasionally, until chorizo is browned and onions are softened, about 8–10 minutes. Pour off any excess fat.
2. To poach the egg: Bring a pan of water with a splash of vinegar to a gentle boil. Crack the egg into a small cup or ladle, and gently transfer the egg to the pan. Don't touch the egg until it turns white and you can see the yolk. Cook approximately 4–5 minutes. Use a slotted spoon or spatula to remove the poached egg.
3. Brush both sides of bread with olive oil and toast in a hot pan or under broiler for just a few minutes. Keep a close eye so as not to burn the bread.

Arrange toasted bread on plate, cover with chorizo, then top with poached egg. Squeeze fresh lemon juice and add a splash of olive oil if desired.

PER SERVING› **Energy** 483 cal • **Fat** 29 g • **Sodium** 1,085 mg • **Carbs** 28 g • **Fiber** 3 g • **Protein** 25 g
Nutrition for optional additions can be found in Appendix A.

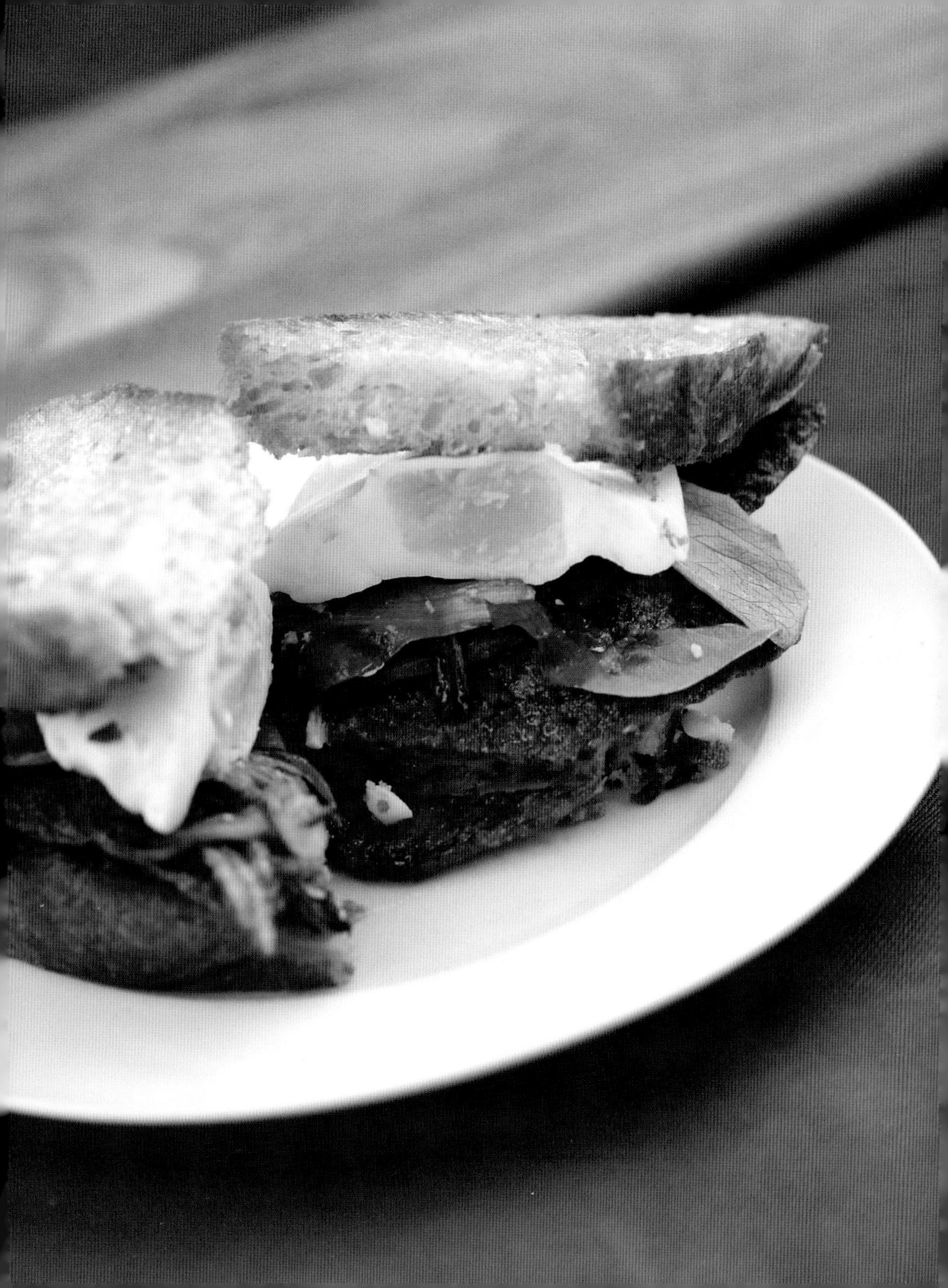

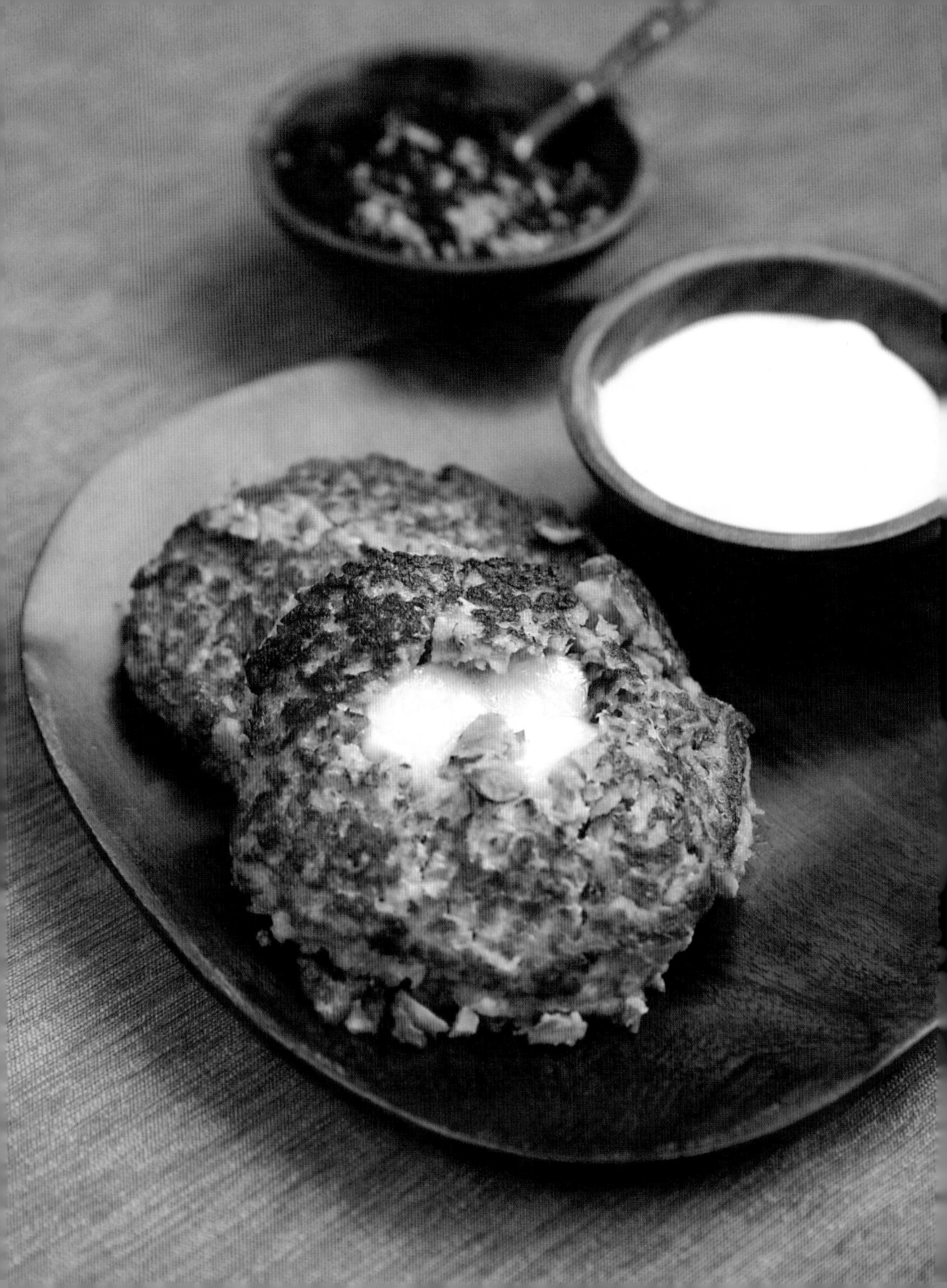

SERVINGS› 4
TIME› 20 minutes

Sweet Potato Cakes

These cakes are more savory than sweet. For a light breakfast, top them with your favorite jam or yogurt. For the perfect brunch following a workout, cook up some bitter greens to accompany the cakes (see page 285). When you have the time, make a double batch and stock up the freezer.

COOKED 2 cups cooked sweet potatoes (peeled)

2 eggs

½ cup (2 slices) cubed bread

2 tablespoons chopped fresh parsley

2 tablespoons chopped red onion

dash of ground nutmeg

¼ cup cubed Swiss cheese

OPTIONAL ADDITIONS

jam

plain yogurt

1. In a bowl or food processor, combine all ingredients except the cheese.
2. Using your hands, form thick patties about 3–4 inches in diameter. Press a cube or two of cheese into the middle of each patty, covering the cheese with the potato mixture.
3. Bring a lightly oiled sauté pan to medium-high heat. Add as many cakes as will comfortably fit in the pan and sauté until crisp and golden, turning once. Repeat with remaining cakes.
4. Finish cakes by putting in the oven for 10 minutes at 350 degrees to help cook all the way through and melt the cheese throughout.

Top with jam, plain yogurt, or olive oil, if desired. Makes about 4 cakes.

TIP Gluten-free bread works great.

PER SERVING (1 cake)› **Energy** 275 cal • **Fat** 6 g • **Sodium** 303 mg • **Carbs** 45 g • **Fiber** 3 g • **Protein** 10 g
Nutrition for optional additions can be found in Appendix A.

SERVINGS› 8
TIME› 25 minutes

Bacon Potato Cakes

Unlike the sweet potato cakes, these are baked in a pan, so the hands-on time is less. This is another dish that packs up for training or an easy midday snack. Before you wrap up a slice, give it a hit of Sriracha (hot sauce).

1 medium onion, coarsely chopped

COOKED 4 cups cooked potatoes (peeled)

COOKED ¼ cup chopped cooked bacon

¼ cup chopped fresh herbs (parsley, basil, thyme, tarragon—any or all)

6 eggs, lightly beaten with a sprinkle of salt and pepper

OPTIONAL ADDITIONS

½ cup grated cheese

Sriracha sauce

1. Heat oven to 350 degrees.
2. Bring a lightly oiled sauté pan to medium-high heat. Add the chopped onion and sauté until translucent and tender, about 5 minutes. Remove from heat.
3. Crush potatoes in a large bowl, leaving some small chunks. Add remaining ingredients (including optional additions, if using) and stir to combine.
4. Transfer mixture to a greased 9-inch square baking pan and bake until set, about 20 minutes. Let dish rest 5 minutes before serving.

TIP Baking pans can be hard to come by if you don't have a kitchen full of options. Use what you have, but keep in mind that a smaller dish will make a thicker cake and take a bit longer to bake.

PER SERVING› **Energy** 206 cal • **Fat** 5 g • **Sodium** 141 mg • **Carbs** 33 g • **Fiber** 3 g • **Protein** 8 g
Nutrition for optional additions can be found in Appendix A.

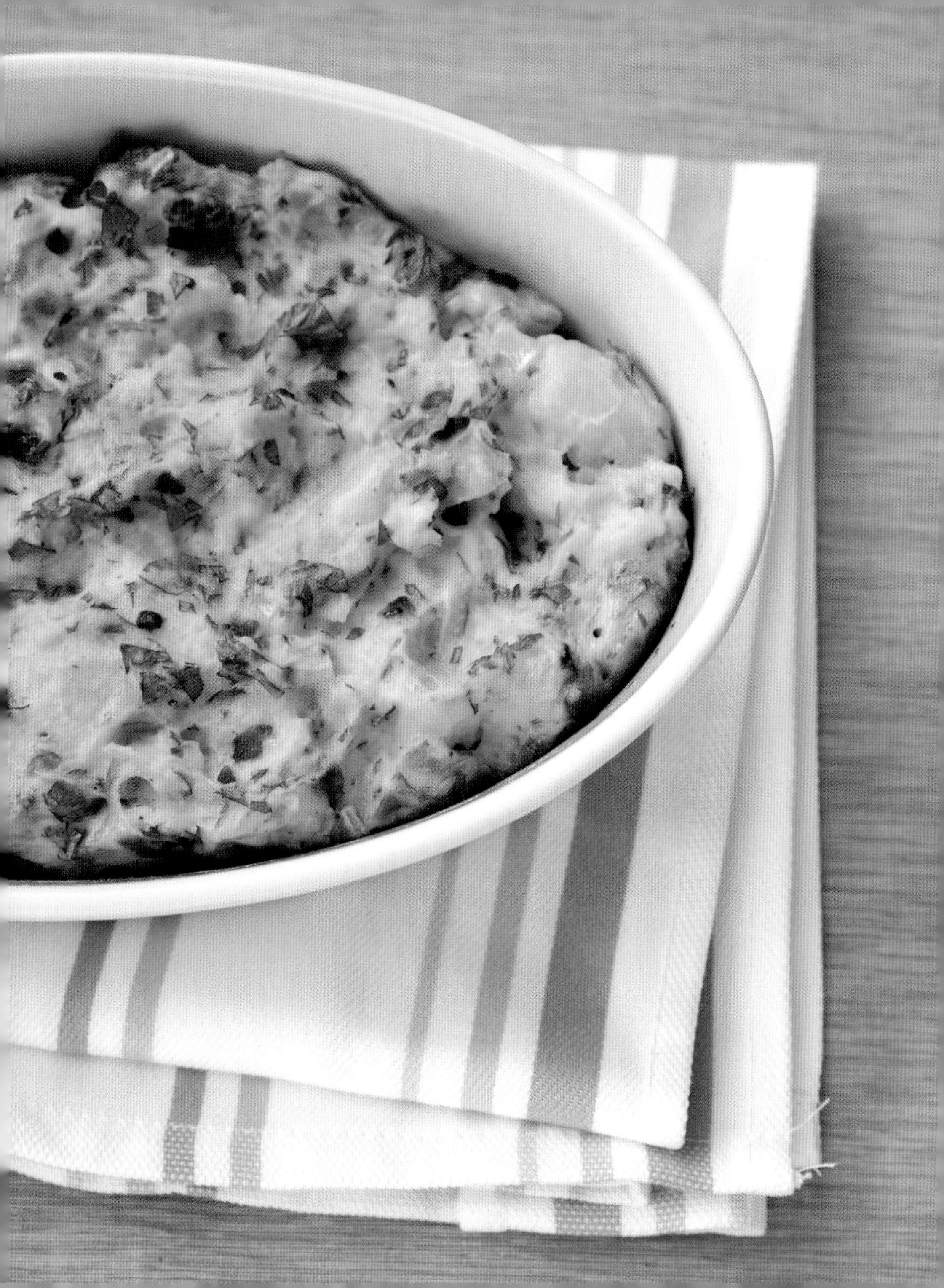

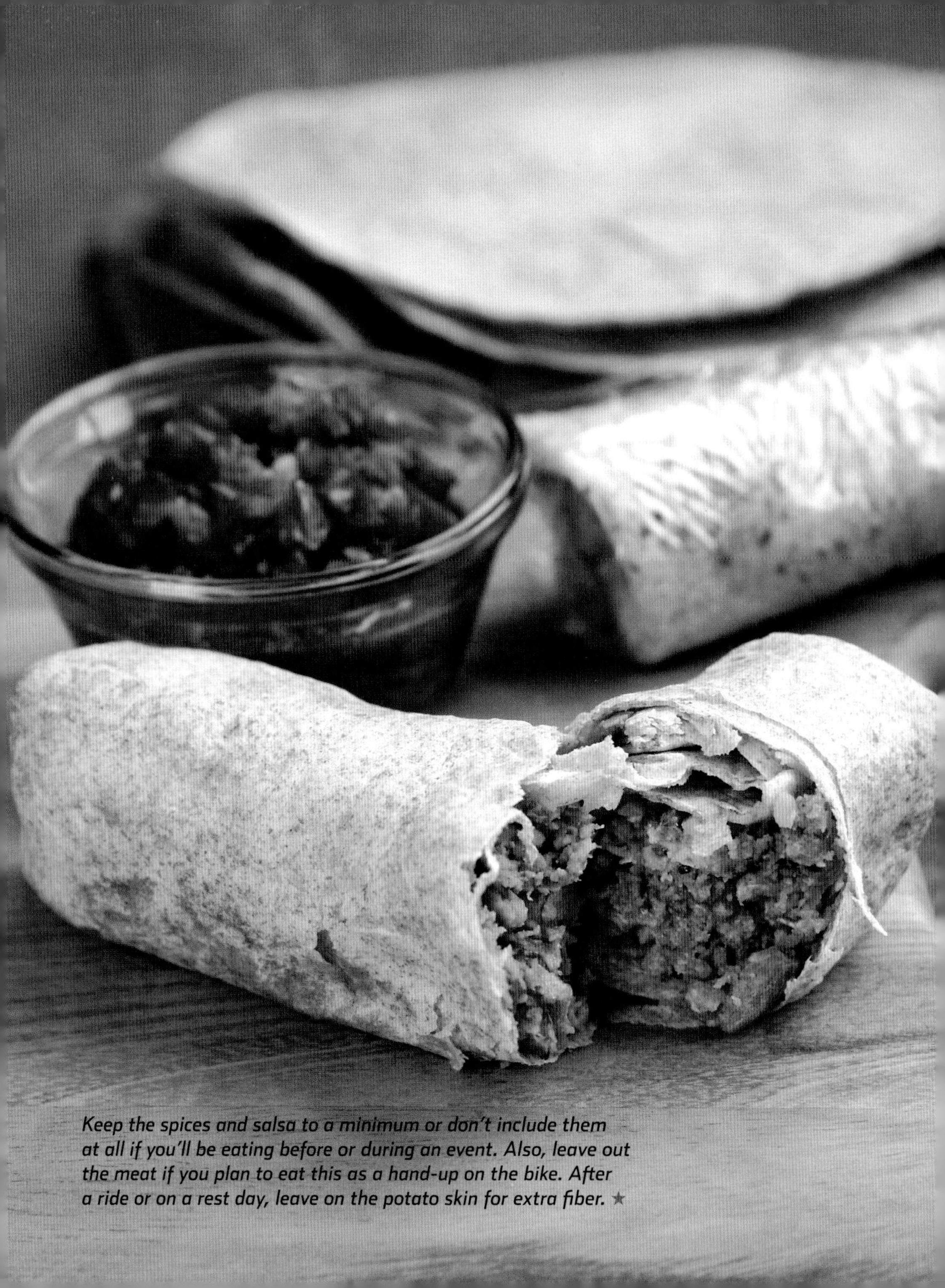

Keep the spices and salsa to a minimum or don't include them at all if you'll be eating before or during an event. Also, leave out the meat if you plan to eat this as a hand-up on the bike. After a ride or on a rest day, leave on the potato skin for extra fiber. ★

SERVINGS› 6
TIME› 20 minutes

Sweet Potato and Egg Burritos

When we are working with the pros we pack a cooler full of these burritos and hand them up to the guys a few hours into the training ride. Most of us don't enjoy the perk of support vehicles, so you can simply stuff a wrapped burrito in your pocket on your next cool morning ride.

COOKED **1 cup cooked sweet potato, packed**

8 ounces lean ground turkey

6 eggs, lightly beaten

1 tablespoon liquid amino acids

½ tablespoon brown sugar

½ cup shredded cheddar cheese

6 large (10-inch) whole wheat tortillas, warmed

OPTIONAL ADDITIONS

6 tablespoons prepared salsa

2 cups cooked red kidney or adzuki beans, drained and rinsed

2 teaspoons Taco Spice (page 295)

chopped cilantro or chives

1. Mash the cooked sweet potato (peeled or not; your choice).
2. Bring a lightly oiled sauté pan to medium-high heat. Add the ground turkey and brown.
3. Add mashed sweet potato and eggs, plus optional additions, if using; stir until the eggs have set to a soft scramble. Remove from heat.
4. Add liquid amino acids, brown sugar, and salt and pepper to taste.

Divide mixture among warmed tortillas. Top with shredded cheese and roll up as burritos, being sure to tuck in both short edges before folding the long ones (this will keep the contents from spilling out). Wrap in plastic and refrigerate or freeze.

PER SERVING (1 burrito)› **Energy** 352 cal • **Fat** 5 g • **Sodium** 896 mg • **Carbs** 58 g • **Fiber** 4 g • **Protein** 19 g

Nutrition for optional additions can be found in Appendix A.

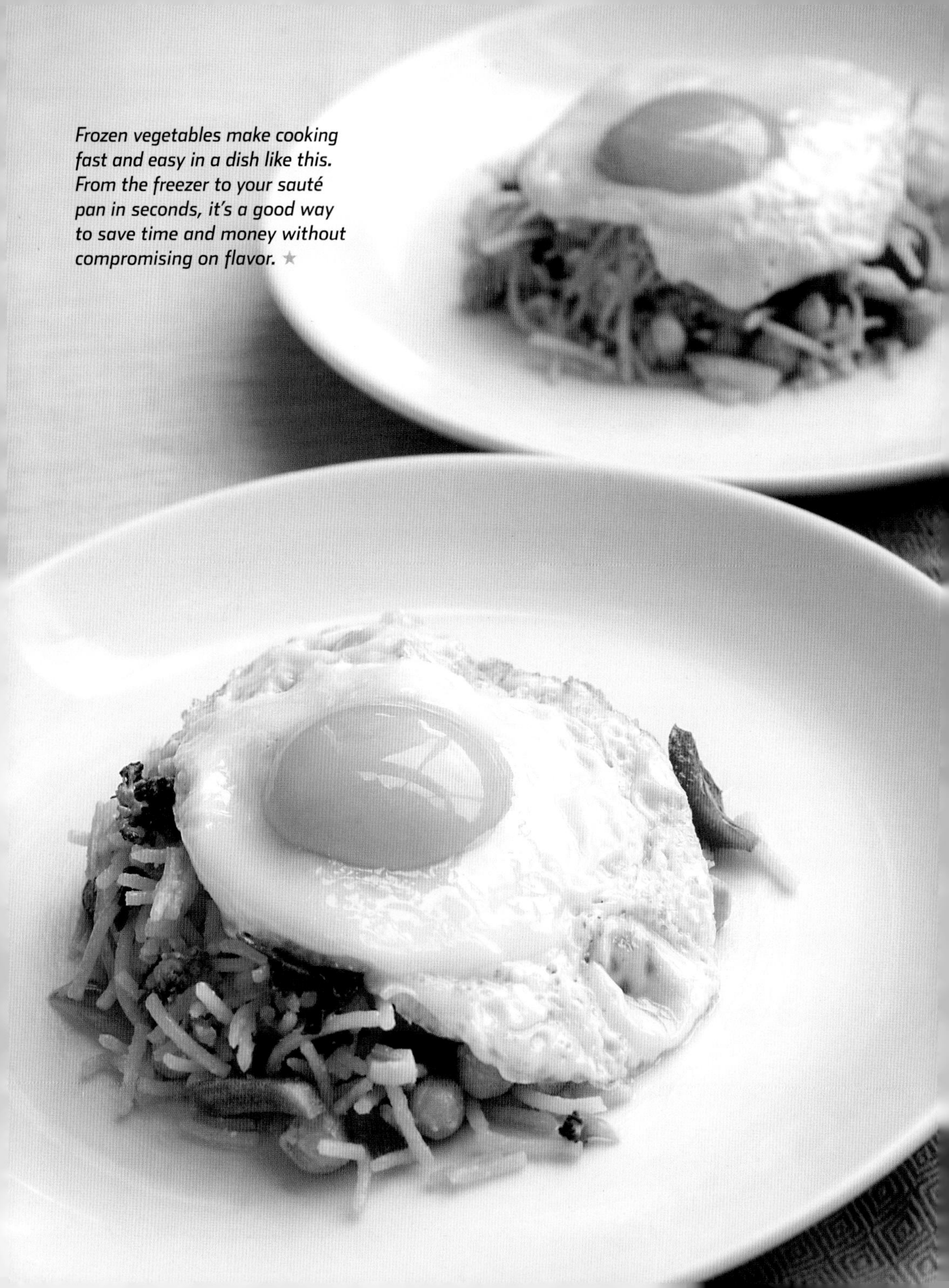

Frozen vegetables make cooking fast and easy in a dish like this. From the freezer to your sauté pan in seconds, it's a good way to save time and money without compromising on flavor. ★

SERVINGS› 2
TIME› 8–10 minutes

Pasta and Eggs

Many of the big plates we serve at breakfast could work well at any time of day. Pasta and eggs is one of our favorite dishes, especially before a big ride. We've kept it vegetarian here, but you can add cooked bacon, chicken, or canned tuna for some extra protein.

COOKED 4 cups cooked pasta
2 tablespoons cream cheese
1 cup mixed vegetables, cut small
1 cup canned garbanzo beans
¼ cup chopped fresh parsley
¼ cup grated parmesan
2 eggs

1. Bring a lightly oiled sauté pan to medium-high heat and add the cooked pasta, stirring to heat through. Add the cream cheese in small pieces, combine thoroughly, and remove from heat.
2. Add vegetables, beans, parsley, and parmesan; mix thoroughly.
3. In a separate pan, cook the eggs as you like.

Divide the pasta onto two plates. Top with the cooked eggs. Add salt and pepper to taste.

TIP Try using gluten-free quinoa pasta as shown here.

PER SERVING› **Energy** 560 cal • **Fat** 16 g • **Sodium** 432 mg • **Carbs** 78 g • **Fiber** 12 g • **Protein** 28 g

Shake up the flavor with Japanese seasoning made up of seaweed and dried fish.

SERVINGS› 2
TIME› 5 minutes

Rice and Eggs

This simple dish is a staple for most pro cyclists, especially on race days. During the 2010 Tour de France, the RadioShack team ate rice and eggs for breakfast every day. If you make a habit of it, vary the flavors with your favorite condiments (most notably Sriracha sauce and amino acids).

COOKED **4 cups cooked white rice**

4 eggs

1 teaspoon salt

OPTIONAL ADDITIONS

Sriracha sauce

liquid amino acids or low-sodium soy sauce

Japanese dry seasoning mix

toasted sesame seeds

1. Add a splash of water to the cooked rice and warm in a sauté pan over medium-high heat.
2. Cook the eggs however you like: sunny-side up, over easy, or scrambled.
3. In a large bowl, combine the rice and eggs and add the salt, along with your favorite seasoning.

TIP If you are watching your sodium intake, cut the salt to ½ teaspoon and use liquid amino acids or low-sodium soy sauce instead of soy sauce or Japanese seasoning.

PER SERVING› **Energy** 530 cal • **Fat** 11 g • **Sodium** 1,473 mg • **Carbs** 88 g • **Fiber** 2 g • **Protein** 18 g

Nutrition for optional additions can be found in Appendix A.

SERVINGS› 8
TIME› 20–30 minutes

Spanish Tortilla

If you've traveled or ridden through Spain, you've definitely had this dish. An all-time favorite of pros and amateurs alike, it's a simple and filling frittata of potatoes, eggs, and onions. You can top it with any type of grated cheese and enjoy it hot or cold most any time of day.

½ cup or more of olive oil

4 cups potatoes, sliced ¼-inch thick

2 medium sweet onions, cut into ¼-inch-thick slices

8 eggs

dash each of ground nutmeg, salt, and pepper

OPTIONAL ADDITIONS

grated parmesan

tomatoes

1. In a deep nonstick sauté pan, bring ¼ cup of olive oil to medium-high heat. Add the potatoes in two or three batches, cooking until slightly crisp. Remove cooked potatoes with a slotted spoon and drain on a plate covered with paper towels while you cook the onions. Add olive oil to the pan as needed to prevent sticking.
2. Meanwhile, in a large bowl, lightly beat the eggs with the nutmeg, salt, and pepper. Add the cooked potatoes and onions and combine.
3. Drain most of the oil from pan, leaving just enough to coat the bottom. Return the egg-and-potato mixture to the pan and cook over medium-high heat. Push contents around until they are just starting to cook through and the edges have set, about 5 minutes.
4. Invert a large dinner plate over the pan. Carefully flip the contents of the pan onto the plate, then return the tortilla with uncooked side down in pan. Let cook for 2–3 minutes, until bottom is crispy. Top with cheese or tomatoes, if desired.

Serve warm, or let cool and take along for your next ride.

PER SERVING› **Energy** 305 cal • **Fat** 19 g • **Sodium** 203 mg • **Carbs** 27 g • **Fiber** 3 g • **Protein** 9 g
Nutrition for optional additions can be found in Appendix A.

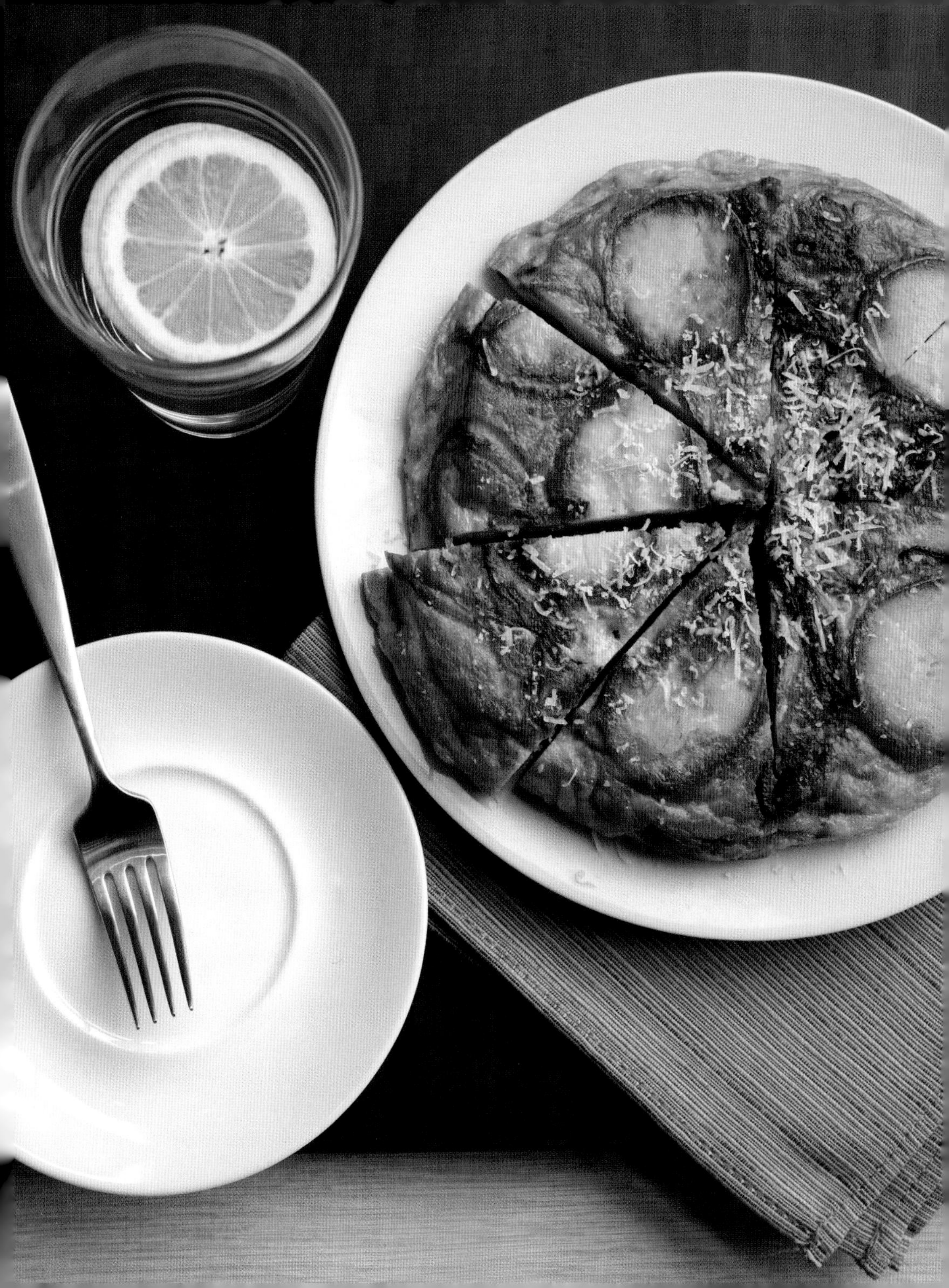

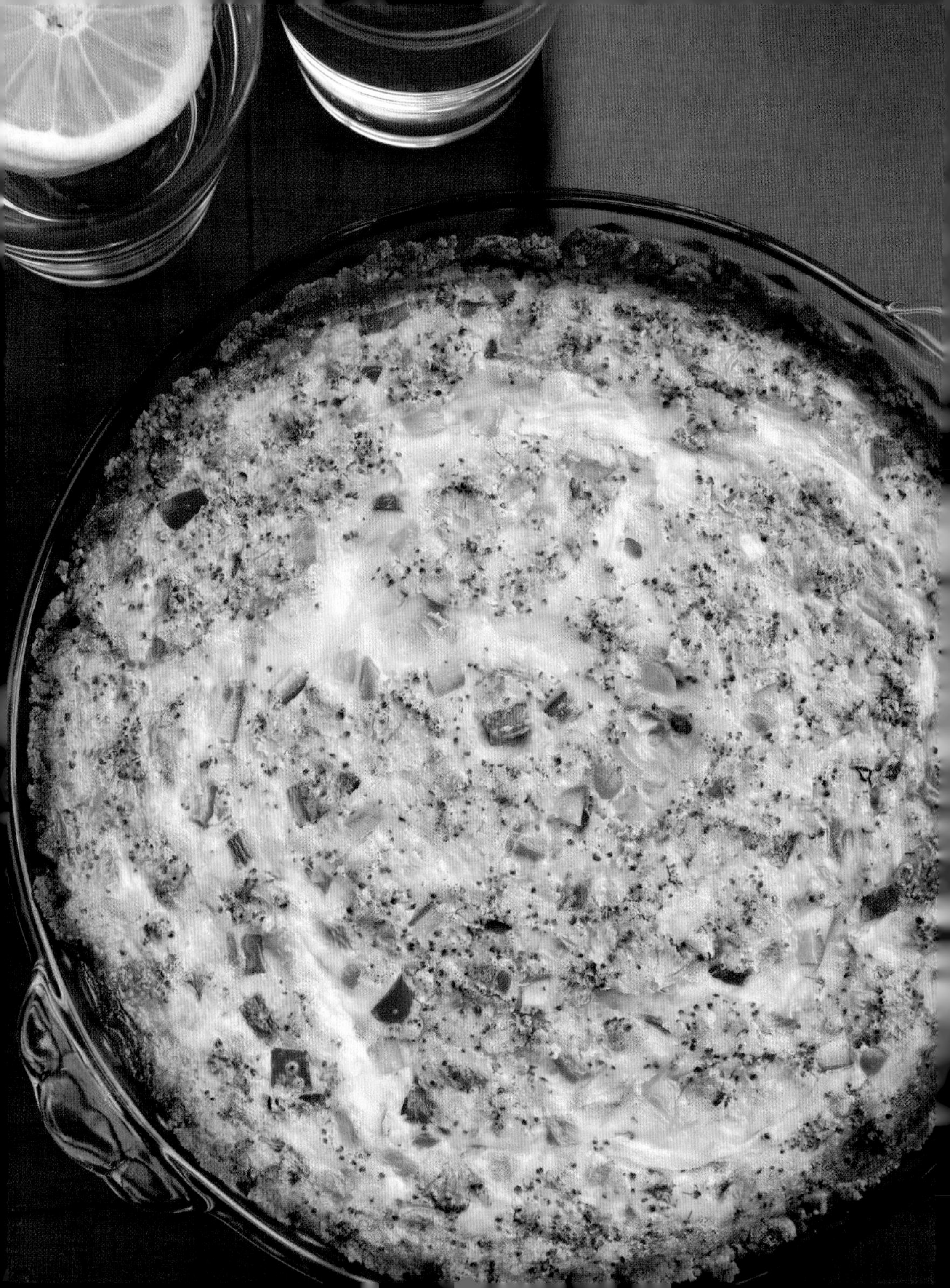

SERVINGS› 6
TIME› 20 minutes prep,
bake 35 minutes

Quiche

Most quiche recipes call for a classic pie crust, which, though delicious, is made of wheat flour and shortening. Our healthier recipe is quick and satisfying—and, if you like, gluten-free. Quiche is not quick, but when you have the time, it's well worth the wait.

CRUST

3–4 slices (2 cups) regular or gluten-free bread

2 tablespoons butter

FILLING

8 eggs

¼ cup almond or dairy milk

½ cup shredded Swiss cheese

½ teaspoon salt

½ teaspoon ground nutmeg (optional)

½ cup thinly sliced vegetables (onions, bell peppers, and/or broccoli)

COOKED **¼ cup chopped cooked meat (bacon, shaved ham, sausage, or roasted chicken)**

1. Heat oven to 325 degrees.
2. Use a food processor or blender until bread slices are cut into fine crumbs. If using a blender, pulse small amounts at a time. Add the butter and whirl again until mixture begins to hold together. Press into a 9-inch pie tin.
3. Bake crust for 8–10 minutes.
4. In a large bowl, whisk eggs and milk together. Then add cheese, salt, and nutmeg, if using. Add desired veggies and cooked meat; stir. Pour into pie shell.
5. Bake for 35–40 minutes, until center of quiche is set (you can test it with a knife blade).

Let the quiche sit for a few minutes before cutting into it. Serve warm or at room temperature. Refrigerate any leftovers.

PER SERVING› **Energy** 258 cal • **Fat** 17 g • **Sodium** 584 mg • **Carbs** 12 g • **Fiber** 1 g • **Protein** 13 g

Nutrition for optional additions and alternatives can be found in Appendix A.

SERVINGS› 2
TIME› 10 minutes

Quinoa and Vegetable Hash with Eggs

This nutritious hash can be served chilled or hot off the stove. Save time in the morning by cooking the quinoa and sweet potatoes in advance. Change the ingredients to use what you have on hand—hash shouldn't be fussy!

- 2 tablespoons olive oil
- 1 medium onion, sliced
- COOKED 2 cups cubed cooked sweet potatoes
- ¼ cup chopped fresh parsley
- COOKED 3 cups cooked quinoa
- salt, pepper, and grated parmesan
- 2 eggs

1. Bring a lightly oiled sauté pan to medium-high heat. Add onion slices and sauté until browned slightly.
2. Add cooked sweet potatoes and parsley; sauté until the edges of the potatoes begin to brown.
3. Add cooked quinoa. Add salt, pepper, and cheese to taste.
4. In a separate pan, cook the eggs as you like.

Divide hash onto two plates and top with cooked eggs. A squeeze of fresh lemon juice and a bit of olive oil or hot sauce complete the dish.

PER SERVING› **Energy** 725 cal • **Fat** 26 g • **Sodium** 830 mg • **Carbs** 101 g • **Fiber** 11 g • **Protein** 25 g

Instead of topping hash with eggs, add cooked red kidney beans, lentils, or black beans to the pan. If you are looking for a lower-calorie, higher-fiber option (i.e., you are not training after breakfast), substitute carrots or squash for the sweet potatoes. ★

Romesco is a traditional Spanish sauce commonly used in food of the Catalan. There are numerous versions, based on family preferences and local ingredients. The basic idea is to toast scraps of bread along with nuts—most commonly almonds—add in some red peppers, tomatoes, garlic, and onions; finish with a bit of vinegar; and blend it all into a hearty, earthy, chunky sauce. * See page 288 for full recipe.

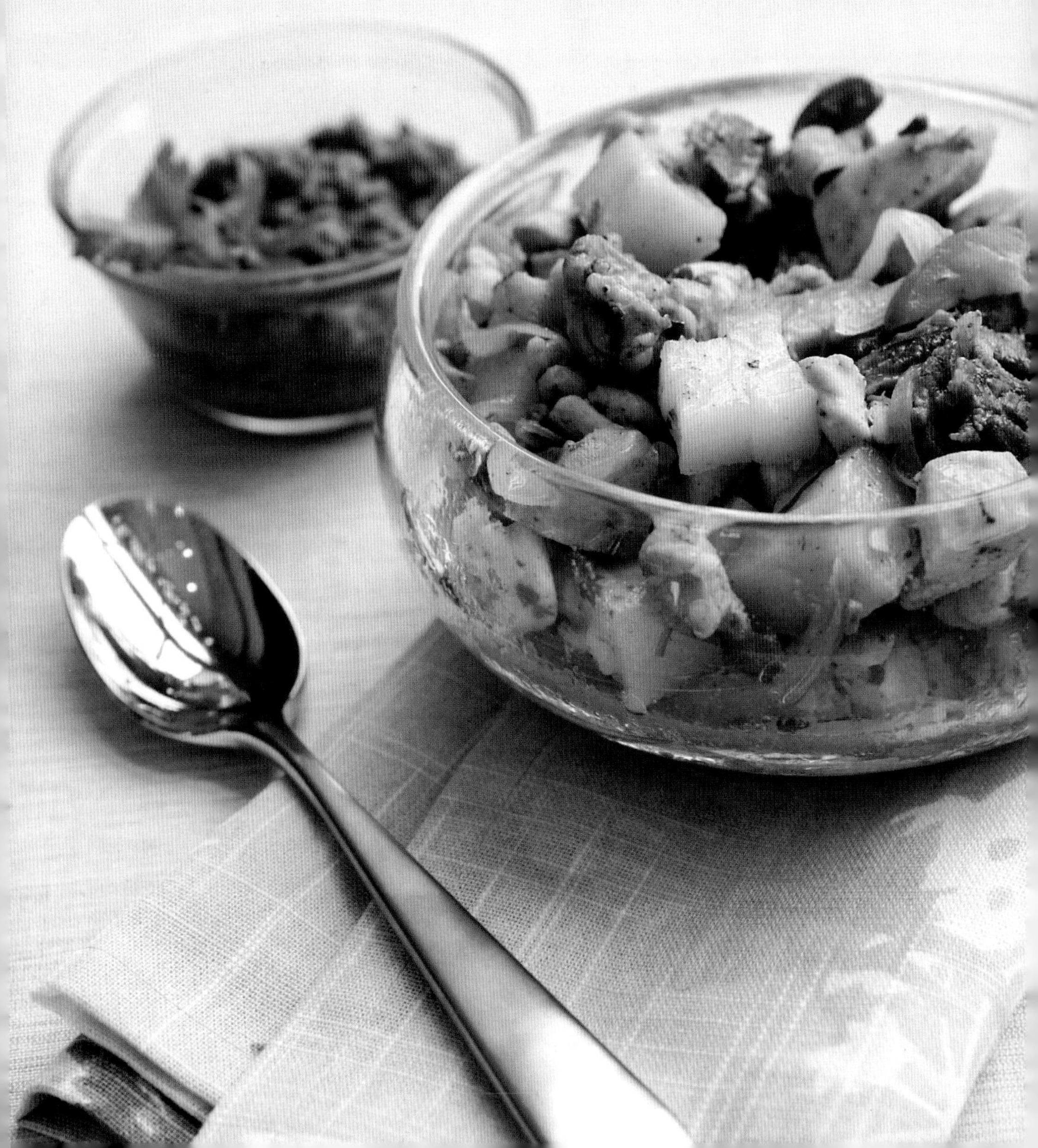

SERVINGS› 2
TIME› 20 minutes

Chicken and Bacon Hash

The smoky, sweet bacon and chicken in this hash are perfect when accompanied with a spicy Romesco sauce. When you don't have time to make homemade Romesco, your favorite prepared salsa or hot sauce will be a good substitute.

4 ounces bacon, chopped

8 ounces chicken, cut into cubes

COOKED **2 medium cooked potatoes, peeled and cut into bite-size pieces**

¼ cup thinly sliced onions

¼ cup thinly sliced bell peppers

2 tablespoons chopped fresh parsley

Romesco (page 288)

1. Fry the bacon in a medium-hot sauté pan until crispy; drain most of the fat.
2. Add chicken, then potatoes, onions, and peppers. Cook until the chicken is cooked through and the potatoes are as crispy as you like, about 8–10 minutes. Mix in parsley and add salt and pepper to taste.

PER SERVING› **Energy** 481 cal • **Fat** 11 g • **Sodium** 603 mg • **Carbs** 51 g • **Fiber** 4 g • **Protein** 44 g

★ Breakfast Tacos go great with Cilantro-Mint Yogurt. See page 291 for recipe.

SERVINGS› 4
TIME› 30 minutes

Breakfast Tacos

This is a great, fun way to have breakfast with your family on weekend mornings. Cook each ingredient, one at a time, using the oven to keep the potatoes and bacon warm while you scramble the eggs. The cilantro-mint yogurt takes the place of sour cream and goes together quickly.

4 ounces bacon, chopped

½ cup diced potatoes

COOKED **½ cup cooked pinto beans**

¼ cup shredded cheese

chopped scallions or onions

4 scrambled eggs

4 corn tortillas or taco shells

4 tablespoons salsa

Cilantro-Mint Yogurt (page 291)

1. Bring a lightly oiled sauté pan to medium-high heat, and cook the bacon. Set bacon aside.
2. In the same pan, cook the potatoes and beans until they are soft and the potatoes are brown. Set aside when finished.
3. While your potatoes and beans are cooking, shred the cheese and chop the onions.
4. In sauté pan, scramble eggs.
5. Wrap the tortillas in foil and warm them in a heated oven, or arrange taco shells on a baking tray and heat in oven. (Be careful not to forget these in the oven; they will catch fire!)

Set out all desired ingredients and let your family assemble their own tacos.

PER SERVING (1 taco)› **Energy** 268 cal • **Fat** 13 g • **Sodium** 459 mg • **Carbs** 23 g • **Fiber** 4 g • **Protein** 15 g

SERVINGS› 2
TIME› 20 minutes

Buttermilk Pancakes

Pancakes are a favorite pre-ride meal for American cyclists. During the season, when every bite counts, pancakes are one of the most pleasurable ways to get the carbs you need.

DRY INGREDIENTS

1½ cups all-purpose flour

2 tablespoons brown sugar

1½ teaspoons baking powder

1 teaspoon baking soda

1 teaspoon ground cinnamon

WET INGREDIENTS

1½ cups buttermilk (see note)

2 eggs, lightly beaten

¼ cup butter, melted

1. Combine all the dry ingredients in a large bowl.
2. Fold in the wet ingredients, slowly adding milk to achieve desired thickness. Do not overmix.
3. Bring a lightly oiled sauté pan to medium-high heat. Pour batter onto pan, forming pancakes of your desired size (be sure to allow room for batter to spread). Flip pancakes after bubbles begin to form along the edges or when first side is golden brown; cook on second side until done.

Transfer cooked pancakes to plates or a serving platter. Top them off with fruit of your choice. Makes about 6 pancakes.

NOTE› If you don't have buttermilk on hand, add 1 tablespoon of lemon juice to 1½ cups of regular dairy milk; stir, then allow the milk to sit for 5 minutes before using.

TIP To save time, make a double or triple batch of the dry ingredient mix and store it in an airtight container in your pantry. Scoop out 2 cups of dry mix and then proceed with the recipe.

PER SERVING (3 pancakes)› Energy 771 cal • Fat 32 g • Sodium 519 mg • Carbs 96 g • Fiber 3 g • Protein 25 g

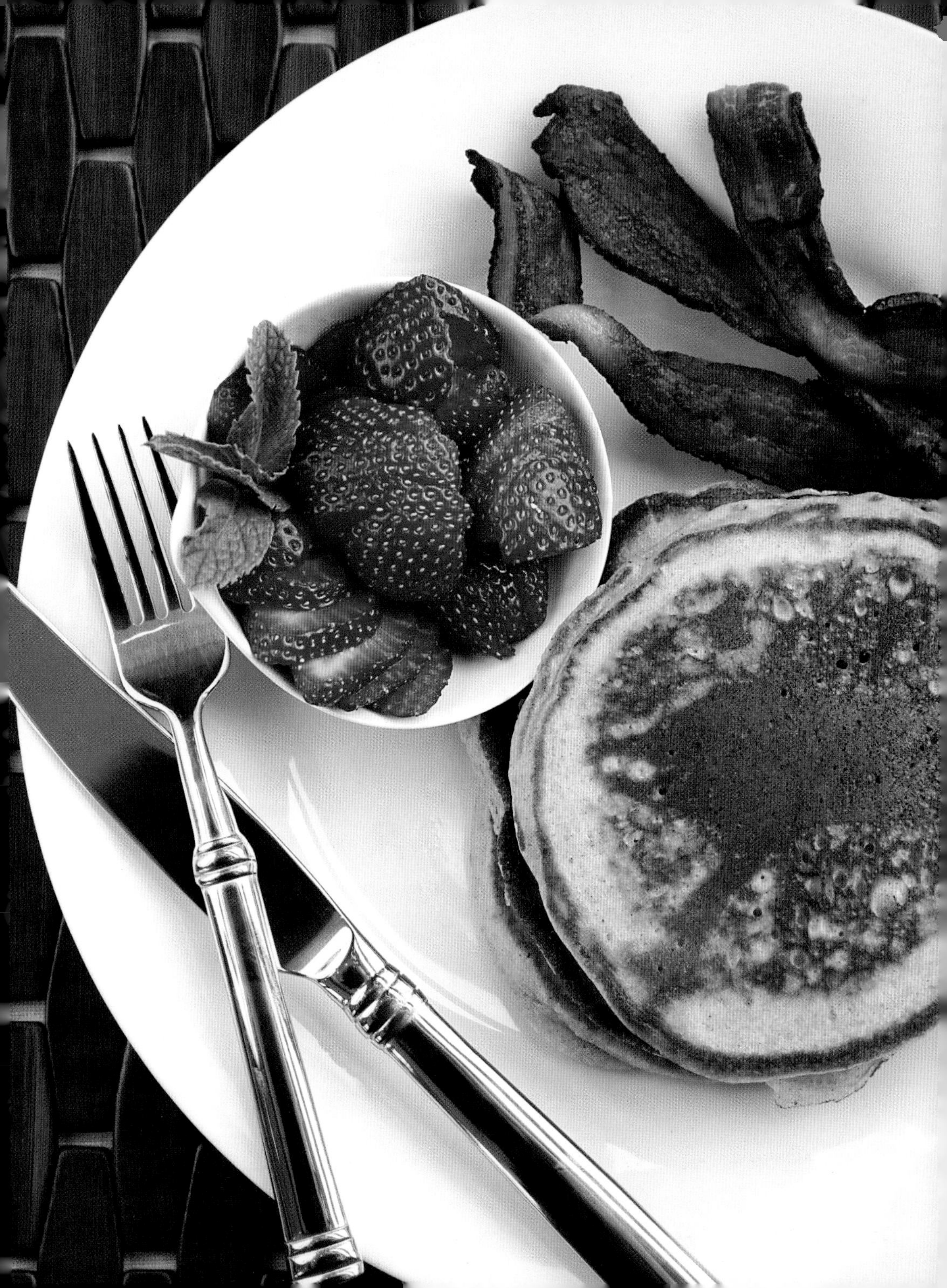

SERVINGS› 2
TIME› 25 minutes

Rice and Banana Pancakes

Rice pancakes are a great source of carbs and are naturally free of wheat gluten. These pancakes take a little longer to cook than regular pancakes but stay super moist and creamy inside.

COOKED 2 cups cooked white rice

2 eggs, lightly beaten

1 ripe banana

2 tablespoons brown sugar

1 tablespoon rice flour or potato flour

1½–2 cups milk

pinch of salt

OPTIONAL ADDITIONS

1 teaspoon vanilla or almond extract

sprinkle each of ground cinnamon and nutmeg

1. Heat oven to 325 degrees.
2. Mix all ingredients in a blender, adding milk slowly to achieve desired thickness. The batter will be slightly thicker than traditional pancakes.
3. Bring a lightly oiled sauté pan to medium-high heat. Pour batter onto pan, forming pancakes of your desired size (be sure to allow room for batter to spread). These take a little longer than regular pancakes to set up before you can safely flip them; plan on about 4 minutes per side.

Transfer cooked pancakes to oven and allow to finish baking while you make the rest of the pancakes. Makes about 6 pancakes.

PER SERVING (3 pancakes) › Energy 405 cal • Fat 7 g • Sodium 100 mg • Carbs 71 g • Fiber 3 g • Protein 16 g

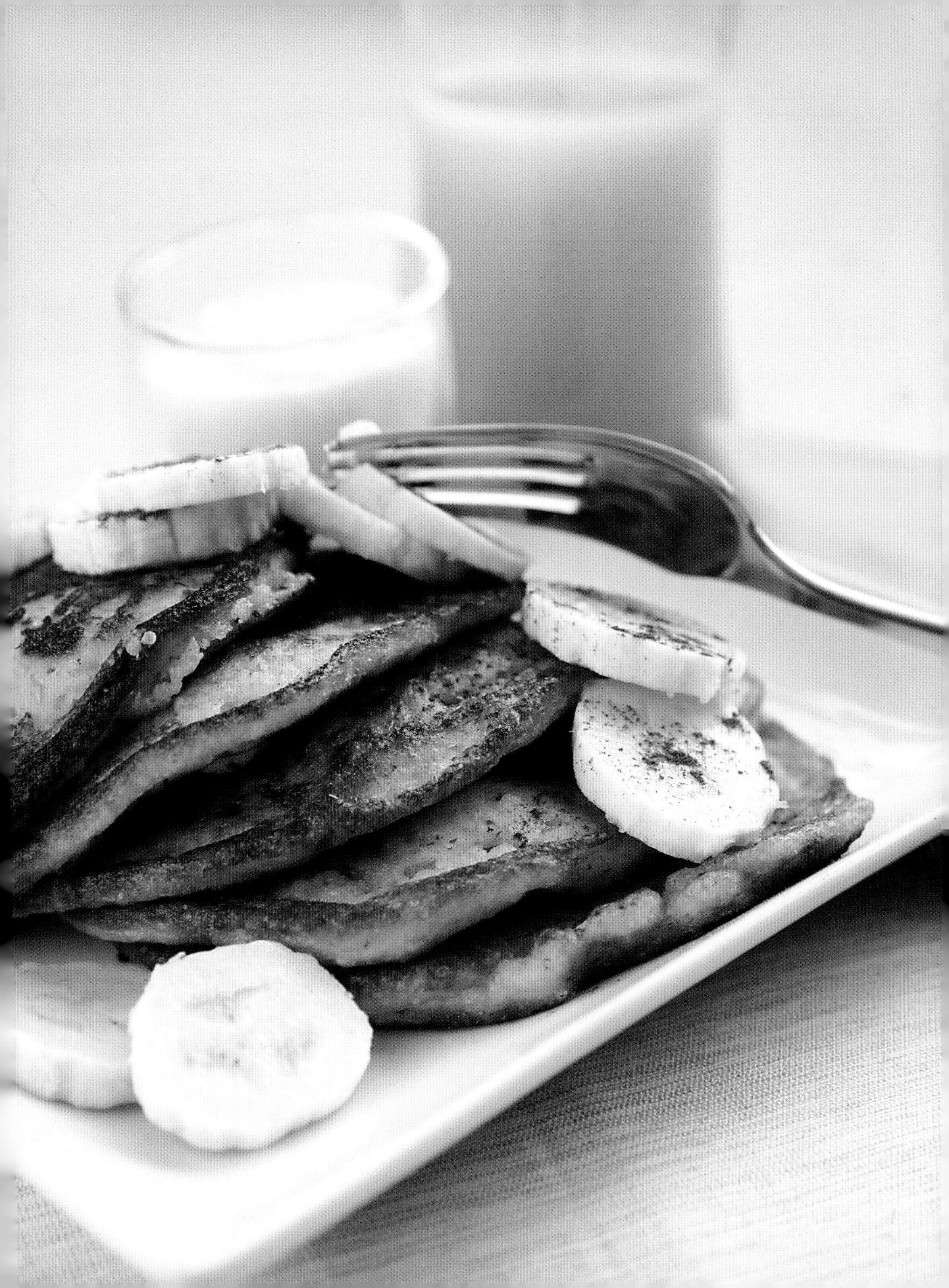

Almond flour is just finely ground whole almonds. Most groceries now stock it in the baking goods aisle or with natural foods (one common brand is Bob's Red Mill). You can make your own using a food processor or blender—just be sure not to grind the nuts too long or you'll end up with almond butter! ★

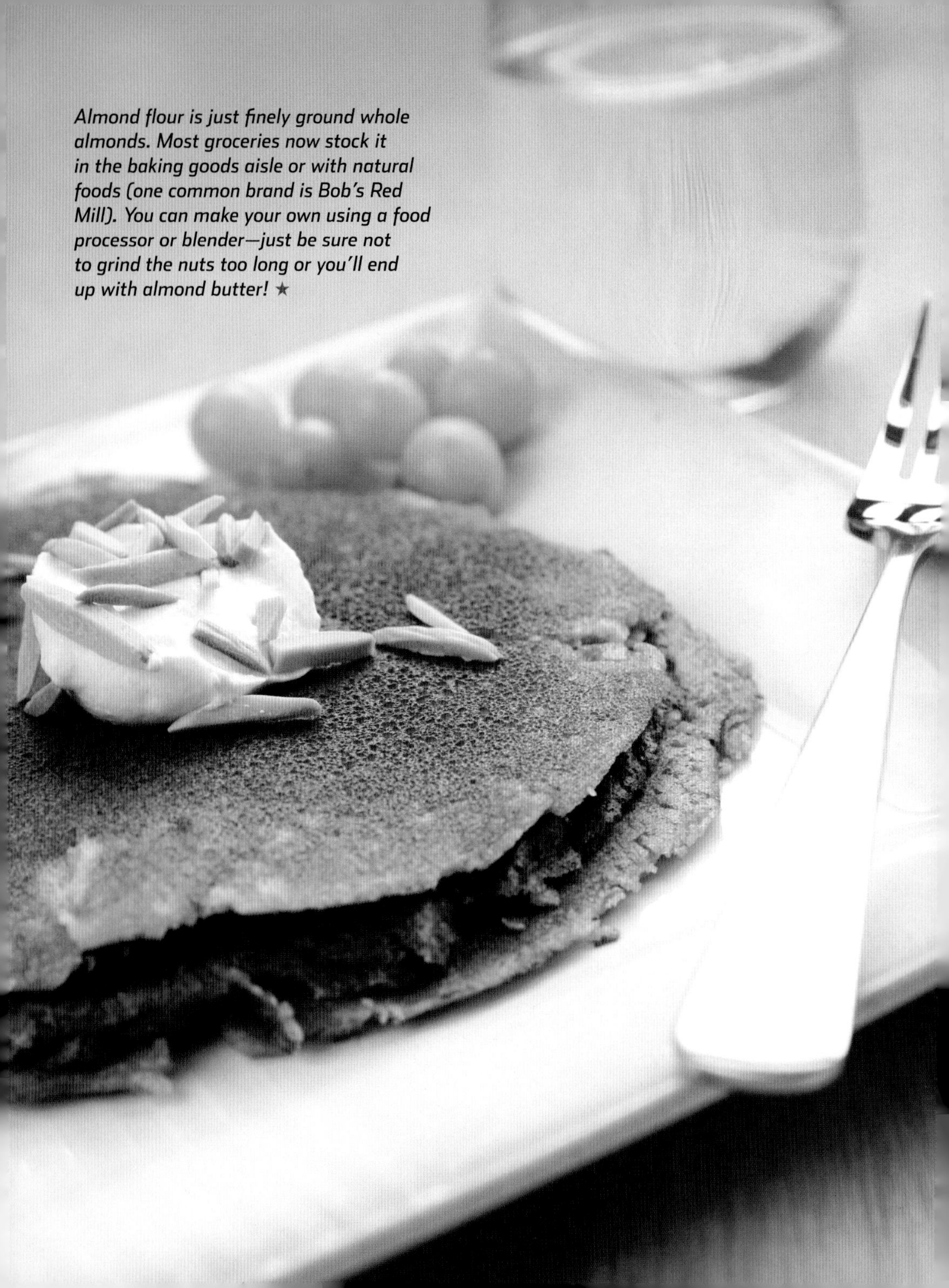

SERVINGS> 2
TIME> 20 minutes

Cinnamon Almond Pancakes

Made with almond flour, these pancakes are gluten-free and lower in carbs than traditional pancakes. The batter will be thin and delicate, more like a crepe than a pancake.

1 cup almond flour
2 eggs
¼ cup milk or water
2 tablespoons cooking oil
1 tablespoon honey or agave nectar
a dash each of ground cinnamon and salt

OPTIONAL ADDITIONS

toasted almonds
plain yogurt

1. Mix together all ingredients in a bowl.
2. Bring a lightly oiled sauté pan to medium-high heat. When pan is hot, pour batter to form pancakes, leaving ample space between each to allow batter to spread. Unlike traditional pancakes these will not bubble, so watch for the edges to brown, then gently flip over and brown the other side.

Serve hot, topped with toasted almonds, yogurt, or fresh fruit. Makes about 6 pancakes.

TIP Even easier: If you're not concerned about gluten, add ground almonds to your usual packaged pancake mix. Follow package directions from there.

PER SERVING (3 pancakes)> **Energy** 557 cal • **Fat** 47 g • **Sodium** 447 mg • **Carbs** 23 g • **Fiber** 6 g • **Protein** 19 g
Nutrition for optional additions can be found in Appendix A.

SERVINGS› 4
TIME› 30 minutes

Sweet Potato Pancakes

There are a few ways to make a basic sweet potato pancake, but this is the simplest. The amount of milk needed to make a thick batter may vary due to the moisture content of the potatoes. For added texture, I top the pancakes with toasted slivered almonds and sometimes add ground almonds to the batter.

DRY INGREDIENTS

2 cups all-purpose flour

3 teaspoons baking powder

1 teaspoon salt

½ teaspoon ground cinnamon

2 tablespoons brown sugar

WET INGREDIENTS

COOKED 2 cups cooked sweet potatoes, mashed

2 eggs, lightly beaten

1½–2 cups almond milk

2 tablespoons melted butter

1. Combine all dry ingredients in a bowl.
2. In another bowl, blend together sweet potatoes, eggs, 1 cup of the milk, and the melted butter. Add the combined dry ingredients, mix thoroughly, and add more milk if needed to make a thick batter.
3. Bring a lightly oiled sauté pan to medium-high heat. Pour batter onto pan. Let cook until the edges turn golden brown, then flip. Cook second side until golden brown.

Top pancakes with the toasted almonds. Serve with yogurt or peanut butter. Makes about 8 pancakes.

TIP You can also use organic canned sweet potatoes. One large can is about equal to 2 whole potatoes.

PER SERVING (2 pancakes) › **Energy** 573 cal • **Fat** 22 g • **Sodium** 798 mg • **Carbs** 81 g • **Fiber** 7 g • **Protein** 16 g
Nutrition for optional additions can be found in Appendix A.

Optional topping: In a small bowl, combine ½ cup slivered almonds and 1 tablespoon brown sugar. Heat a small, dry pan over medium-high heat, then turn off the heat and add the almond-sugar mixture. Stir constantly while the almonds toast and the sugar coats the slivers, about 3 minutes. Remove pan from heat. ★

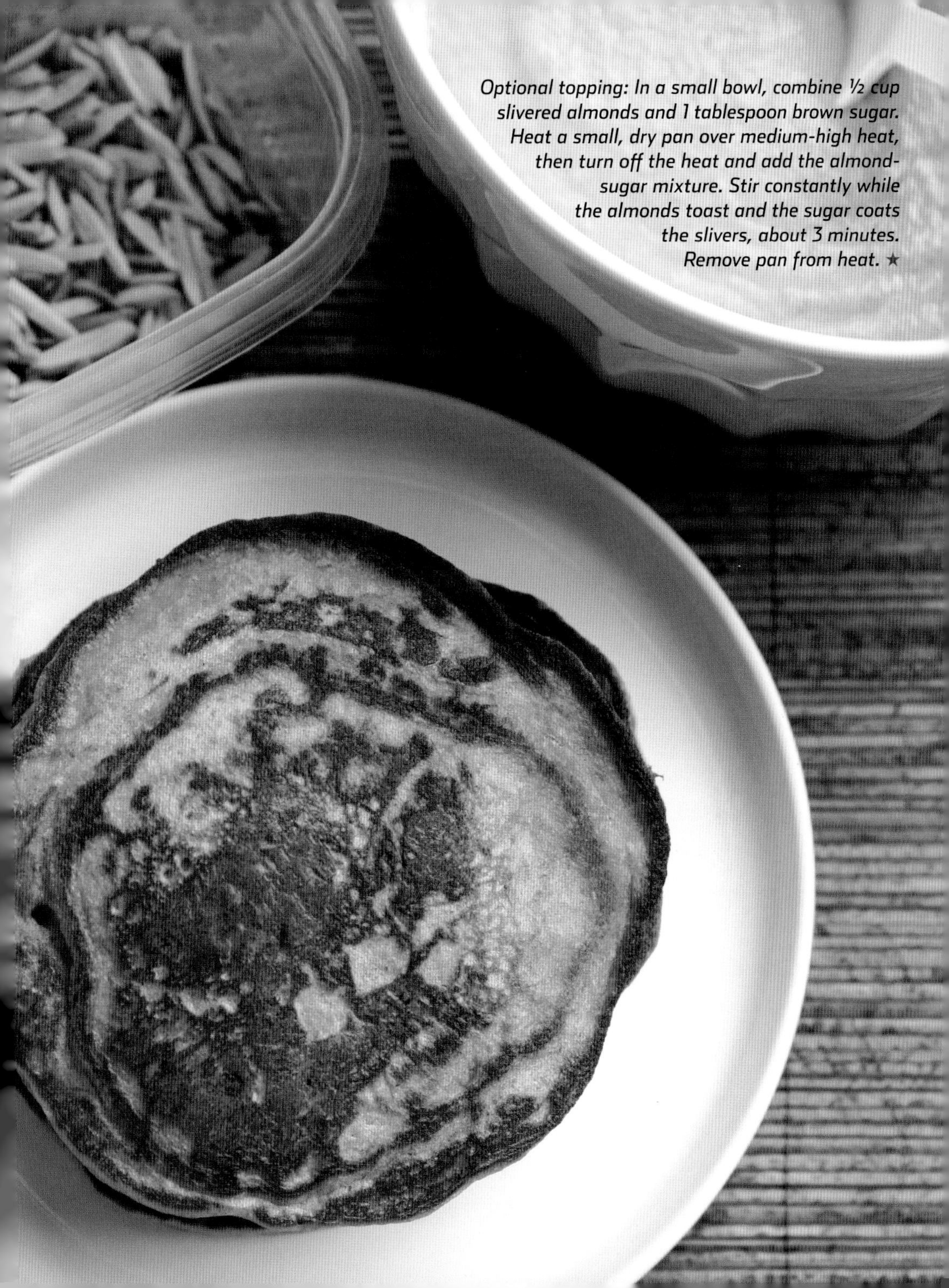

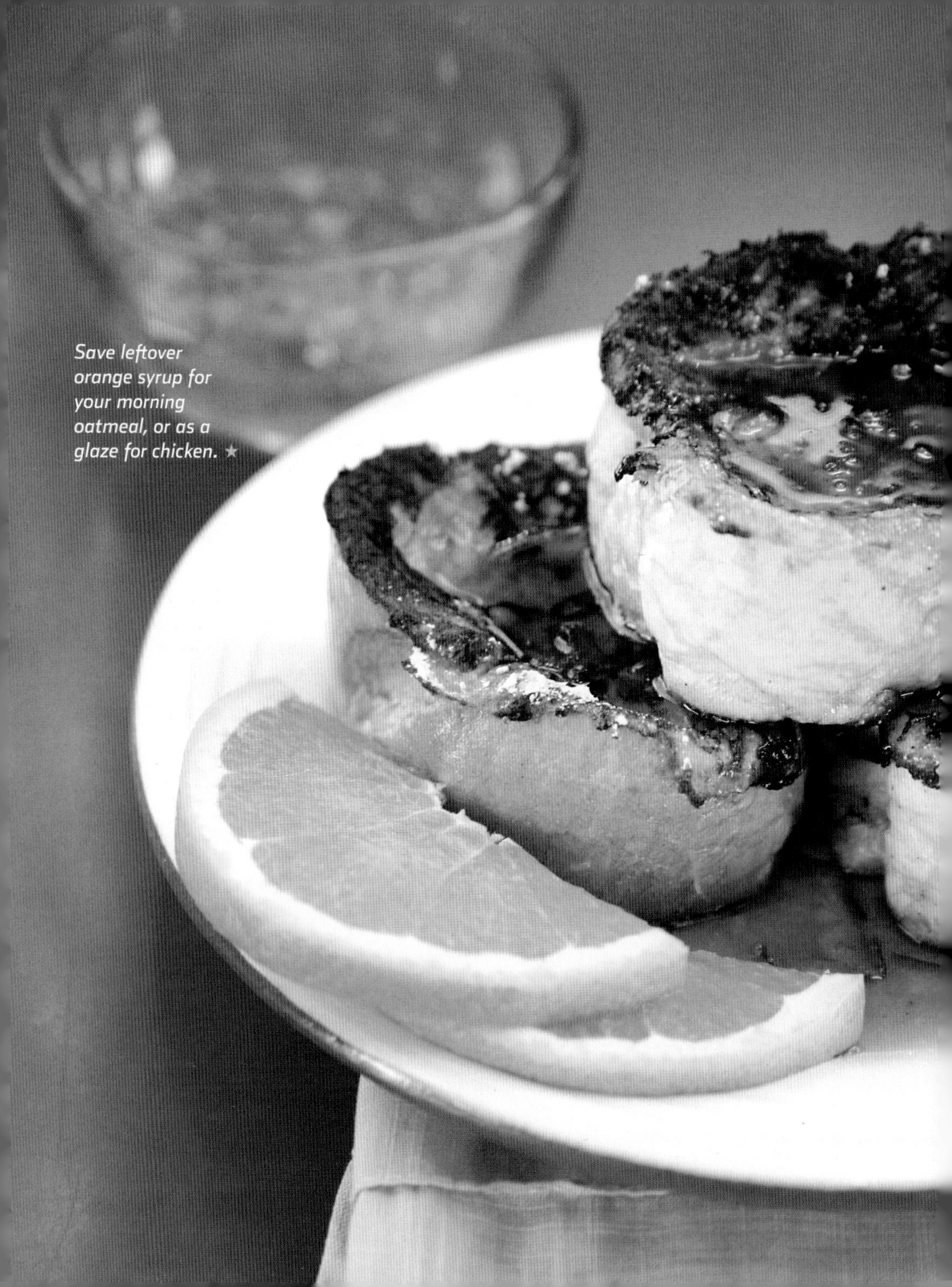

Save leftover orange syrup for your morning oatmeal, or as a glaze for chicken. ★

SERVINGS› 2
TIME› 20 minutes

French Toast

A rustic boule with an orange twist makes this French toast recipe fantastic. Any other dense bread will work well, too—challah, sourdough, French bread, potato bread, or whole wheat. If possible, use day-old bread, which won't soak up the batter too quickly and fall apart before hitting the pan.

4–6 thick slices of bread

3 eggs

1 cup milk

2 tablespoons sugar

1 teaspoon vanilla extract

1 teaspoon ground pumpkin pie spice

1 tablespoon butter

ORANGE SYRUP

1 cup maple syrup

1 teaspoon vanilla extract

1 tablespoon orange marmalade

1. If desired, slice the crusts off the bread slices (they make good bread crumbs). Combine the eggs, milk, sugar, vanilla, and spice in a bowl or blender. Soak the bread slices in the batter, turning slices once so that both sides are soaked through.
2. Bring a lightly oiled sauté pan to medium-high heat. Add a tablespoon or so of butter and swirl it over the surface of the pan. Add bread slices. Turn them over when the bottom is the desired shade of golden brown and cook the second side.
3. To make the orange syrup: Mix ingredients together. Serve warm. Refrigerate any leftover syrup.

Garnish with powdered sugar and fresh fruit, and serve orange syrup alongside.

TIP Pumpkin pie spice is a combination of ground nutmeg, cinnamon, and allspice. Use what you have on hand.

PER SERVING (3 pieces)› **Energy** 456 cal • **Fat** 12 g • **Sodium** 857 mg • **Carbs** 66 g • **Fiber** 3 g • **Protein** 22 g
SYRUP (2 tbsp.)› **Energy** 110 cal • **Fat** 0 g • **Sodium** 0 mg • **Carbs** 28 g • **Fiber** 0 g • **Protein** 0 g

SERVINGS› 3
TIME› 20 minutes

Stuffed French Toast

Take French toast from basic to decadent with your favorite fruits, nut butters, and other good things. We have suggested some of our favorite pairings, but you should experiment to find your own stuffing of choice.

- 4–6 thick slices of bread
- 3 eggs
- 1 cup milk
- 2 tablespoons agave nectar or honey
- 2 teaspoons almond or vanilla extract
- ½ teaspoon salt
- 1 tablespoon butter

STUFFING

- 2 tablespoons cream cheese
- 2 slices ham

OR

- 4 tablespoons Nutella
- 1 ripe banana, sliced

OR

- 1 apple, sliced
- 2 tablespoons honey

1. Heat oven to 350 degrees. If desired, trim crusts from bread (keep for bread crumbs).
2. In a large mixing bowl, combine eggs, milk, agave nectar, extract, and salt. Have ready your desired stuffing ingredients.
3. Soak two slices of bread in egg mixture. While bread is soaking, melt butter in a sauté pan over medium-high heat.
4. Transfer the soaked bread to the sauté pan and cook until golden brown, flipping once. Soak two more slices while the first batch is cooking.
5. Remove cooked French toast to a baking sheet. Pile one slice with your favorite stuffing ingredients; cover with second slice, pressing down lightly. Place in oven while you fry the rest of the French toast. Leave all toast in the oven 5 minutes more, then serve. If you're pressed for time, skip the oven. The stuffing ingredients won't be as softened but will still taste great.

PER SERVING (ham & cheese)› Energy 385 cal • Fat 12 g • Sodium 1,151 mg • Carbs 50 g • Fiber 2 g • Protein 19 g
PER SERVING (banana & Nutella)› Energy 424 cal • Fat 11 g • Sodium 891 mg • Carbs 66 g • Fiber 4 g • Protein 16 g
PER SERVING (apple & honey)› Energy 388 cal • Fat 7 g • Sodium 1,272 mg • Carbs 67 g • Fiber 3 g • Protein 15 g

Gluten-free bread works well, but let it soak in the batter a bit longer. ★

★★★

The foods in the Portables section were originally designed to give riders an alternative to pre-packaged bars and food. We found that if the riders only ate sweet, dense energy bars, they would develop a bad stomach, or "gut rot," toward the end of the race—the time when being able to digest food and absorb fluids is most critical. Riders were also bored and simply not satisfied by the taste of the food that was available to them. They often did not eat enough as a result. **To address these problems, we started making many of our race foods from scratch, including little sandwiches and rice-based bars.**

Among the team's favorite foods is a savory rice cake made with calrose rice, scrambled eggs, and bacon, based on Zong Zi, a portable savory Chinese rice dish that is typically wrapped in bamboo leaves. Unlike Zong Zi, **our portables are wrapped in a paper foil to keep them fresh and accessible while out training or racing.** You can cut up and wrap almost anything you like to eat if it's easily digested and contains primarily carbohydrate. So feel free to turn any sweet or savory food into a portable snack for training and racing.

PORTABLES

HOW TO MAKE BOILED POTATOES

One portable found in the peloton requires just 3 ingredients: potatoes, olive oil, and parmesan. Wash 12–13 potatoes that are under 1½ inches in diameter. Put potatoes, with skin on, into a pot of boiling water for about 10 minutes. (The skins prevent the potatoes from getting soggy.) Drain the water, and while the potatoes are still warm, begin gently peeling the skins. Immediately roll each potato in a small bowl of olive oil, and then in a small bowl of parmesan. Set on a plate to cool. Parmesan will crust over. Wrap up individual potatoes and enjoy this salty carb as you train.

HANDHELDS

V **VEGETARIAN**
G **GLUTEN-FREE**

Wrap It Up

Instead of eating a pre-packaged energy bar, wrap up your food for a ride or a quick snack to go. This works great for rice cakes and other portable snacks as well as for little sandwiches, boiled potatoes, or sweet pastries.

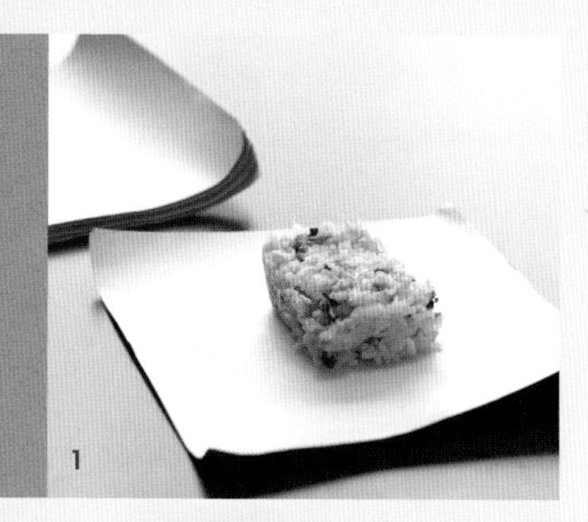

STEP 1

Cut your food item 3 inches long and 2½ inches wide, or roughly the size and shape of a brownie. (Of course, feel free to cut your food or your paper a little bigger or smaller to suit your preference or appetite.) Place the food in the center of a square sheet of paper foil (roughly 8 inches square), with the parchment side up.

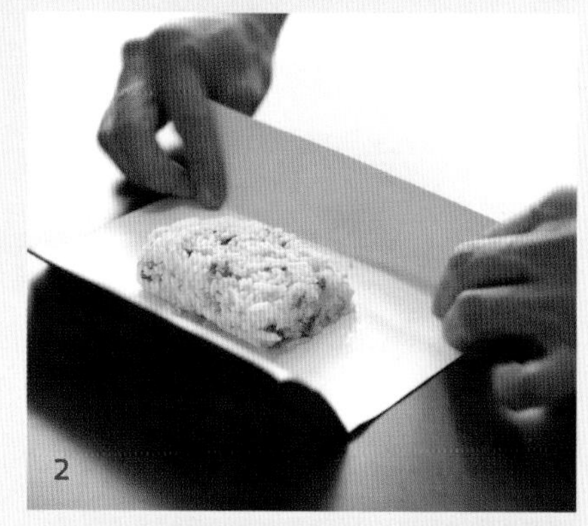

***

STEP 2

Fold in the two sides of paper foil along the long edge of the rice cake with the edges overlapping.

***

STEP 3

Make a crease on the outside edge of the top layer of foil. This will help you open the wrapper and create a little pocket to help you hold the food without getting your hands dirty.

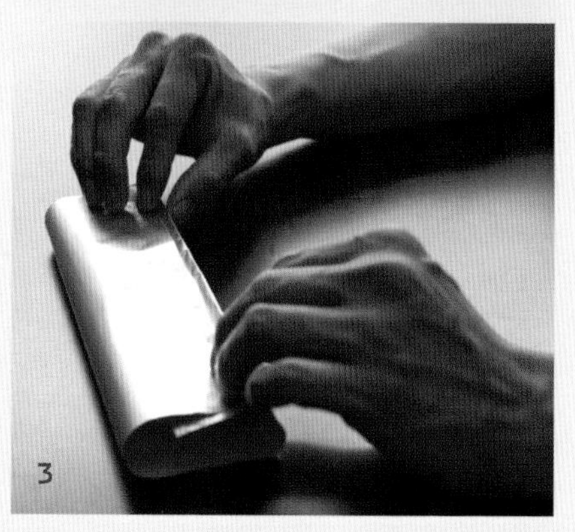

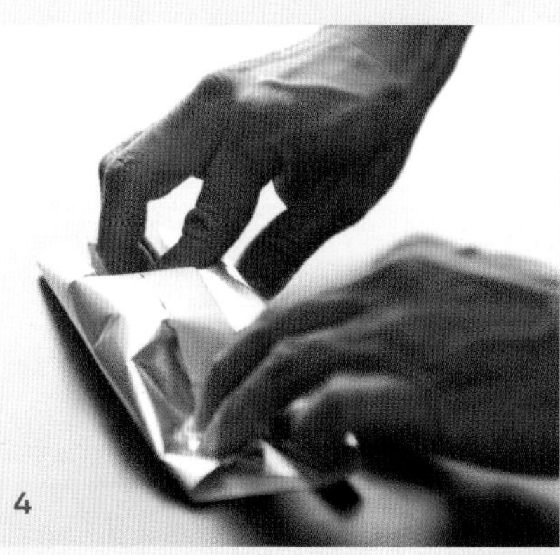

STEP 4

Fold the two open sides of the foil into triangle tabs as you would to wrap a gift.

★★★

STEP 5

Tuck the triangular tabs at each end underneath the wrapped edges.

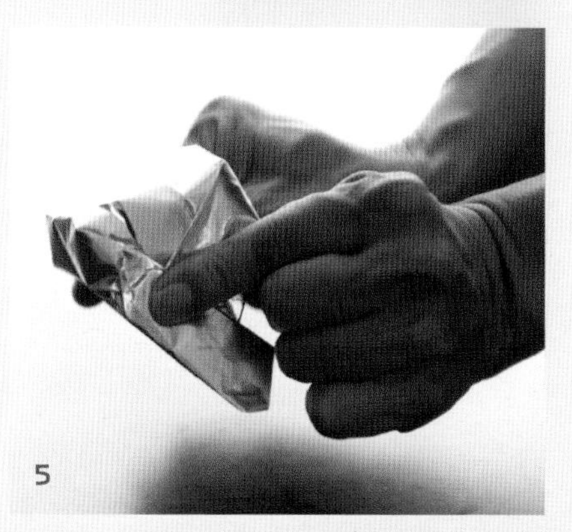

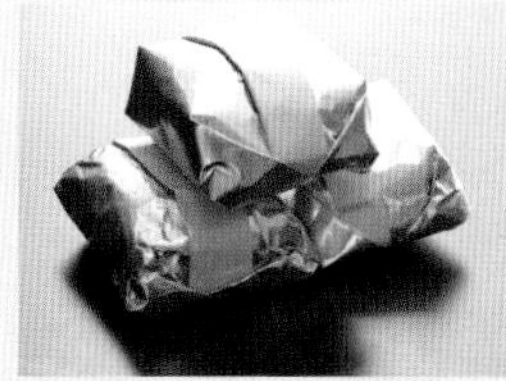

TIP Rice- and potato-based cakes will keep fresh longer if you individually wrap them. Cut and wrap cooled slices and store them in the fridge in a sealed plastic bag. Grab and go!

PAPER FOIL

In Europe, our *soigneurs* buy packages of 8 x 8-inch wrapping paper that is effectively parchment-lined aluminum foil. The parchment foil holds its shape incredibly well, proving durable enough to securely store food in a jersey pocket while still being easy to open and eat quickly. In the United States, the only paper that we have found that is remotely similar is a product called Martha Wrap™, a parchment foil available in some grocery chains and online. If you don't have paper foil, you can get by with heavyweight aluminum foil.

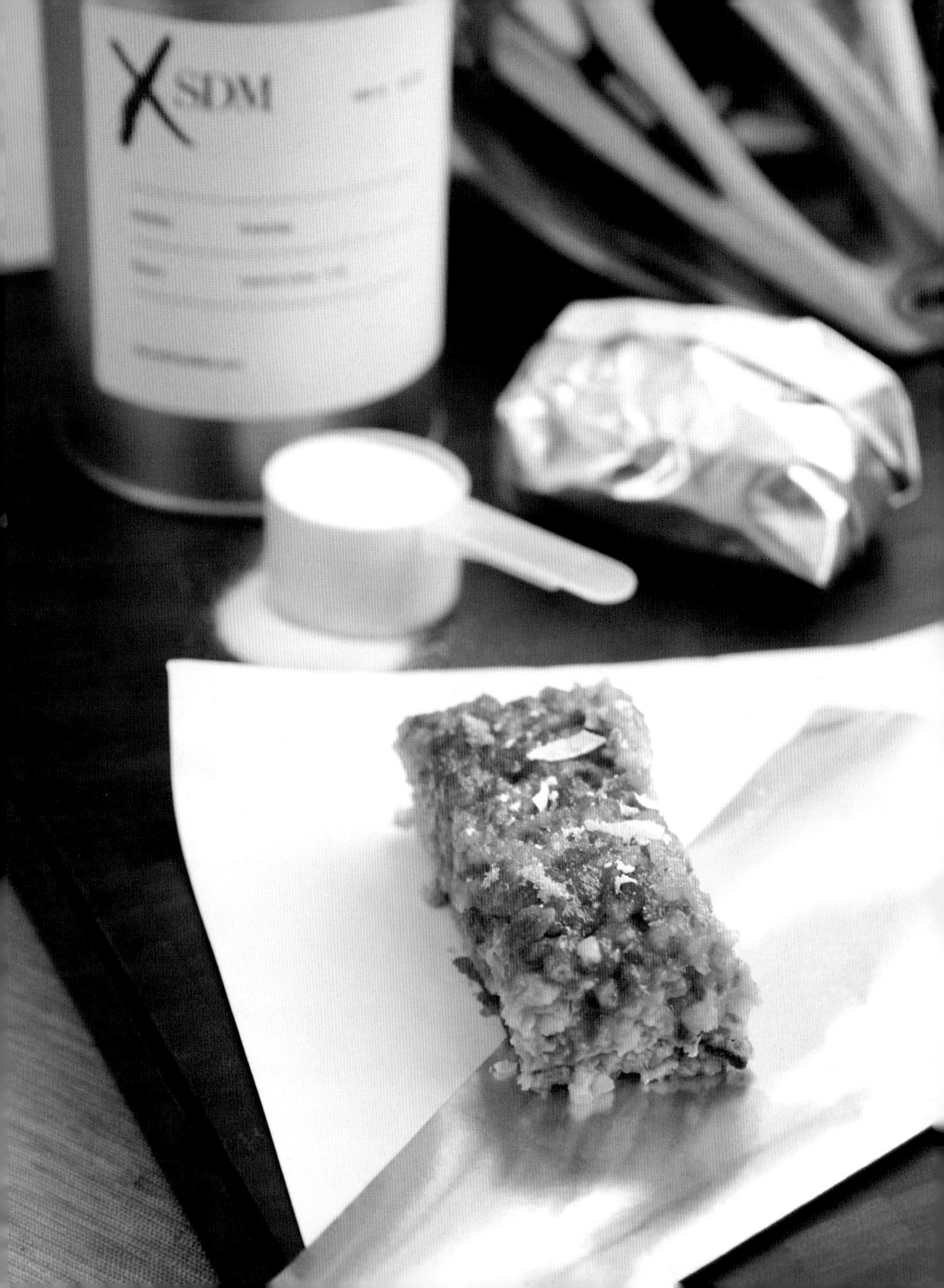
SDM

SERVINGS› 10
TIME› 30 minutes

Allen's Rice Cakes

I started making these rice cakes at training camps and races to give riders something savory and fresh to eat while on the bike. They became a huge hit since almost everything the riders ate was pre-packaged and sweet. Not only are these rice cakes delicious, they also provide a consistent energy source that doesn't upset the stomach.

2 cups uncooked calrose or other medium-grain "sticky" rice

3 cups water

8 ounces bacon

4 eggs

2 tablespoons liquid amino acids or low-sodium soy sauce

brown sugar

salt and grated parmesan (optional)

TIP We always use calrose rice, a strain of medium-grain rice common in Asian cooking. This variety cooks fast (in 20 minutes or less), retains a nutty flavor, and is just sticky enough to hold our cakes together. If you can't find it, use another medium-grain rice or any kind marked "sushi rice."

1. Combine rice and water in a rice cooker.
2. While rice is cooking, chop up bacon before frying, then fry in a medium sauté pan. When crispy, drain off fat and soak up excess fat with paper towels.
3. Beat the eggs in a small bowl and then scramble on high heat in the sauté pan. Don't worry about overcooking the eggs as they'll break up easily when mixed with the rice.
4. In a large bowl or in the rice cooker bowl, combine the cooked rice, bacon, and scrambled eggs. Add liquid amino acids or soy sauce and sugar to taste. After mixing, press into an 8- or 9-inch square baking pan to about 1½-inch thickness. Top with more brown sugar, salt to taste, and grated parmesan, if desired.

Cut and wrap individual cakes. Makes about 10 rice cakes.

PER SERVING (1 cake)› **Energy** 225 cal • **Fat** 8 g • **Sodium** 321 mg • **Carbs** 30 g • **Fiber** 1 g • **Protein** 9 g

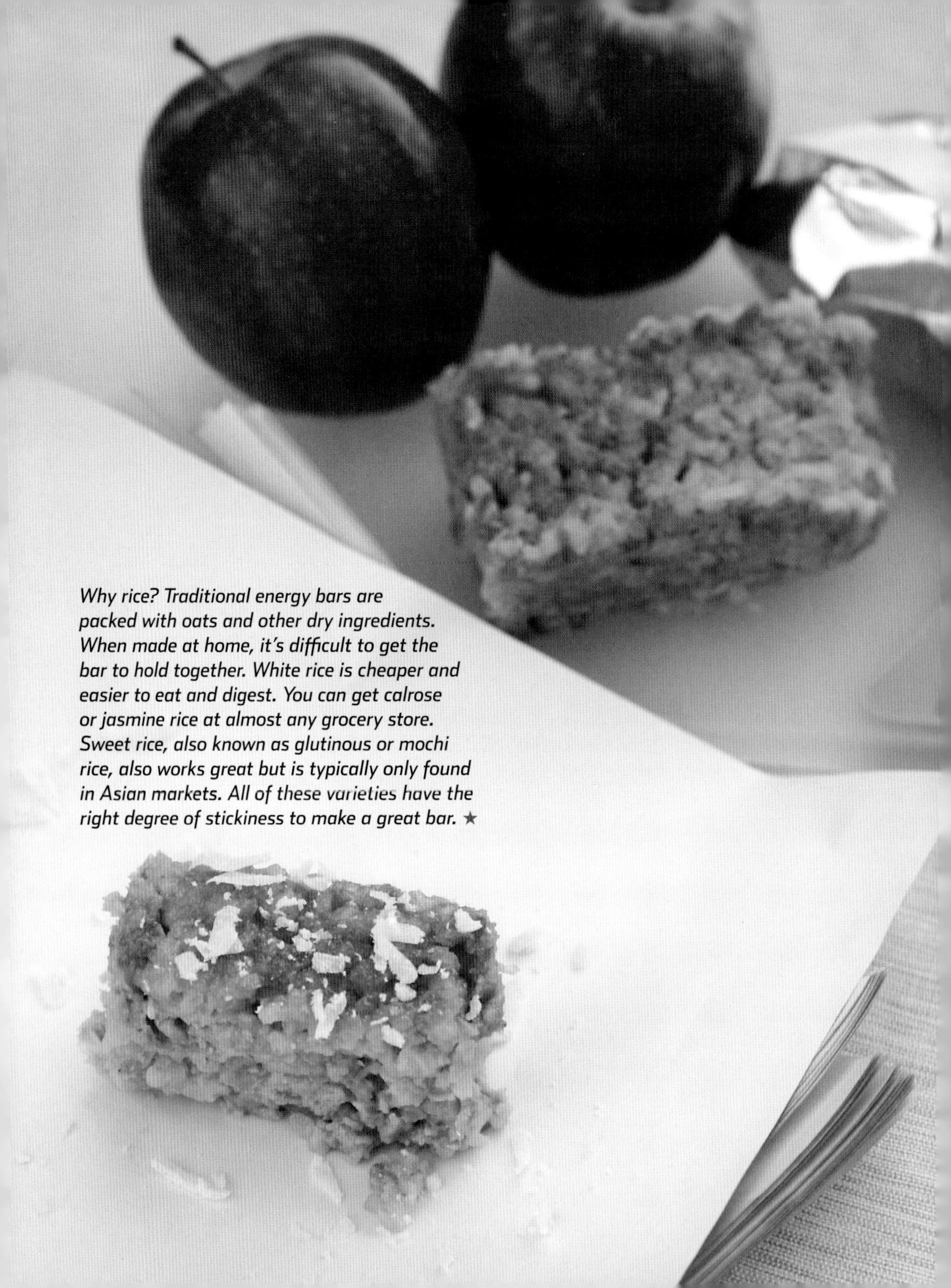

Why rice? Traditional energy bars are packed with oats and other dry ingredients. When made at home, it's difficult to get the bar to hold together. White rice is cheaper and easier to eat and digest. You can get calrose or jasmine rice at almost any grocery store. Sweet rice, also known as glutinous or mochi rice, also works great but is typically only found in Asian markets. All of these varieties have the right degree of stickiness to make a great bar. ★

SERVINGS› 10
TIME› 30 minutes

Chicken Sausage Rice Cakes

We made this rice cake especially for Levi Leipheimer because he does not eat bacon. We like the taste of chicken apple sausage best—it's a slightly sweet flavor that is easy on the stomach when training. We tested some Italian sausage varieties as well, but more neutral flavors work best for eating while training.

2 cups uncooked calrose rice or other medium-grain "sticky" rice

3 cups water

1 pound mild chicken sausage

2 tablespoons brown sugar

1 tablespoon low-sodium soy sauce

3 eggs

1. Combine rice and water in a rice cooker.
2. While the rice is cooking, in a sauté pan over medium-high heat, cook the sausage until no pink remains. Drain the fat. Add brown sugar and soy sauce. Adjust flavor if needed. (You may not need to add anything to the sausage.)
3. Lightly beat the eggs and scramble them in a sauté pan. Don't let the eggs overcook; you want some moisture in them still.
4. Put the cooked rice in a large bowl. Add the cooked sausage and the scrambled eggs; mix to combine. Press into an 8- or 9-inch square baking pan to about 1½-inch thickness.

Cut and wrap individual cakes. Makes about 10 rice cakes.

PER SERVING (1 cake)› **Energy** 228 cal • **Fat** 5 g • **Sodium** 343 mg • **Carbs** 33 g • **Fiber** 1 g • **Protein** 11 g

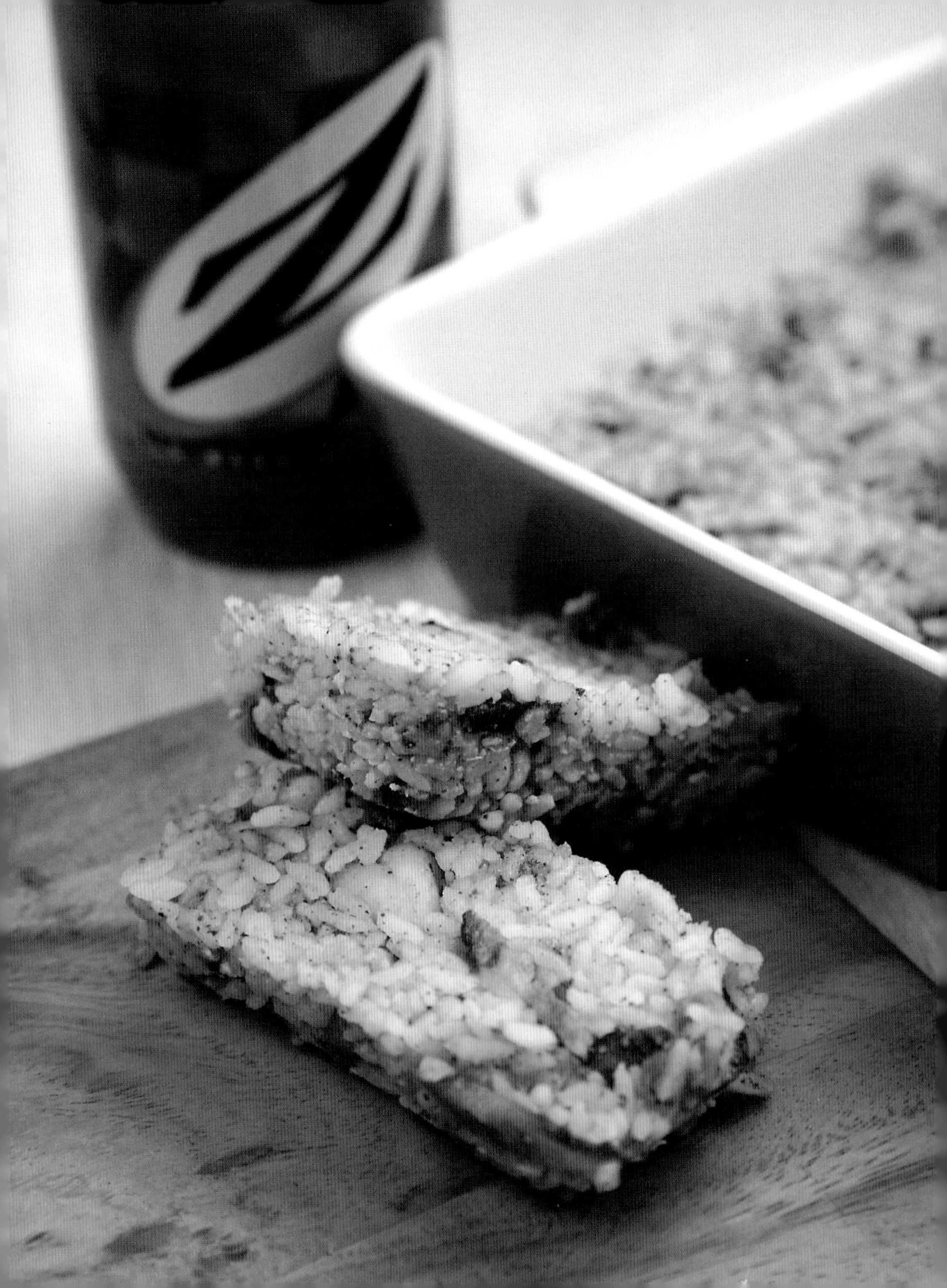

SERVINGS› 10
TIME› 30 minutes prep, chill 30 minutes

Cashew and Bacon Rice Cakes

This variation of Allen's original is the favorite of our friends at Velo *magazine. Together with the bacon, the cashews and nut butter give these rice cakes a salty-sweet taste. The extra boost of protein makes this portable great for longer training sessions.*

- **2 cups uncooked calrose rice or other medium-grain "sticky" rice**
- **3 cups water**
- **8 ounces bacon**
- **3 eggs**
- **½ cup cashews, raw or roasted**
- **¼ cup nut butter**
- **½ cup raisins (optional)**

1. Combine rice and water in a rice cooker.
2. While the rice is cooking, fry the bacon in a medium sauté pan over medium-high heat. Drain off fat and wrap the bacon in paper towels; then press on the towels to crumble the bacon.
3. Lightly beat the eggs in a small bowl and softly scramble them in your sauté pan over medium heat.
4. In a large bowl, combine the cooked rice, bacon, scrambled eggs, cashews, nut butter, and raisins, if using. Mix well. Press mixture into an 8- or 9-inch square pan to about 1½-inch thickness.

Let cool thoroughly in fridge before cutting and individually wrapping individual cakes. Makes about 10 rice cakes.

PER SERVING (1 cake)› **Energy** 286 cal • **Fat** 14 g • **Sodium** 246 mg • **Carbs** 31 g • **Fiber** 1 g • **Protein** 10 g

Nutrition for optional additions can be found in Appendix A.

SERVINGS› 8
TIME› 10 minutes prep, bake 20–30 minutes

Savory Bread Cakes

Here's another great savory food for training rides, this time with bread. You can make these by the truckload, individually wrap them, and store them in the freezer.

4 cups of your favorite bread, cut into cubes

2 cups milk

4 eggs, lightly beaten

½ cup grated cheese (such as parmesan, mozzarella, or cheddar)

COOKED ½ cup bacon or other cooked meat, chopped into small pieces

brown sugar

1. Heat the oven to 350 degrees.
2. Put the bread cubes in a large bowl. In a saucepan, bring the milk to a simmer. Pour the hot milk over the bread cubes and mix. Let rest for just a minute until the bread is soaked. (Gluten-free breads will take a bit longer to absorb the liquid.)
3. Add eggs, cheese, and bacon, and stir to combine. Pour into a loaf pan and bake until firm, about 20 minutes.

Sprinkle some brown sugar and salt on top, and let cool before wrapping. Makes about 8 cakes.

PER SERVING (1 cake)› **Energy** 141 cal • **Fat** 6 g • **Sodium** 307 mg • **Carbs** 11 g • **Fiber** 1 g • **Protein** 9 g

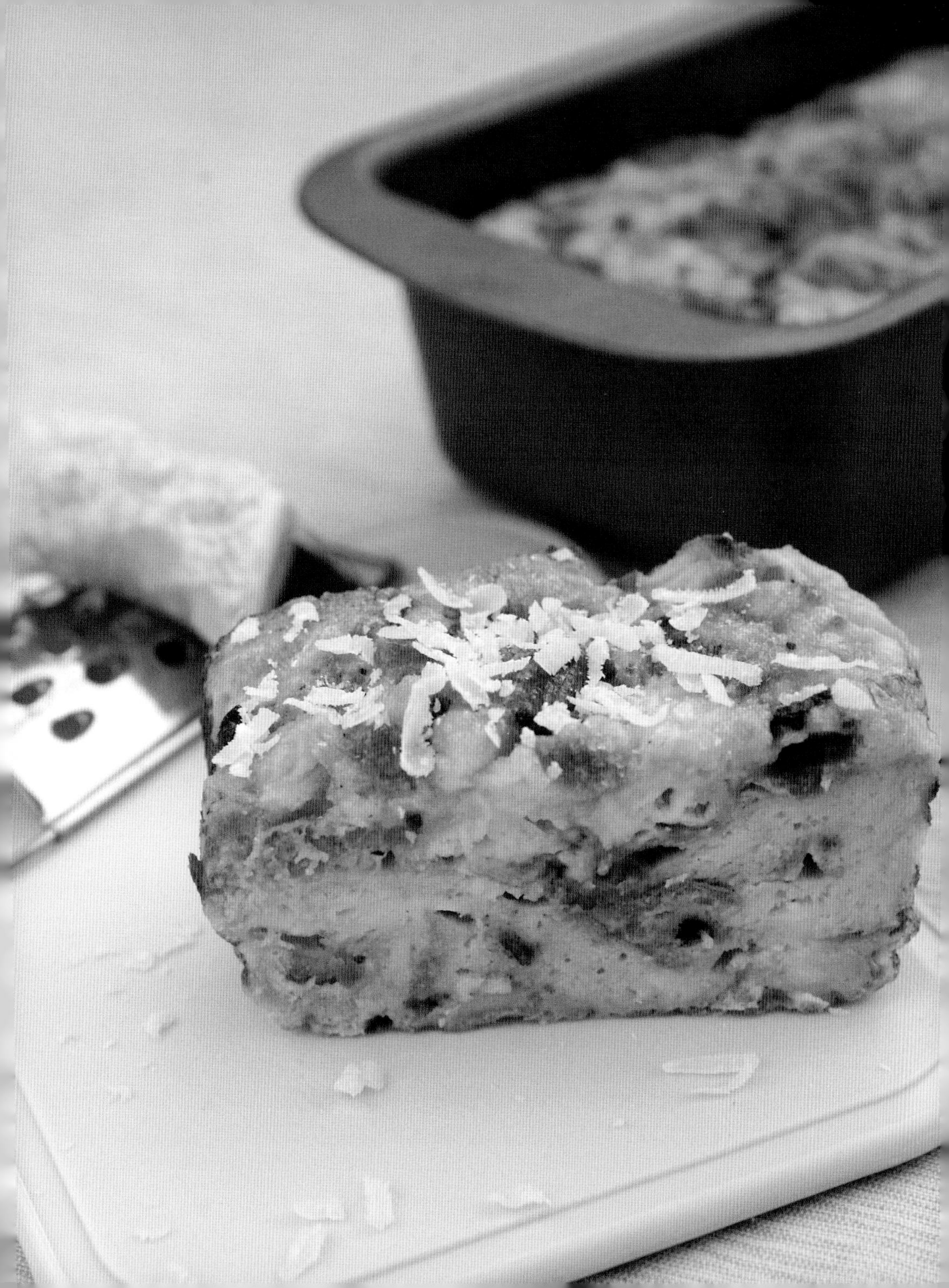

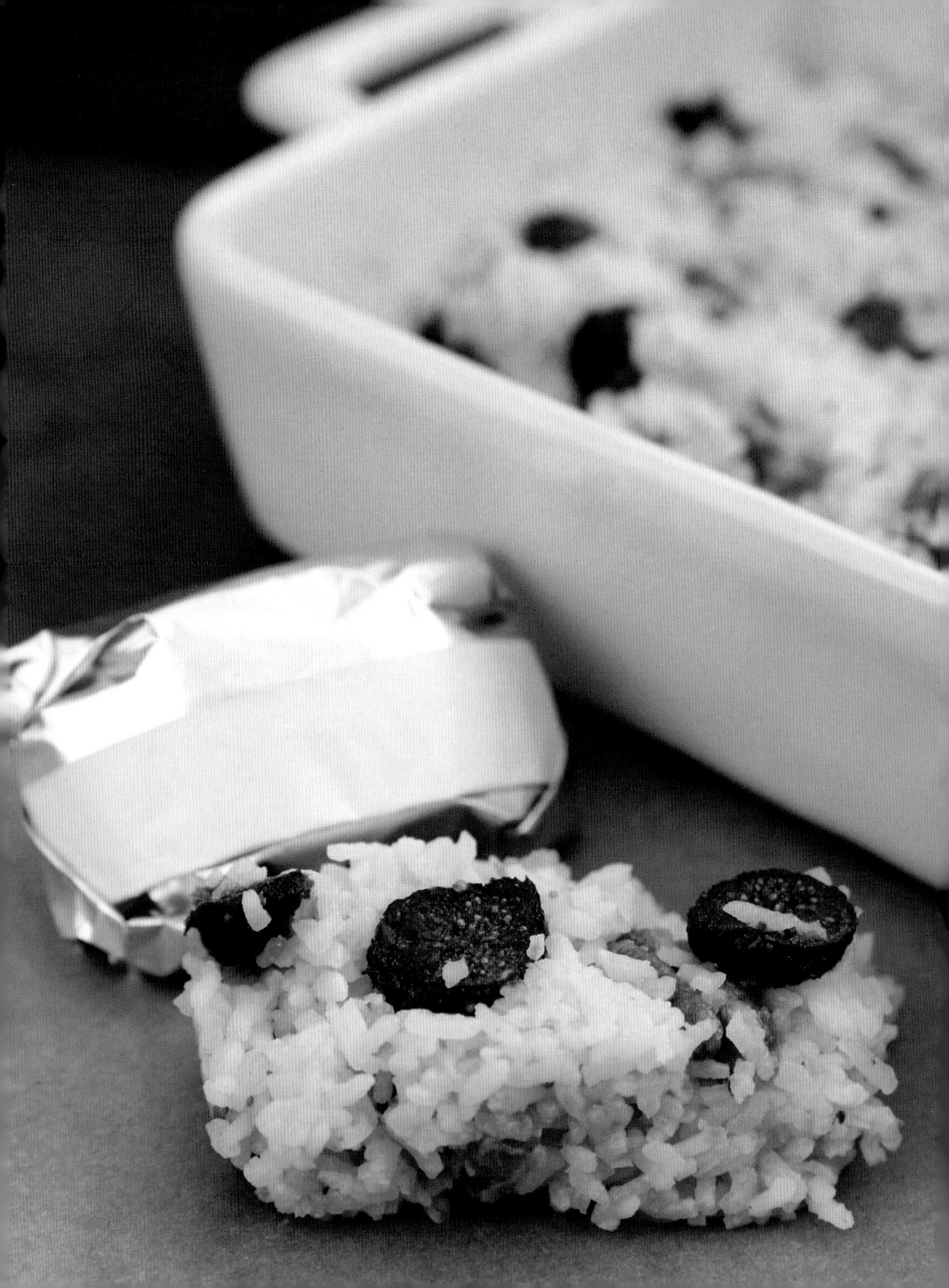

SERVINGS› 10
TIME› 25 minutes

Fig and Honey Rice Cakes

We've put a gluten-free spin on the classic fig cookies that many of us grew up eating. Because of the excellent fiber that is in the dried fruit, these rice cakes work best as a snack following a workout or most any other time of the day. If figs aren't your favorite, try raisins or dates instead.

2 cups uncooked calrose rice or other medium-grain "sticky" rice

3 cups water

1 cup toasted pecans

1 cup chopped dried figs

2 tablespoons honey

brown sugar (optional)

1. Combine rice and water in a rice cooker.
2. To toast the nuts: Heat oven to 350 degrees. Place the pecans on a baking sheet and toast 8–10 minutes, stirring after 5 minutes.
3. In a large bowl, combine the cooked rice, pecans, and figs. Add the honey and stir thoroughly.
4. Press mixture into an 8- or 9-inch square pan to about 1½-inch thickness and sprinkle with brown sugar, if desired.

Cut and wrap individual cakes. Makes about 10 rice cakes.

TIP To make a more compact rice cake, place the rice, pecans, and figs in the food processor and pulse the mixture several times to combine.

PER SERVING (1 cake)› **Energy** 268 cal • **Fat** 10 g • **Sodium** 20 mg • **Carbs** 41 g • **Fiber** 3 g • **Protein** 6 g

SERVINGS> 10
TIME> 20 minutes prep, chill 1 hour

Chocolate Peanut Coconut Rice Cakes

Many athletes are comfortable eating sweet bars, often dipped in some kind of chocolate, while training. We think these rice cakes improve on that concept. They satisfy your craving for peanuts and chocolate, and best of all, they will not end up a melted, gooey mess on a hot day.

- 2 cups uncooked calrose rice or other medium-grain "sticky" rice
- 3 cups water
- 1 cup raw or roasted peanuts
- 1 cup unsweetened shredded coconut
- 2 tablespoons brown sugar
- 1 tablespoon salt
- honey or molasses (if needed)
- ½ cup chocolate chips

1. Combine rice and water in a rice cooker.
2. Once the rice is cooked, put all ingredients except chocolate chips in a food processor and pulse together into a thick, crumbly paste. Add a bit of honey or molasses if mixture is too dry.
3. Add the chocolate chips to the mixture and pulse until the chocolate melts and incorporates into the mixture.
4. Transfer mixture to an 8- or 9-inch square baking pan and press to be about 1 inch thick. Top with more peanuts and chocolate chips if desired.

Let cool before cutting and wrapping individual cakes. Makes about 10 rice cakes.

PER SERVING (1 cake)> Energy 323 cal • Fat 14 g • Sodium 700 mg • Carbs 44 g • Fiber 3 g • Protein 6 g

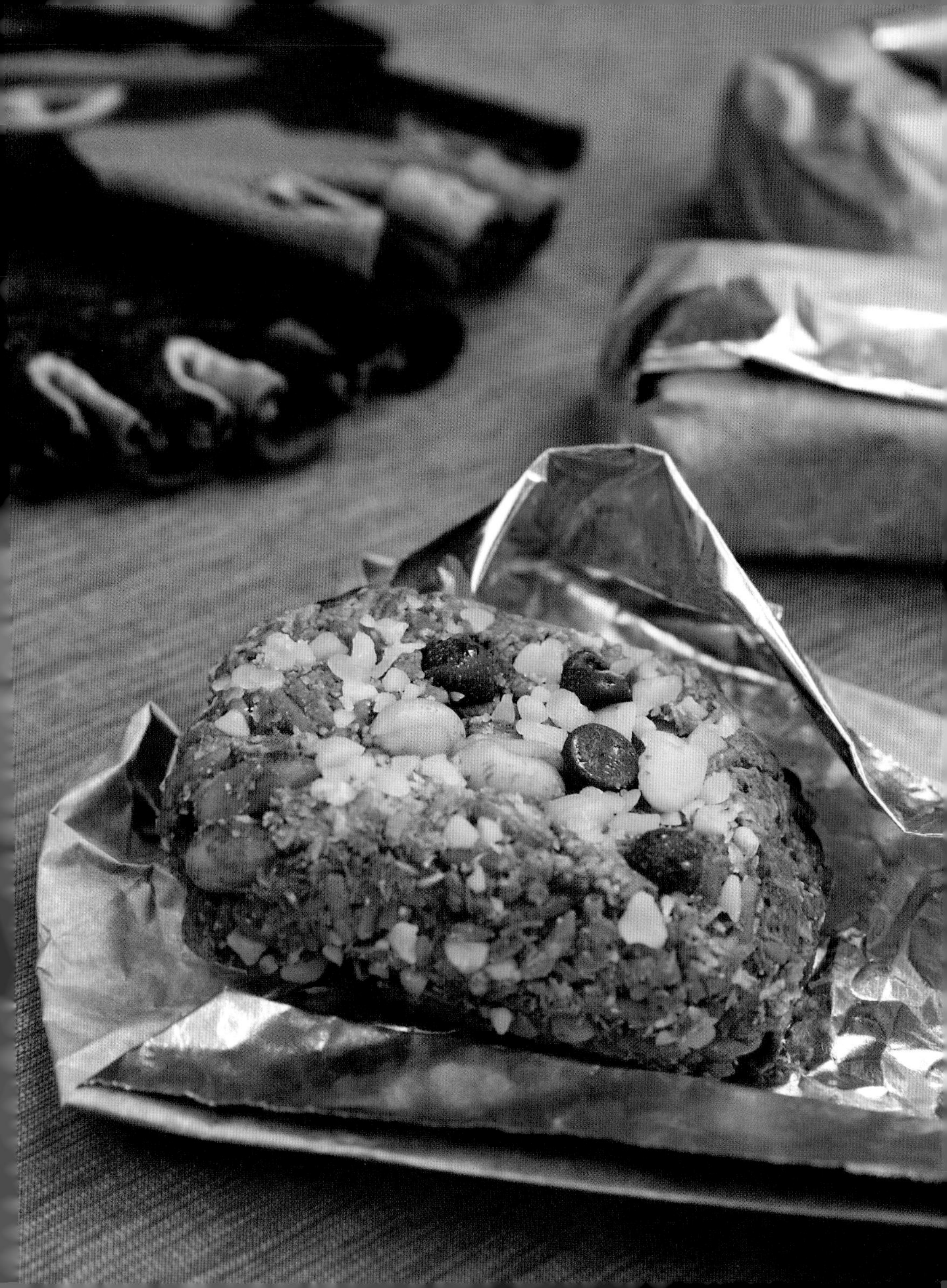

SERVINGS> 10
TIME> 20 minutes

Almond and Date Rice Cakes

Now this is a hearty rice cake. Full of fiber, this portable is not for training, but it's perfectly suited for a post-workout snack thanks to the sugary dates. We like to cut these rice cakes a little smaller than the others since they are good and dense.

2 cups uncooked calrose rice or other medium-grain "sticky" rice

3 cups water

1 cup pitted dates

1 cup raw almonds

2 tablespoons brown sugar

½ tablespoon coarse salt

honey or agave nectar (if needed)

1. Combine rice and water in a rice cooker.
2. Once the rice is cooked, put all ingredients in a food processor and pulse until a very thick and crumbly paste is formed. Add a touch of honey or agave nectar if mixture is dry.
3. Transfer mixture to an 8- or 9-inch square baking pan and press to be about 1 inch thick.

Cut and wrap individual cakes. Makes about 10 rice cakes.

TIP Fruit and nut rice cakes can be stored in the fridge for up to one week if covered or wrapped well.

PER SERVING (1 cake)> **Energy** 234 cal • **Fat** 6 g • **Sodium** 349 mg • **Carbs** 41 g • **Fiber** 3 g • **Protein** 5 g

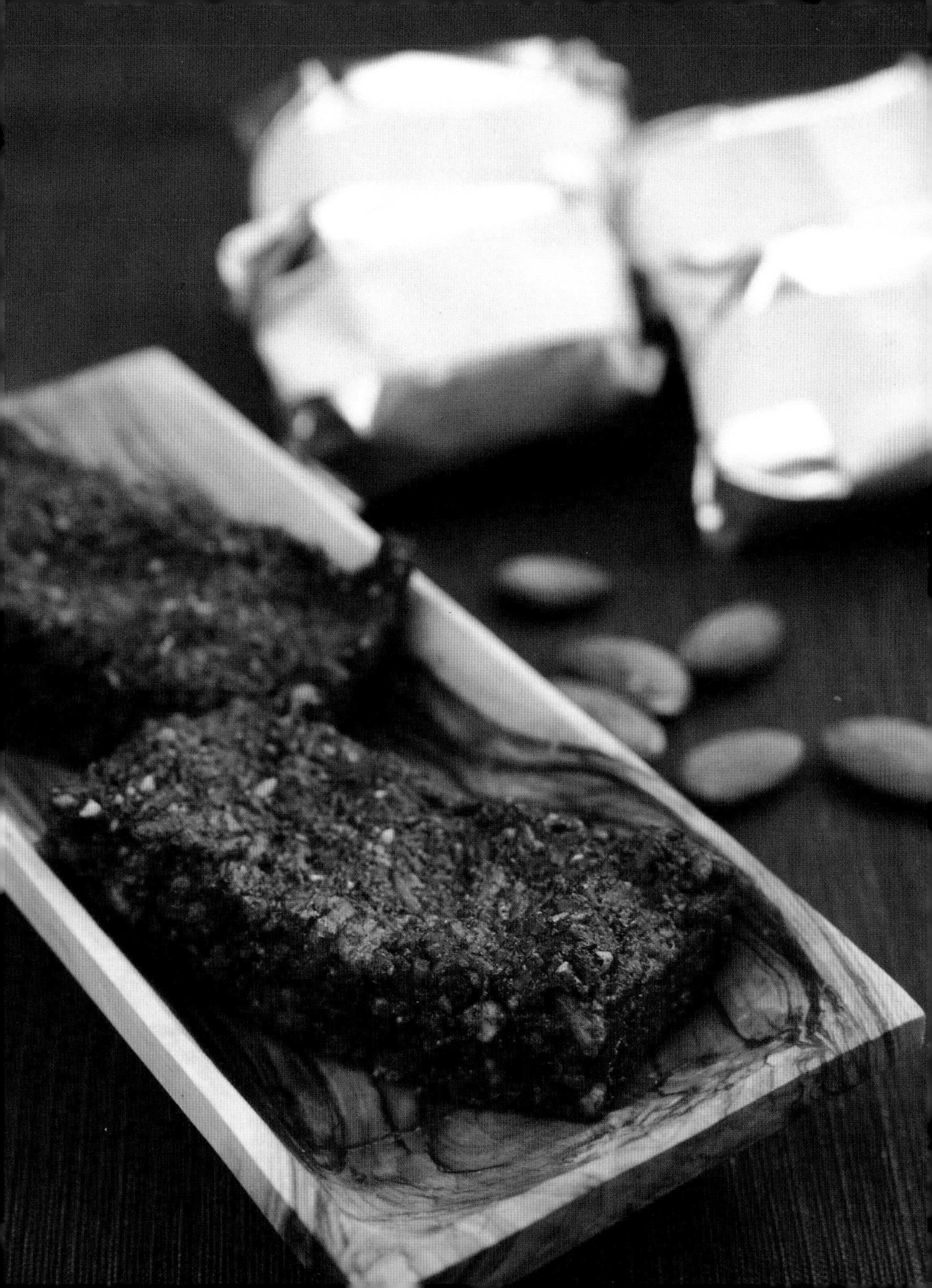

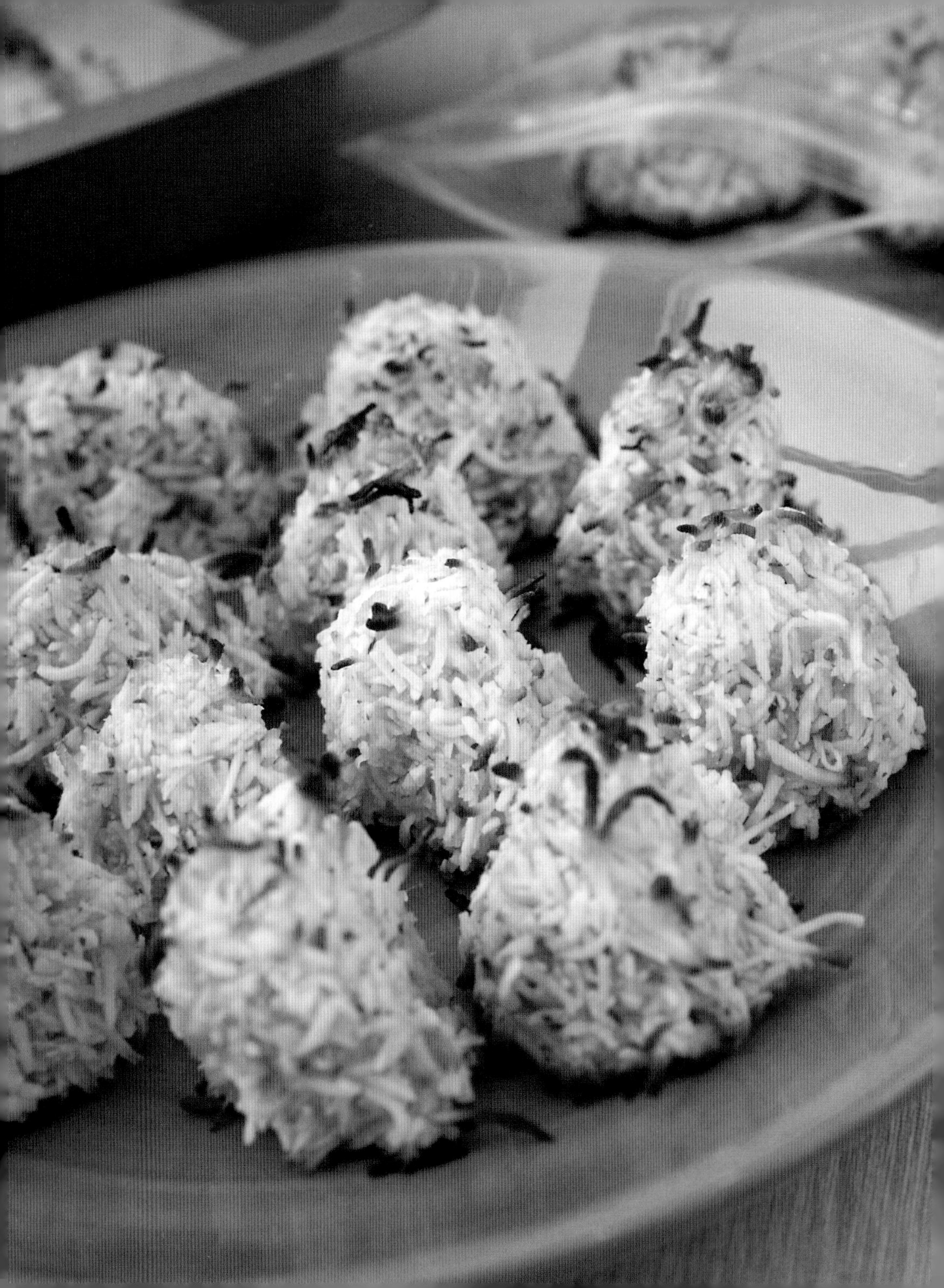

SERVINGS› 18
TIME› 20 minutes

Orange Almond Macaroons

Riders in the European peloton are fond of putting small pastries and sweets in their musette bags for a hit of sugar during the race. These bite-size treats pack in ground almonds and a hint of orange marmalade—but just enough to keep you light on the pedals.

1 cup raw almonds

1 pound (about 4 cups) shredded unsweetened coconut

1 teaspoon vanilla extract

¼ cup honey

¼ cup orange marmalade

1–2 tablespoons applesauce or additional honey

4 egg whites

1. Heat oven to 350 degrees.
2. Place almonds in food processor and process until finely ground. Add coconut, vanilla, honey, marmalade, and 1 tablespoon applesauce. Pulse until a thick paste is formed. If mixture is too dry, add another tablespoon of applesauce or honey.
3. In a bowl, whisk egg whites until stiff.
4. Combine coconut mixture and egg whites and gently blend together in a bowl. Use a teaspoon to drop macaroons onto a baking sheet lined with parchment paper.
5. Bake for 15–20 minutes or until golden brown on the outside.

Let cool completely before serving. Store macaroons in an airtight container. If you live in a humid climate, store in the fridge. Makes about 18 macaroons.

PER SERVING (1 macaroon)› **Energy** 131 cal • **Fat** 9 g • **Sodium** 15 mg • **Carbs** 11 g • **Fiber** 2 g • **Protein** 3 g

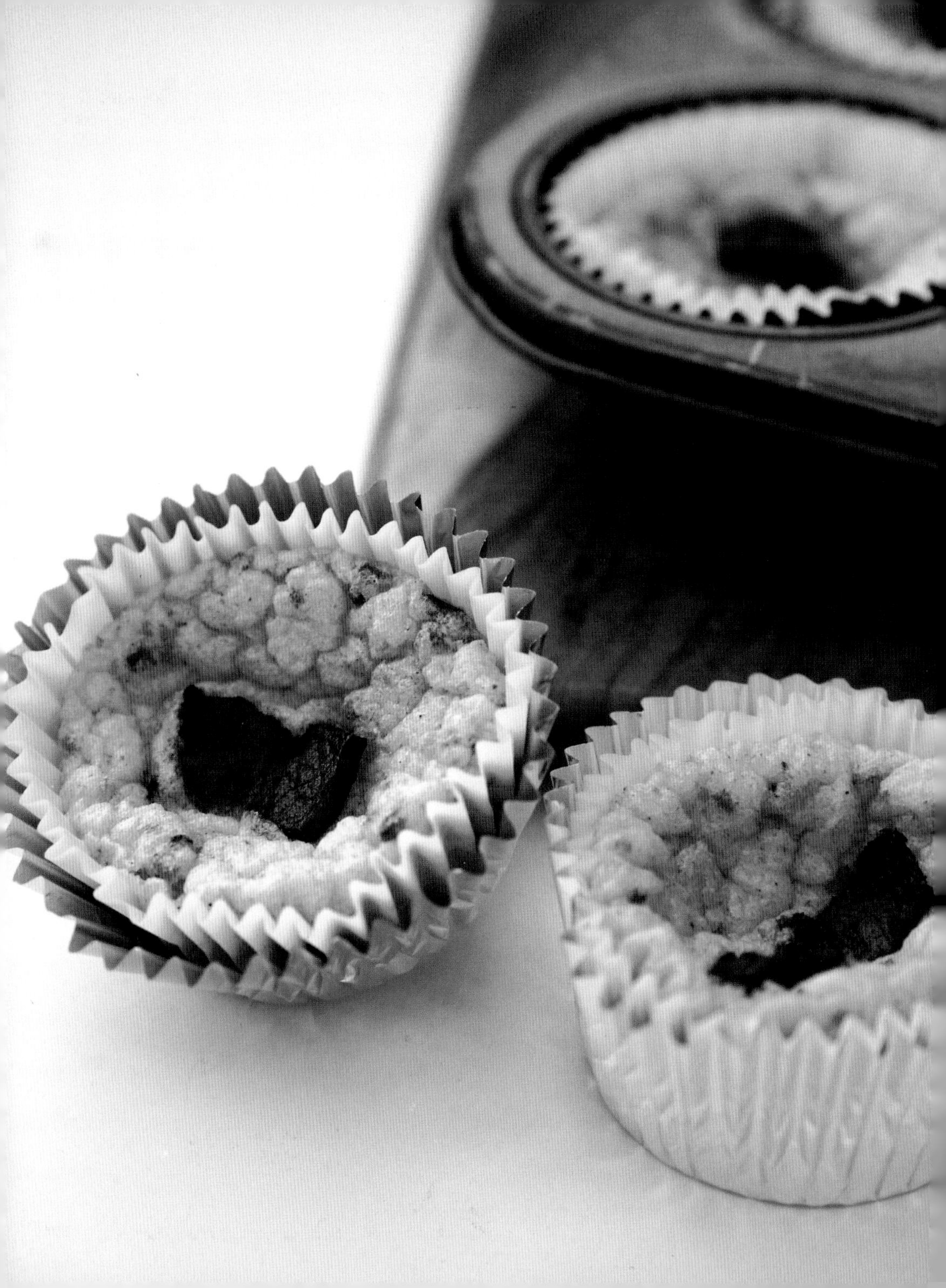

SERVINGS› 12
TIME› 30 minutes

Bacon Muffins

These are slightly salty, slightly sweet, and very portable little muffins that pack well as a "hand-up" or to keep in your pocket on a cool day. We like to add semi-sweet chocolate chips.

- COOKED 2 cups cooked white rice
- 2 eggs
- 2 tablespoons honey
- 1 tablespoon rice or potato flour
- ½ teaspoon salt
- 1 cup milk
- COOKED ¼ cup chopped cooked bacon
- 1 cup semi-sweet chocolate chips (optional)

1. Heat oven to 325 degrees.
2. Place rice, eggs, honey, flour, and salt in blender. Process quickly to combine ingredients. Add milk slowly to make a thick batter, pulsing between additions. Fold in bacon and chocolate chips, if using.
3. Fill greased muffin tins or cupcake liners ¾ full with batter. Bake 15–20 minutes or until centers are firm (test with a toothpick). Muffins will not rise much.

Let cool completely, then use a knife to gently loosen the muffins from the pan. Store in the fridge in a sealed container. Makes about 12 muffins.

NOTE› If you are using fresh rice, reduce the milk to ½ cup.

TIP Cupcake liners save you the trouble of cleaning a muffin tin, and unless you splurged on the chocolate, there's no further wrapping required!

PER SERVING (1 muffin)› **Energy** 126 cal • **Fat** 3 g • **Sodium** 300 mg • **Carbs** 22 g • **Fiber** 0 g • **Protein** 5 g
Nutrition for optional additions can be found in Appendix A.

SERVINGS› 10
TIME› 10 minutes prep, bake 15 minutes

Rice and Banana Muffins

We'll let you in on a little secret: This batter is very similar to our Rice and Banana Pancakes (page 72), but a muffin is much easier to eat on-the-go than pancakes. The rice batter keeps the muffin light and moist, so even though this muffin does not rise like the traditional flour varieties, it's every bit as good.

COOKED 2 cups cooked white rice
2 eggs
1 ripe banana
2 tablespoons brown sugar
1 tablespoon rice or potato flour
¼–½ cup milk (see note)
pinch of salt

OPTIONAL ADDITIONS

1 teaspoon vanilla or almond extract
1 teaspoon each of ground cinnamon or nutmeg

1. Heat oven to 325 degrees. Lightly grease or butter a muffin tin.
2. Combine rice, eggs, banana, brown sugar, and flour in a blender. Process quickly to combine ingredients and slowly add milk to make a thick batter.
3. Fill muffin tin halfway with batter. Bake 15–20 minutes or until centers are firm (test with a toothpick). Muffins will not rise much.

Let cool completely, then use a knife to gently loosen the muffins from the pan. Store in the fridge in a sealed container. Makes about 10 muffins.

NOTE› You will need to adjust the milk depending on how much banana is added and how dry your rice is. If your batter is runny, just let it sit for 5 minutes so the rice can absorb the extra liquid.

PER SERVING (1 muffin)› Energy 77 cal • Fat 1 g • Sodium 36 mg • Carbs 15 g • Fiber 1 g • Protein 2 g

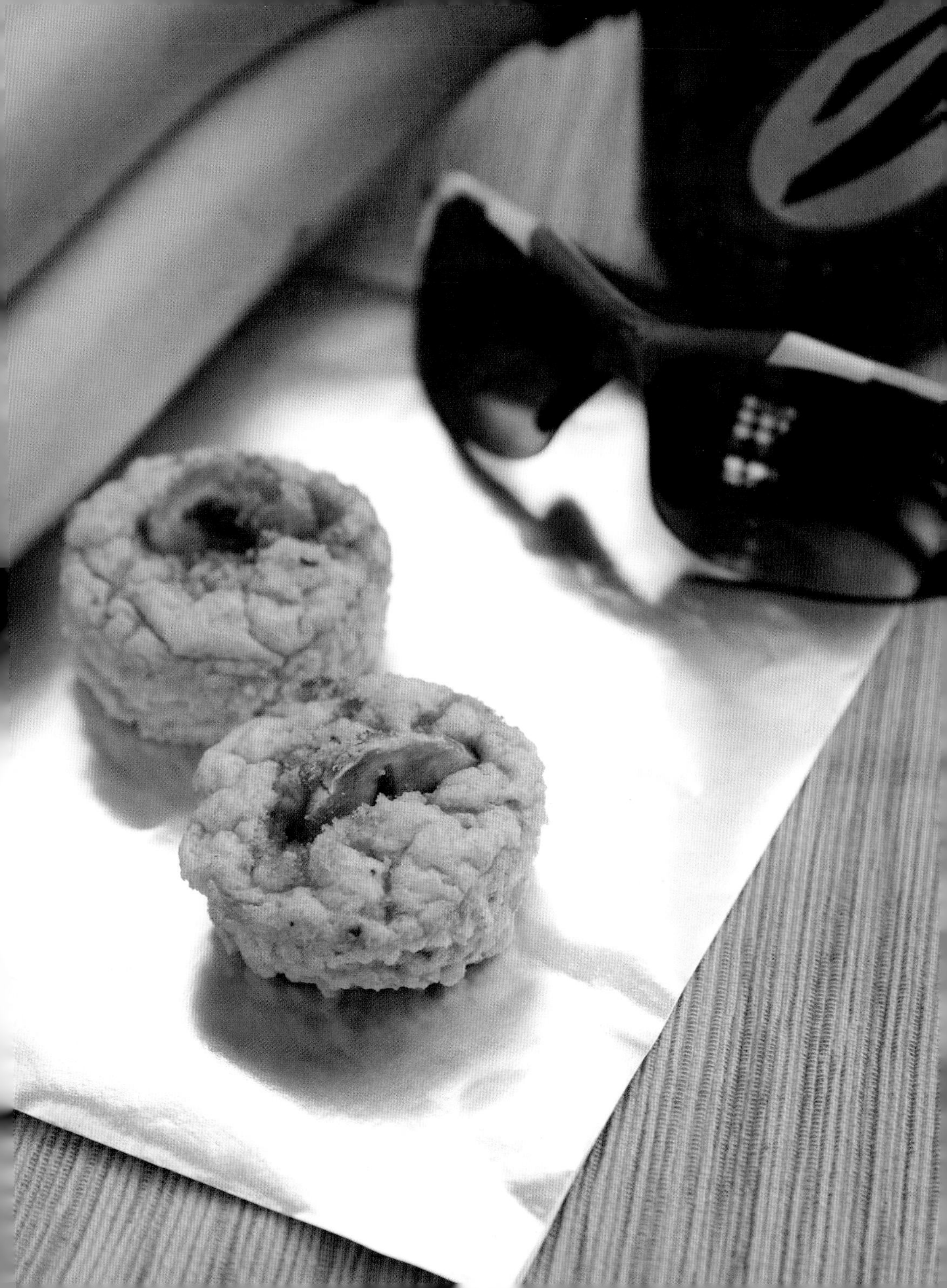

SERVINGS> 10
TIME> 10 minutes prep, bake 15 minutes

Brown Rice Muffins

Most of our recipes use white rice simply because it cooks faster and has a higher glycemic index. If you want to pack a bit more nutrition into your portable, try this brown rice muffin.

- COOKED 2 cups cooked brown rice
- 3 eggs
- ½ cup applesauce
- 2 tablespoons molasses
- 2 tablespoons rice or potato flour
- ¼–½ cup milk (see note)
- pinch of salt

OPTIONAL ADDITIONS

- 1 teaspoon vanilla or almond extract
- 1 teaspoon each of ground cinnamon and nutmeg

1. Heat oven to 325 degrees. Lightly grease a muffin tin.
2. Combine all ingredients in a blender. Fill prepared muffin tin ¾ full.
3. Bake 15 minutes or until centers are firm (test with a toothpick). Muffins will not rise much.

Let cool thoroughly, then wrap and take along for great ride food. Makes about 10 muffins.

NOTE> Add the milk slowly, starting with ¼ cup. More milk may be needed if the rice is dry from being in the fridge.

PER SERVING (1 muffin)> Energy 248 cal • Fat 3 g • Sodium 52 mg • Carbs 49 g • Fiber 2 g • Protein 25 g

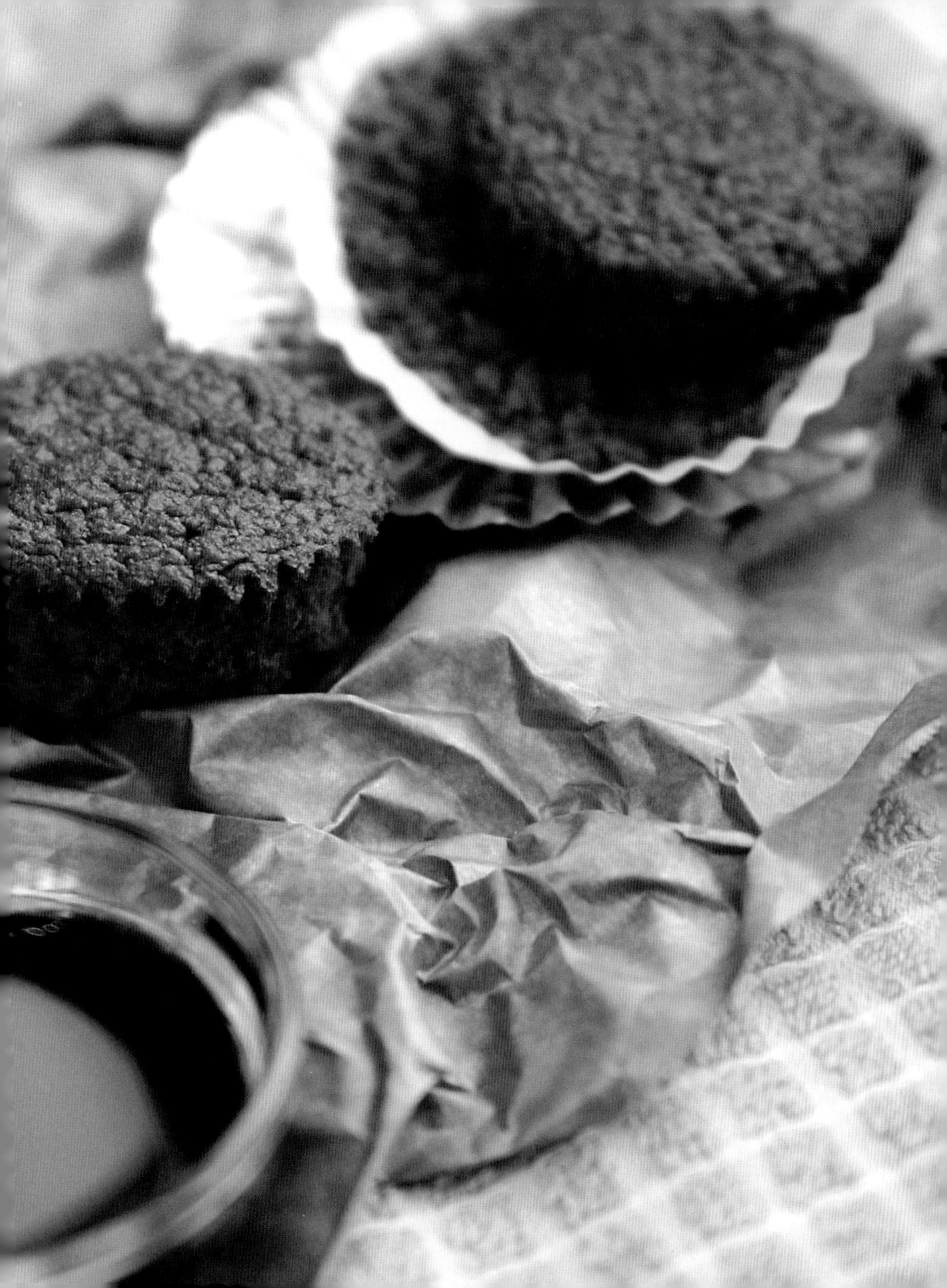

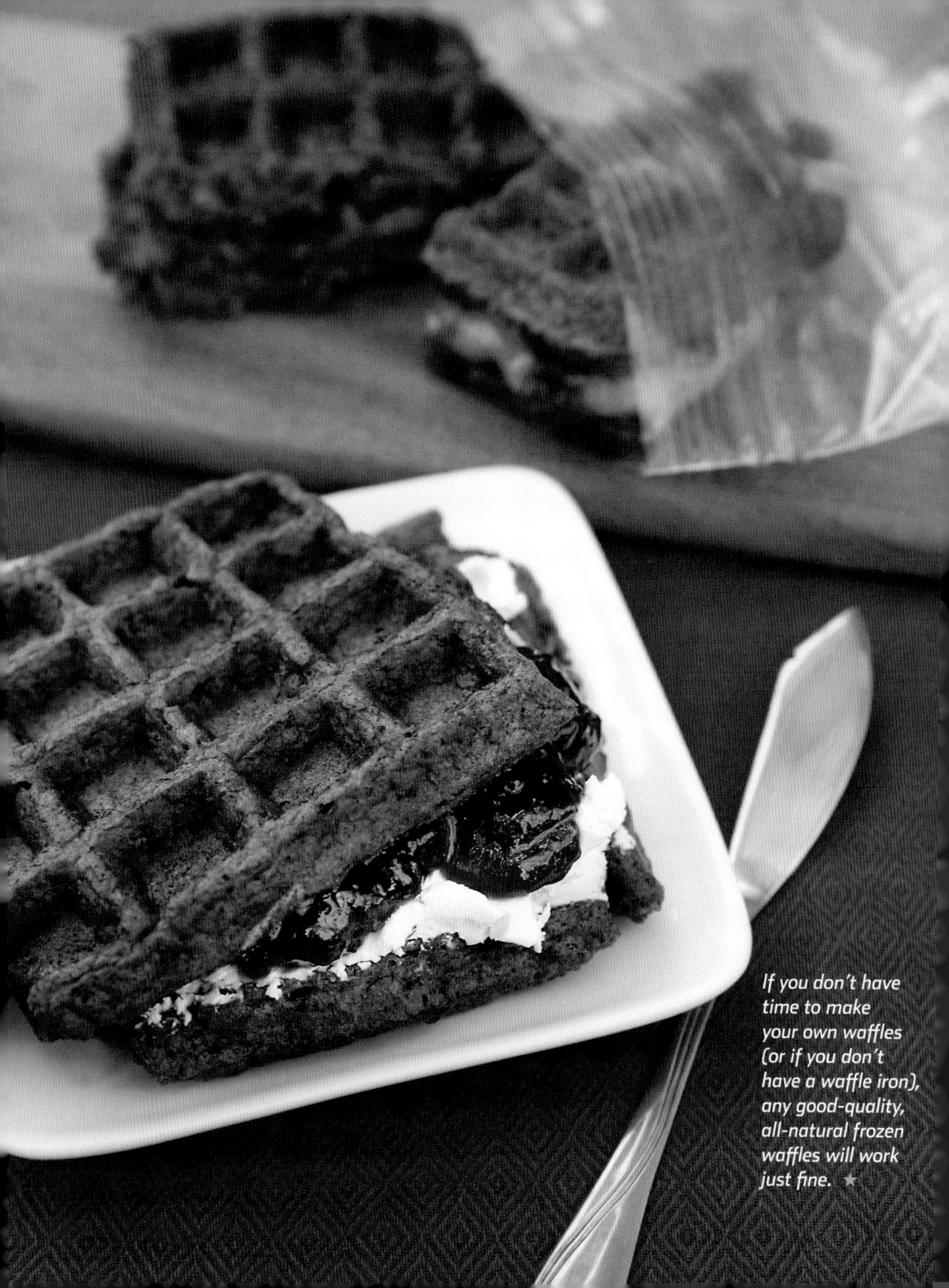

If you don't have time to make your own waffles (or if you don't have a waffle iron), any good-quality, all-natural frozen waffles will work just fine. ★

SERVINGS› 3
TIME› 25 minutes

Waffle Ride Sandwich

Waffles are a practical solution for an otherwise messy portable sandwich. The waffle squares help keep peanut butter or Nutella and fruit jams in place while stuffed into jersey pockets during rides. If you use white rice in place of brown, it typically requires more milk to get the consistency of the batter thick enough.

COOKED 2 cups cooked brown or white rice

3 eggs, lightly beaten

1 ripe banana

2 tablespoons molasses

2 tablespoons rice flour or potato flour

½–1 cup milk (see note)

pinch of salt

FILLINGS
(2 tablespoons of any of the following)

cream cheese

peanut butter, almond butter, or Nutella

jam

TIP Any of the muffin or pancake recipes will work in this recipe. The waffle shown uses brown rice.

1. Heat waffle iron.
2. Mix all ingredients in a blender, adding milk slowly to achieve desired thickness. The batter should be thick.
3. Pour batter into waffle iron, nearly filling the area (be sure to allow room for batter to spread). When the surface of the waffle looks crisp, remove the waffle gently using a fork.
4. Allow the waffle to cool while you cook the rest of the batter.
5. Once the waffles are cool, spread wth your favorite jams, cream cheese, and/or nut butters. Cut into squares or wedges and wrap to enjoy during your ride.

If you are not using them right away, separate waffles with sheets of wax paper and store in a sealed plastic bag in the freezer. To quickly defrost waffles, place in toaster and cool before adding filling.

NOTE› This batter will be slightly more thick than the rice pancake batter.

PER SERVING› Energy 346 cal • Fat 5 g • Sodium 153 mg • Carbs 61 g • Fiber 1 g • Protein 11 g

★★★

There is an overwhelming amount of evidence that eating within 30 minutes of exercise is vital to properly restoring muscle glycogen stores and speeding up the recovery process. This information has spawned an entire category of pre-packaged food products and protein shakes purported to optimize recovery. However, by eating real food you can achieve the same level of nutrition, if not better.

Our Après menu is designed to be highly nutritious and require little prep time. For example, the salads in small plates can be thrown together quickly after a shorter ride or if you're trying to make weight. Big plates like Angel Hair with Bacon and Sweet Corn or Chicken Fried Rice are items that we regularly eat after a long day on the road.

Our "one pots" are designed for a slow cooker. While they sometimes require a longer initial prep time, these nutritious stews can be quickly reheated and served over pre-made pasta or rice.

Be resourceful—last night's dinner can be re-purposed for a great meal after training.

APRÈS

QUICK RECOVERY

SMALL PLATES

HANDHELDS

BIG PLATES

ONE POTS

V **VEGETARIAN**
G **GLUTEN-FREE**

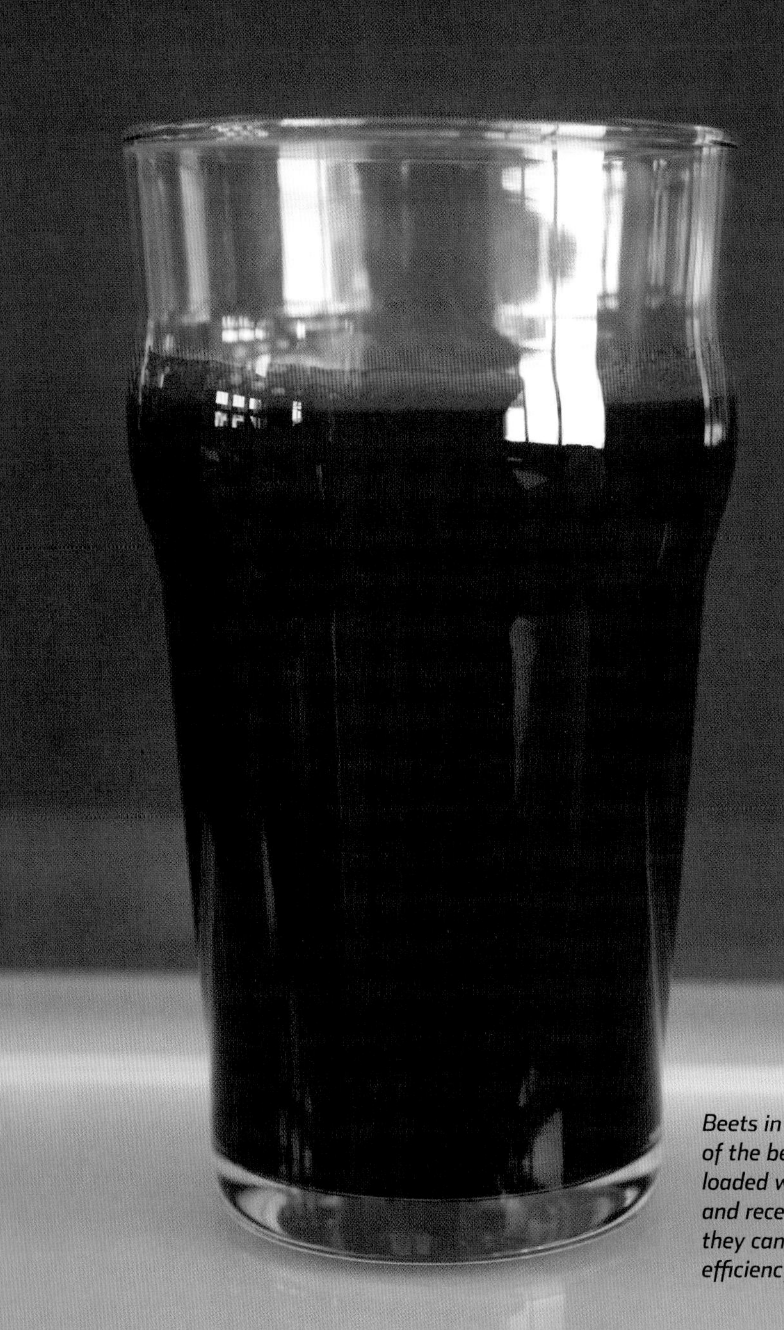

Beets in all their forms are one of the best foods for us. They are loaded with vitamins and minerals and recent research has shown that they can even help improve the efficiency of exercising muscles. ★

SERVINGS› 2
TIME› 5 minutes

Beet Juice

We started athletes juicing to increase the nutrient density of their diets without adding a lot of bulk. Beet juice has been used to treat ailments ranging from anemia to constipation. To maximize the entire nutrient value of the beet, save the pulp and blend it into dishes with a red sauce or use it as a base for veggie burgers (see page 213).

3 medium beets, peeled
1 apple, cored
4 medium carrots, peeled

OPTIONAL ADDITIONS
¼ of a fresh pineapple
1 cup chopped kale
½ cup packed fresh parsley
1 cup chopped celery

1. Cut the vegetables to whatever size works best in your juicer. Process according to manufacturer's instructions.

TIP Peeling the vegetables will reduce the bitterness and make the pulp more usable as an ingredient later.

PER SERVING› **Energy** 151 cal • **Fat** 1 g • **Sodium** 146 mg • **Carbs** 36 g • **Fiber** 1 g • **Protein** 4 g
Nutrition for optional additions can be found in Appendix A.

SERVINGS› 2
TIME› 5 minutes

Sweet Rice and Fruit

This quick meal will promote fast recovery after a long training session. Many of the athletes we've worked with also enjoy this dish as a light dessert. You can use whatever rice you have cooked and ready in this recipe, but "sweet rice" is especially good. Found in Asian supermarkets, sweet rice (also known as glutinous or mochi rice) is a short-grained, extra-sticky rice.

COOKED **3 cups cooked rice**

1 cup plain yogurt

1–2 bananas, sliced

2 tablespoons honey or maple syrup

freshly squeezed lemon or orange juice

OPTIONAL ADDITION

2 tablespoons nut butter (stirred into yogurt)

1. Add a splash of water to the rice and warm in a sauté pan over medium-high heat.

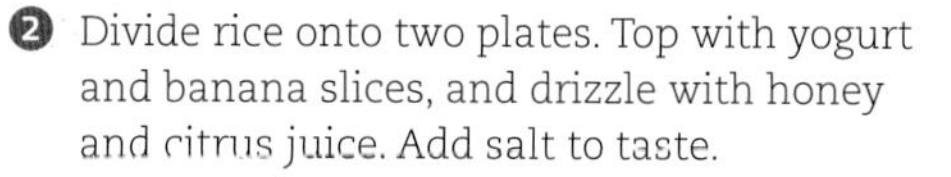

2. Divide rice onto two plates. Top with yogurt and banana slices, and drizzle with honey and citrus juice. Add salt to taste.

TIP If your bananas are plenty ripe, put all of the ingredients into a blender along with 1 cup of ice and 1 cup of milk and you'll have a cool, refreshing smoothie.

PER SERVING› **Energy** 448 cal • **Fat** 5 g • **Sodium** 252 mg • **Carbs** 104 g • **Fiber** 4 g • **Protein** 10 g
Nutrition for optional addition can be found in Appendix A.

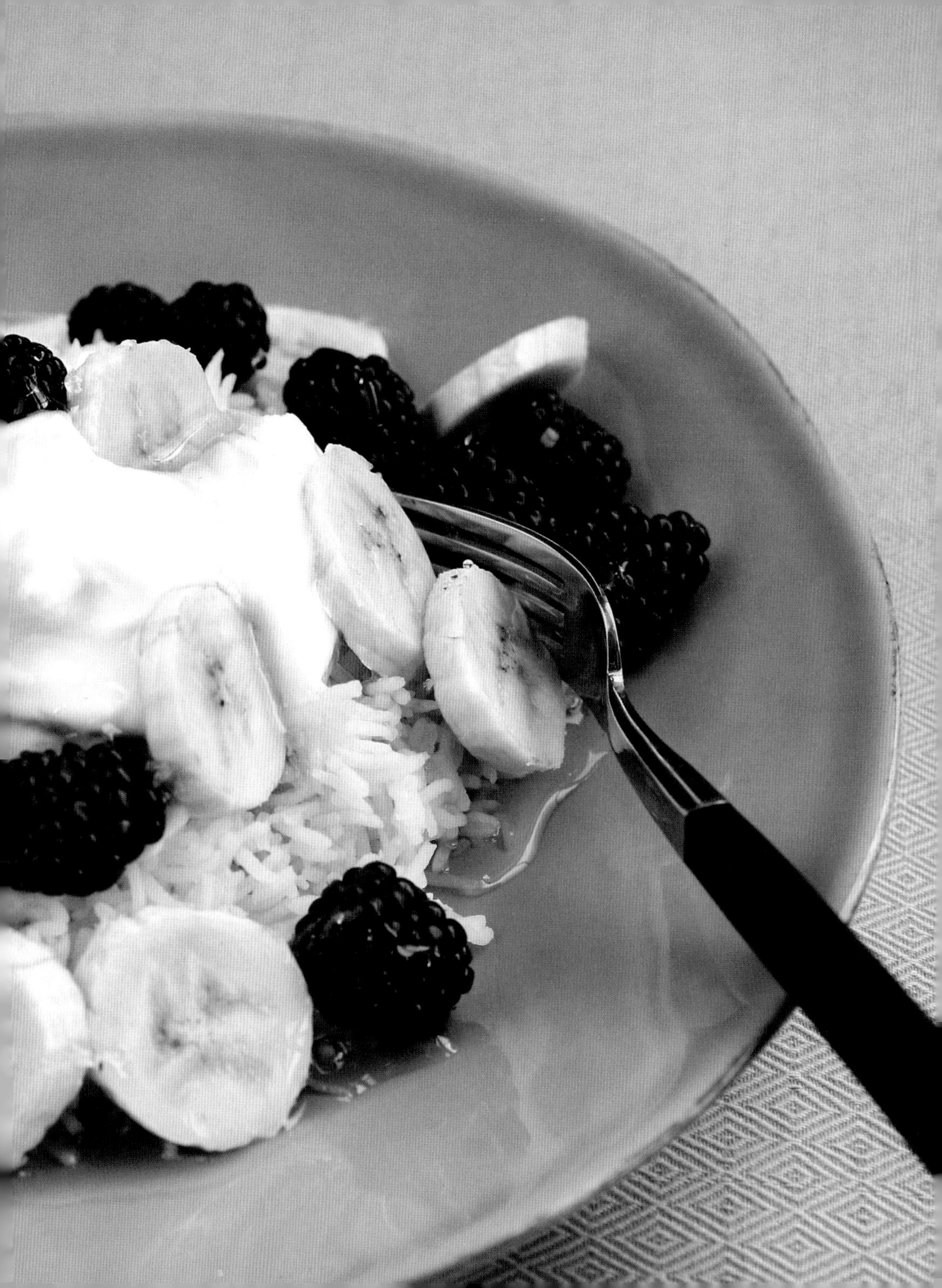

This goes great with poached eggs, fresh mozzarella slices, or some goat cheese. ★

SERVINGS> 2
TIME> 5 minutes

Tomatoes on Toast

I grew up eating ripe tomatoes sprinkled with coarse sugar. Now this is one of my favorite snacks immediately following a long workout because it takes the edge off my hunger while I look for something else to eat.

4 slices of rustic bread

2 ripe tomatoes, thickly sliced

about 2 tablespoons of coarse sugar

small handful of fresh mint leaves

½ tablespoon olive oil

salt

1. Toast the bread.
2. While bread is toasting, place tomatoes in a bowl and sprinkle evenly with coarse sugar. Use as little as you'd like.

To serve, stack tomato slices on toast, top with mint, drizzle a little olive oil, and add a sprinkle of salt.

PER SERVING> **Energy** 252 cal • **Fat** 6 g • **Sodium** 433 mg • **Carbs** 90 g • **Fiber** 5 g • **Protein** 7 g

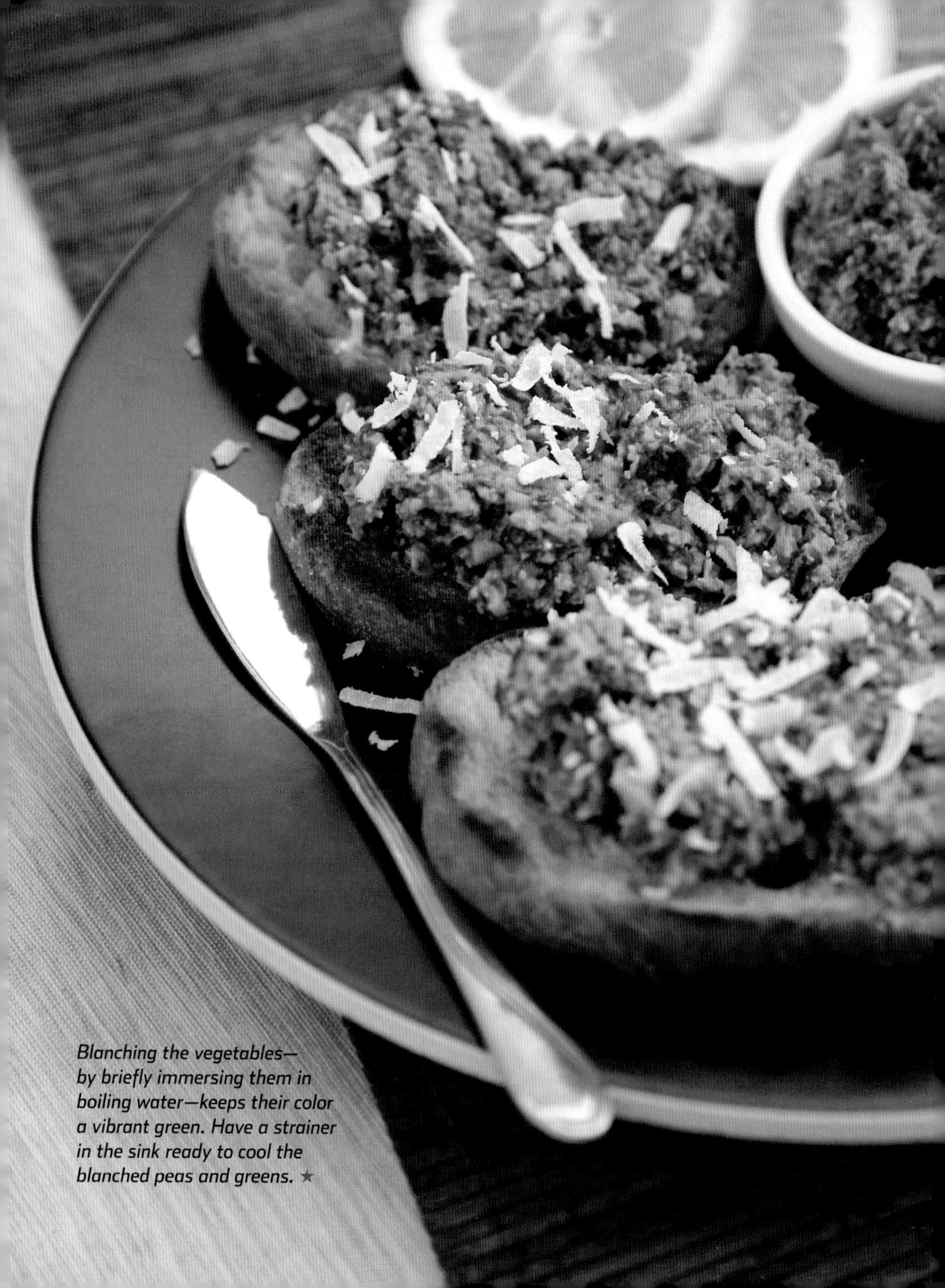

Blanching the vegetables—by briefly immersing them in boiling water—keeps their color a vibrant green. Have a strainer in the sink ready to cool the blanched peas and greens. ★

SERVINGS› 4
TIME› 10 minutes

Spring Pea and Herb Bruschetta

This is a fun alternative to traditional tomato bruschetta. We use frozen peas along with fresh herbs, spinach, and pesto to enjoy the bright green springtime flavor of this dish all year-round.

1 fresh baguette, cut into thick slices

olive oil or butter

TOPPING

1 cup peas (fresh or frozen)

1 cup loosely packed spinach or other greens

½ cup chopped fresh parsley, basil, and/or thyme

1 tablespoon prepared pesto

grated parmesan

fresh lemon juice

1. Brush baguette slices on both sides with olive oil or butter, and toast under the broiler for 2–3 minutes on each side.
2. To make the topping: Blanch the vegetables by bringing a pot of water to a gentle boil and adding a teaspoon of salt. Add the peas, spinach, and parsley and let cook for about 1 minute, until the vegetables turn bright green. Immediately remove, dunk in iced water, and strain.
3. Put blanched vegetables into food processor with pesto (or 1 tablespoon each olive oil and parmesan); process to a thick paste. Add salt and pepper to taste.

Spread a generous amount of the prepared topping onto bread. Top with fresh grated parmesan and a squeeze of fresh lemon juice just before serving.

TIP If you do not have prepared pesto, use 1 tablespoon each of olive oil and grated parmesan.

PER SERVING› **Energy** 125 cal • **Fat** 5 g • **Sodium** 345 mg • **Carbs** 16 g • **Fiber** 3 g • **Protein** 5 g

SERVINGS› 4
TIME› 20 minutes

Apple Salad on Grilled Bread

This is an easy salad using produce that is readily available year-round. If you plan to enjoy this as an après snack, prepare all of the ingredients except for the apples. You can quickly cut these after you return home. Even the grilled bread can be made in advance—the toasted texture is just as good with the crisp apples when served at room temperature.

8 slices of rustic bread

2–3 apples, cored, cut into bite-size pieces (about 2 cups)

1 green or red bell pepper, cut into bite-size pieces

½ cucumber, cut into bite-size pieces

¼ cup chopped fresh parsley

DRESSING

2 tablespoons olive oil

2 tablespoons red wine or red wine vinegar

1 teaspoon brown sugar

¼ of a green chile, minced (optional)

¼ cup crumbled goat cheese (or ricotta salata)

1. Brush the bread on both sides with olive oil and toast under the broiler for 2–3 minutes on each side.
2. In a medium-sized bowl, combine the apples, pepper, cucumber, and parsley.
3. To make the dressing: Whisk together the olive oil, red wine, and brown sugar in a small bowl. Add green chile, if using, and salt to taste.
4. Pour the dressing over the salad and toss to combine.

Pile the salad on the grilled bread and top with crumbled cheese.

NOTE› Ricotta salata is an inexpensive dry goat's milk cheese.

PER SERVING› **Energy** 398 cal • **Fat** 12 g • **Sodium** 612 mg • **Carbs** 64 g • **Fiber** 6 g • **Protein** 11 g

Nutrition for optional addition can be found in Appendix A.

For a different flavor, add spinach leaves and thinly sliced carrots to the salad. Grilled chicken and pasta are good accompaniments if you need a more filling meal. ★

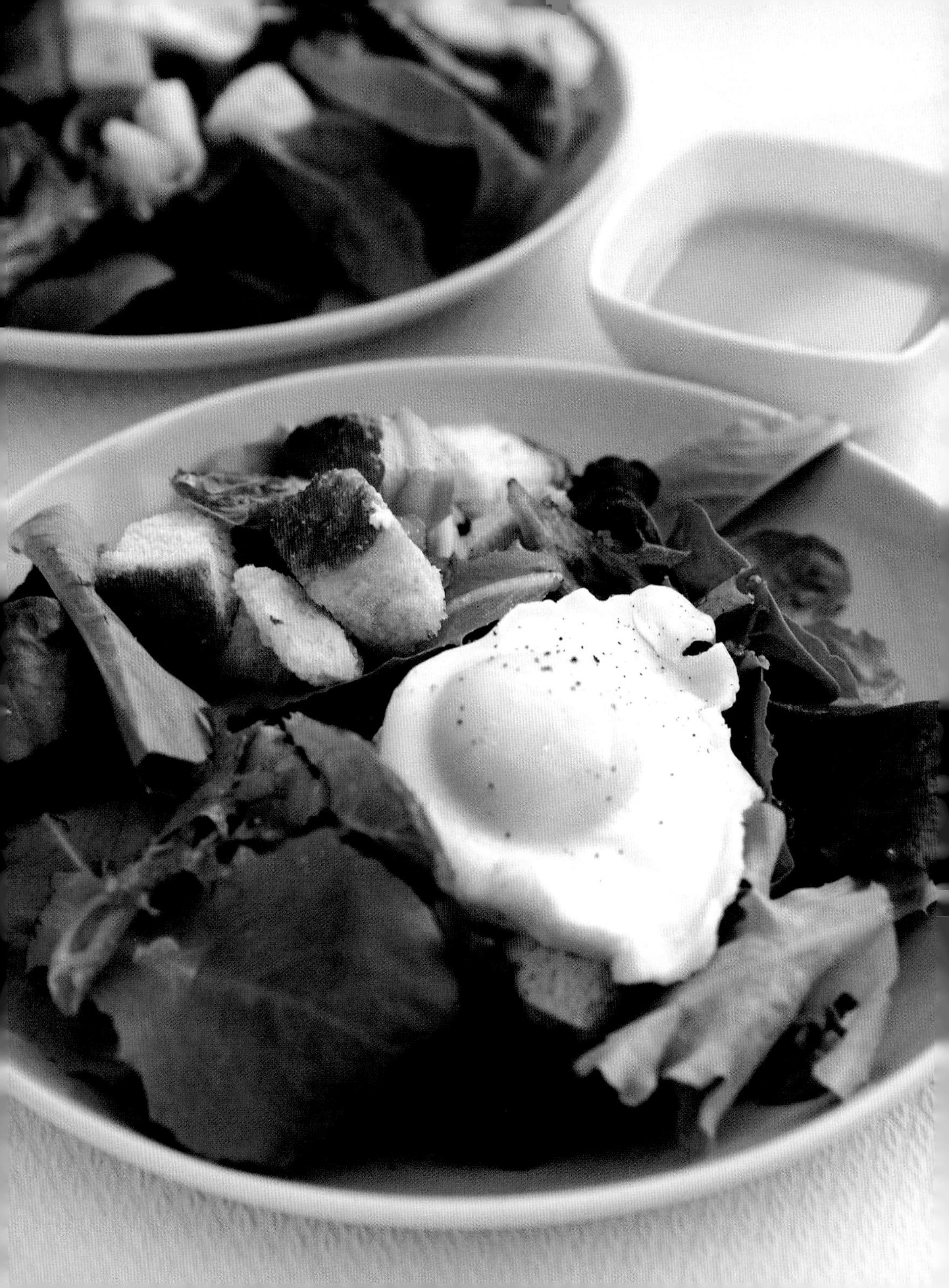

SERVINGS› 2
TIME› 20 minutes

Crouton Salad with Poached Egg

This truly is a very fast and incredibly delicious salad. Unlike pre-packaged croutons, the croutons in this recipe remain chewy inside, giving the salad a wonderful texture. You can use any kind of bread, including gluten-free.

CROUTONS

2–4 slices of bread

2 tablespoons olive oil

grated parmesan

2 eggs

vinegar

2 cups salad greens

DRESSING

2 tablespoons olive oil

juice of ½ a lemon

salt and pepper

1. Heat oven to 350 degrees.
2. To make the croutons: Cut bread into large bite-size pieces. Place bread in a bowl; drizzle with olive oil and stir so that all sides are coated. Sprinkle with parmesan, salt, and pepper. Transfer coated bread pieces to baking sheet. Bake until light golden in color, about 10 minutes. Set aside.
3. While the croutons are baking, poach the eggs: Bring a pan of water with a splash of vinegar to a gentle boil. Crack eggs into individual cups and gently slide each egg into water. Cook approximately 4–5 minutes. Use a slotted spoon or spatula to remove the poached eggs.
4. To make the dressing: In a small bowl, whisk together olive oil, lemon juice, and salt and pepper to taste.

In a large bowl combine greens, warm croutons, and dressing. Divide onto two salad plates and top with poached eggs and more grated parmesan, if desired.

PER SERVING› **Energy** 312 cal • **Fat** 21 g • **Sodium** 489 mg • **Carbs** 21 g • **Fiber** 4 g • **Protein** 13 g

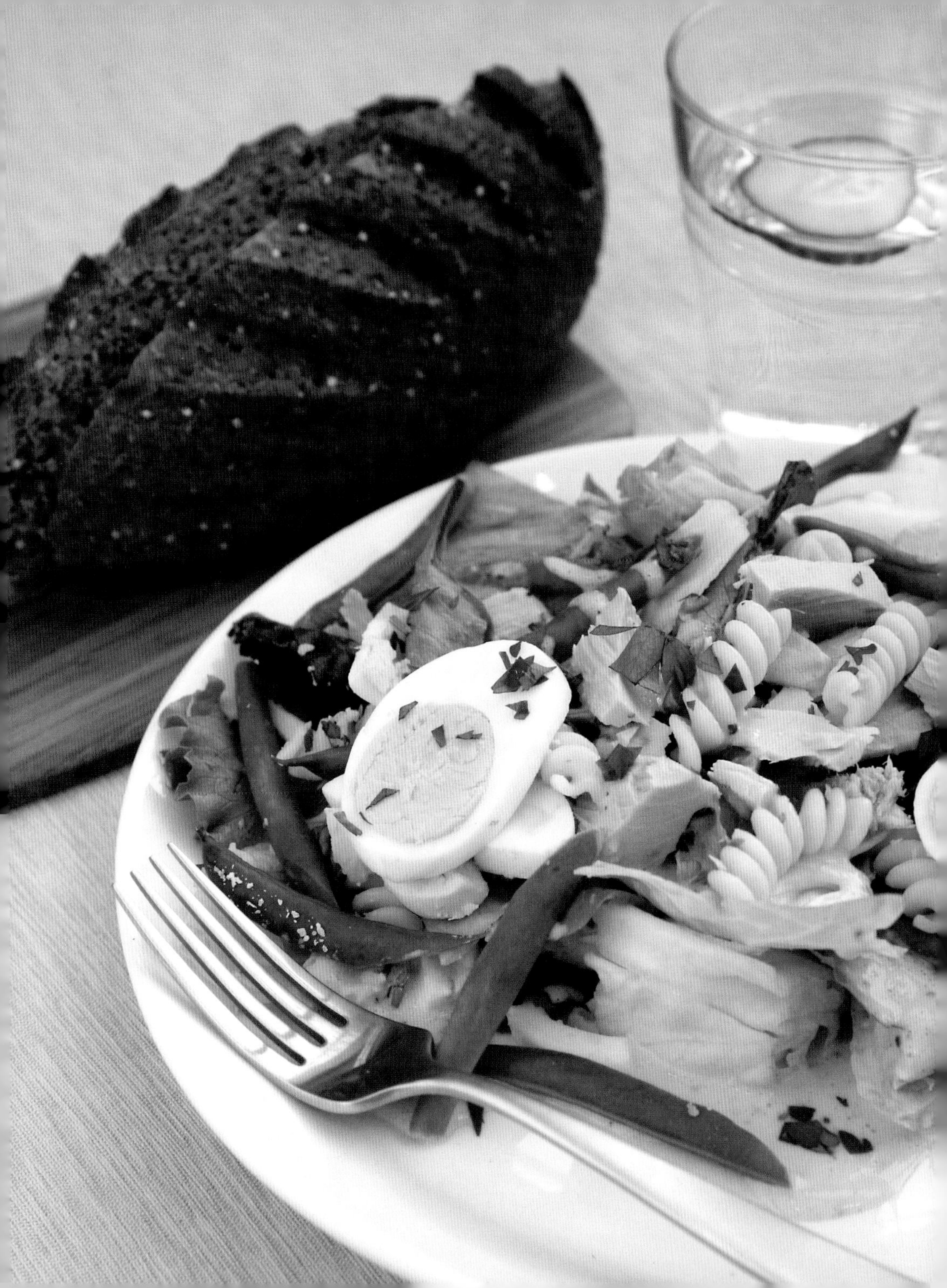

SERVINGS› 2
TIME› 10–15 minutes

Niçoise with Pasta

Classic Niçoise is a combination of crisp romaine and green beans, hard-boiled eggs, tuna, and light lemon aioli. Canned tuna is an economical way to get your protein, but we use it here so you can enjoy a great hassle-free salad.

2 cups romaine or other salad greens

COOKED 1 cup cooked pasta, such as fusilli

1 can (5 ounces) tuna, drained and gently flaked

8 ounces green beans, uncooked or lightly steamed

DRESSING

2 egg yolks, the freshest possible (see note)

1 teaspoon minced garlic

1 tablespoon coarse-ground prepared mustard

1 tablespoon white vinegar

2 tablespoons olive oil

juice of ½ a lemon

COOKED 2 hard-boiled eggs, sliced

1. In a large bowl combine romaine or salad greens, pasta, and tuna.
2. To steam green beans, place ½ cup of water in a sauté pan and cook over medium-high heat until most of the water has evaporated and the beans are bright green. Add to salad.
3. To make the dressing: Put the fresh egg yolks, garlic, mustard, and vinegar in a blender. Turn blender to low speed to incorporate the ingredients, then keep motor running and carefully drizzle in oil and lemon juice. Add more oil if you like a thinner dressing. Add salt and pepper to taste.
4. Add dressing and hard-boiled eggs to salad, toss gently.

Serve with crusty bread and top with fresh grated parmesan.

NOTE› The dressing for this recipe calls for raw egg yolks; if you are pregnant or nursing substitute 2 tablespoons mayonnaise.

PER SERVING› Energy 416 cal • Fat 25 g • Sodium 844 mg • Carbs 18 g • Fiber 3 g • Protein 29 g

SERVINGS› 2
TIME› 5 minutes

Roasted Beets and Greens

We hope that by now we have convinced you of the value of getting more beets into your diet. If you don't have roasted beets cooked and ready, don't hesitate to prepare them in the microwave or use canned beets. Whenever using canned beets, get the best and lowest-sodium ones you can find, drain, and use just after opening.

- 2 tablespoons olive oil
- 1 tablespoon Dijon mustard
- juice of ½ of lemon
- COOKED 1 cup cooked beets, cut into chunks
- 1 cup fresh spinach leaves or other dark greens

OPTIONAL ADDITIONS

- pita bread
- grated parmesan or crumbled goat cheese
- poached egg

1. In a medium serving bowl, whisk together olive oil, mustard, and lemon juice. Gently fold in beets and spinach.

Add salt and pepper to taste, along with desired amount of parmesan or goat cheese, if using.

TIP To prepare this as a warm salad, heat the beets in a sauté pan and then cook the spinach until it becomes slightly wilted but is still a vibrant green color.

PER SERVING› **Energy** 167 cal • **Fat** 14 g • **Sodium** 366 mg • **Carbs** 9 g • **Fiber** 2 g • **Protein** 2 g

Nutrition for optional additions can be found in Appendix A.

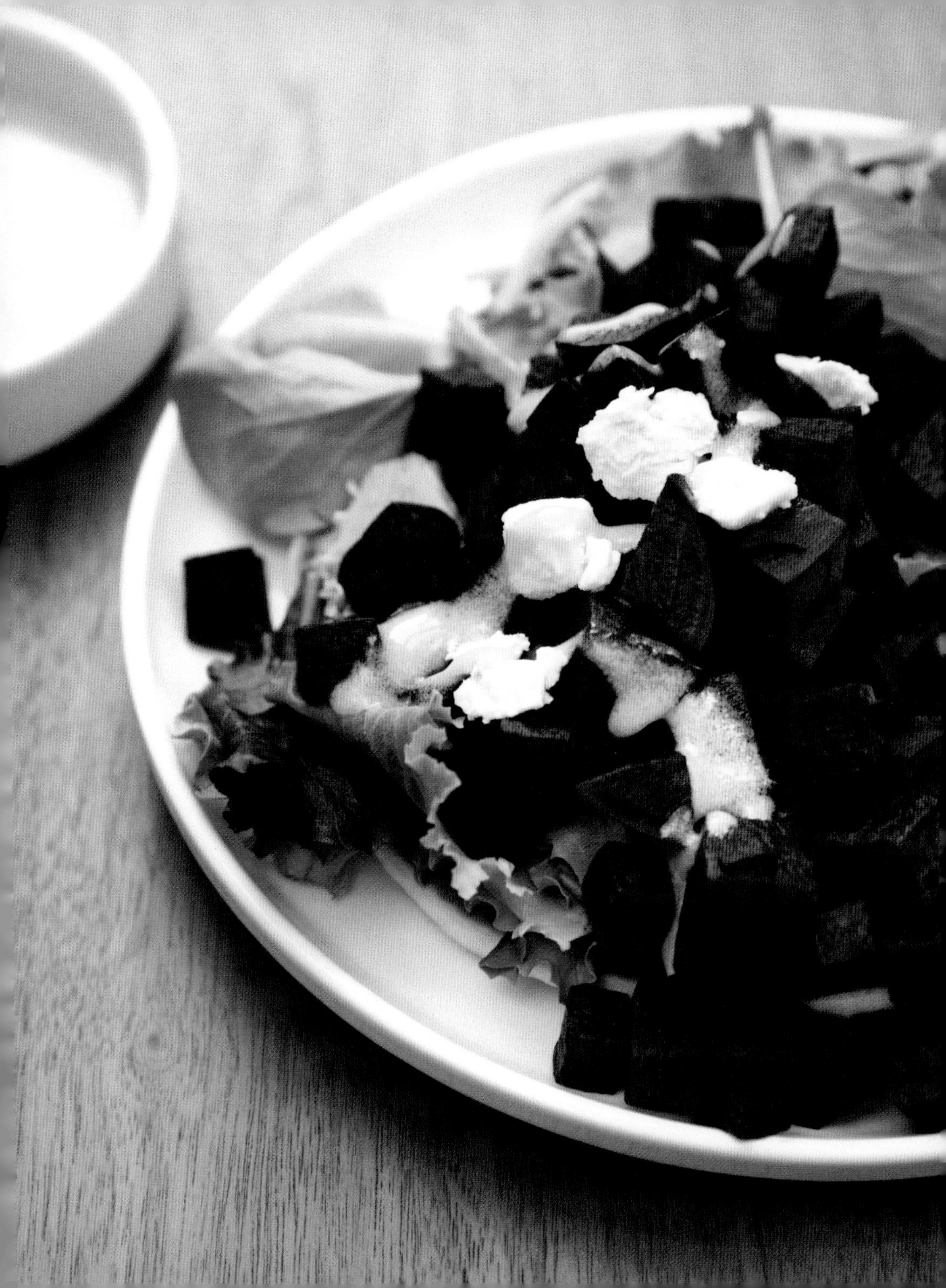

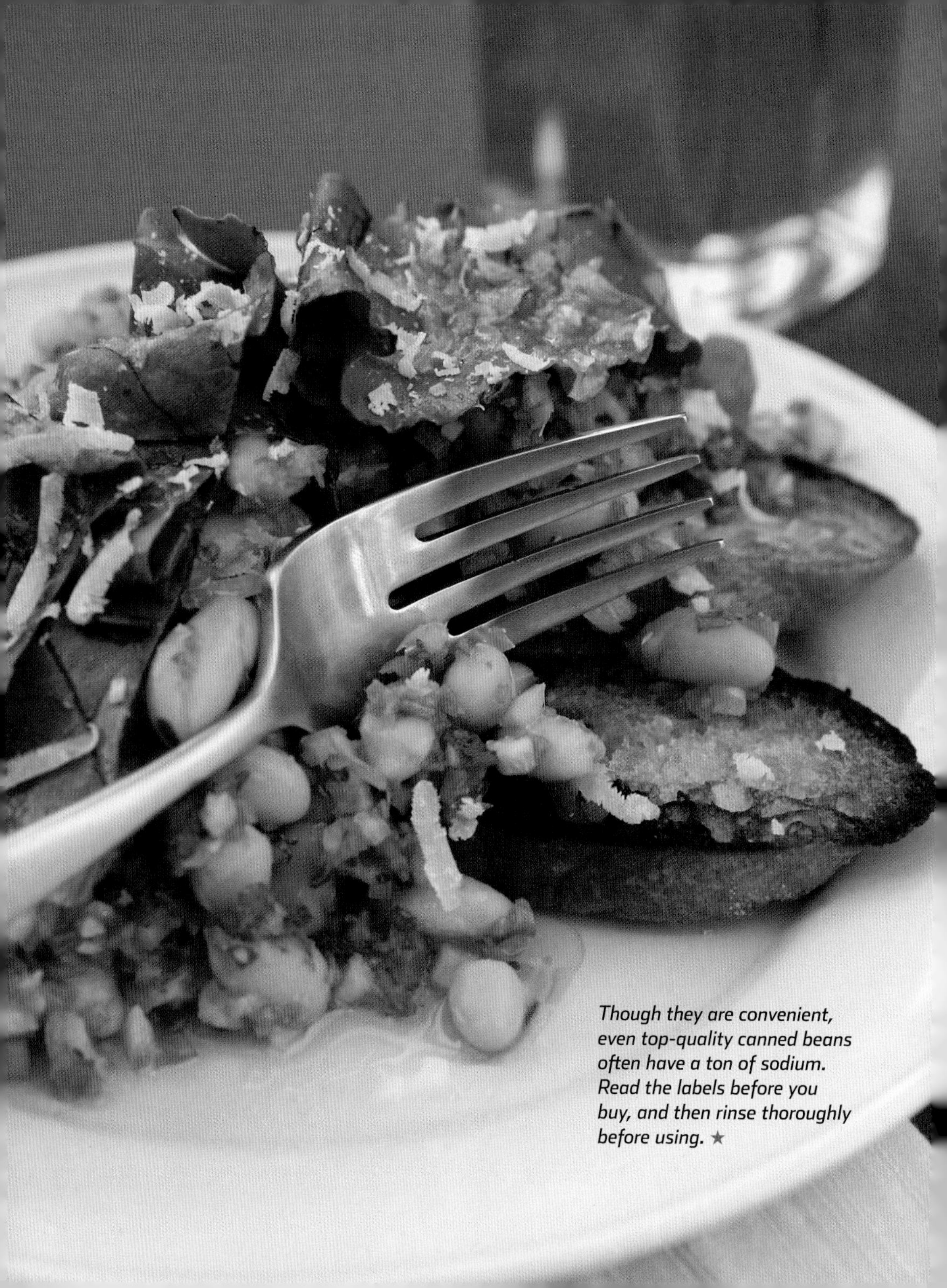

Though they are convenient, even top-quality canned beans often have a ton of sodium. Read the labels before you buy, and then rinse thoroughly before using. ★

SERVINGS› 3
TIME› 15 minutes

White Bean Salad

Grilled bread salads are easy last-minute items that can accommodate most any good hearty leftover bread. As for the beans in this recipe, use your favorite kind—I suggest cannellini, great northern, or butter beans. Of course, adding some crisp bacon or pancetta would make this taste even better!

COOKED **1 cup cooked white beans**

1 large carrot, minced

small handful of fresh parsley, chopped (about ¼ cup)

1 garlic clove, minced

½ of a small onion or shallot, minced

1 lemon

2 tablespoons olive oil, plus extra to brush on the bread

3–6 slices of rustic bread (1 or 2 slices per person)

2 cups loose-leaf bitter greens (chicory, mustard, parsnip, or beet), cut into bite-size pieces

½ teaspoon red pepper flakes

6 tablespoons parmesan

1. Combine beans, carrot, parsley, garlic, onion, juice from ½ a lemon, and oil in a small bowl. Set aside.
2. Brush both sides of bread slices with olive oil. Grill in the oven or in a hot dry pan. Once the bread chars a bit on both sides, remove it from the heat source; it should not be completely dry.
3. Toss greens with the rest of the lemon juice, red pepper flakes, and salt to taste.

Spoon bean mixture over grilled bread. Top with bitter greens and sprinkle with grated parmesan. A dash more of olive oil on top finishes it nicely.

PER SERVING› Energy 459 cal • Fat 15 g • Sodium 719 mg • Carbs 64 g • Fiber 7 g • Protein 18 g

SERVINGS> 4
TIME> 15–20 minutes

Chicken Tacos

Lightly warmed corn tortillas stuffed with spiced chicken and cool salsa are the perfect après-ride food. Bursting with bright flavors and a hint of salt and citrus, these tacos are just what your body craves. To speed things up, prep the chicken in advance.

COOKED 1 cup cooked rice

1 pound boneless, skinless chicken, cut into small chunks (see note)

1 onion, cut into strips

2 mild green chiles, cut into strips

½ teaspoon chili powder and/or ground cumin

fresh lime juice

4–6 corn tortillas

Roasted Salsa (page 286)

Spicy Cabbage Slaw (page 284)

1. Add a splash of water to the cooked rice and warm in a sauté pan over medium-high heat. Put rice aside.
2. Bring a lightly oiled sauté pan to medium-high heat. Add chicken, onion, and chiles. Sauté, sprinkling with spices as desired, until chicken is cooked through and onions have softened and browned, about 10–15 minutes.
3. Add lime juice and salt to taste.
4. Warm the corn tortillas in a dry pan or in the oven, about 3–5 minutes.

Stuff each warmed corn tortilla with a few spoonfuls of cooked rice, chicken, and salsa.

NOTE> Thigh meat will give you a bit more fat and flavor in the summer when you're racking up the training miles. At other times of the year, use chicken breasts.

TIP Feel free to use purchased salsa to save time. But if you want to impress your friends, our fresh option is a great accompaniment.

PER SERVING> **Energy** 274 cal • **Fat** 2 g • **Sodium** 244 mg • **Carbs** 24 g • **Fiber** 1 g • **Protein** 36 g

Tacos can be wrapped and stored in the fridge for up to 3 days. When you get an urge for a snack, reheat one of these tacos in the microwave and you'll be glad you took the time to make them. ★

These tacos go great with Pico de Gallo (page 287).

SERVINGS> 4
TIME> 25–30 minutes

Turkey Tacos

The ground turkey in these easy tacos is a terrific low-fat substitute for beef. Use our Taco Spice (page 295), or purchase a blend that contains no mystery additives. If you are feeling extra hungry, make a fresh pot of rice and pile your taco higher.

- COOKED 2 cups cooked rice
- 1 pound ground turkey
- 1 onion, chopped
- 1–2 tablespoons taco spice or Mexican seasoning mix
- 1 tablespoon low-sodium soy sauce
- ¼ cup tomatoes or cucumbers
- 1 fresh jalapeno, chopped
- small handful of cilantro, chopped
- 12 corn tortillas
- 1 cup salsa or pico de gallo

OPTIONAL ADDITIONS

- grated cheese
- plain yogurt

1. Add a splash of water to the cooked rice and warm in a sauté pan over medium-high heat. Put rice aside.
2. In sauté pan, heat just enough oil to coat the bottom. Add turkey and onion; brown thoroughly, stirring often, about 8–10 minutes.
3. Add seasoning mix, soy sauce, fresh tomatoes or cucumbers, and jalapeno. Remove from heat. Add chopped cilantro, and salt and pepper to taste.
4. Warm the tortillas in a hot, dry pan, one at a time, flipping after 1–2 minutes. Alternatively, heat oven to 375 degrees; lay tortillas flat on the oven rack for about 5 minutes.

Lay out warmed tortillas, top with rice, then add turkey and salsa. If desired, top with grated cheese and plain yogurt.

PER SERVING> **Energy** 457 cal • **Fat** 5 g • **Sodium** 1,036 mg • **Carbs** 71 g • **Fiber** 6 g • **Protein** 34 g

Nutrition for optional additions can be found in Appendix A.

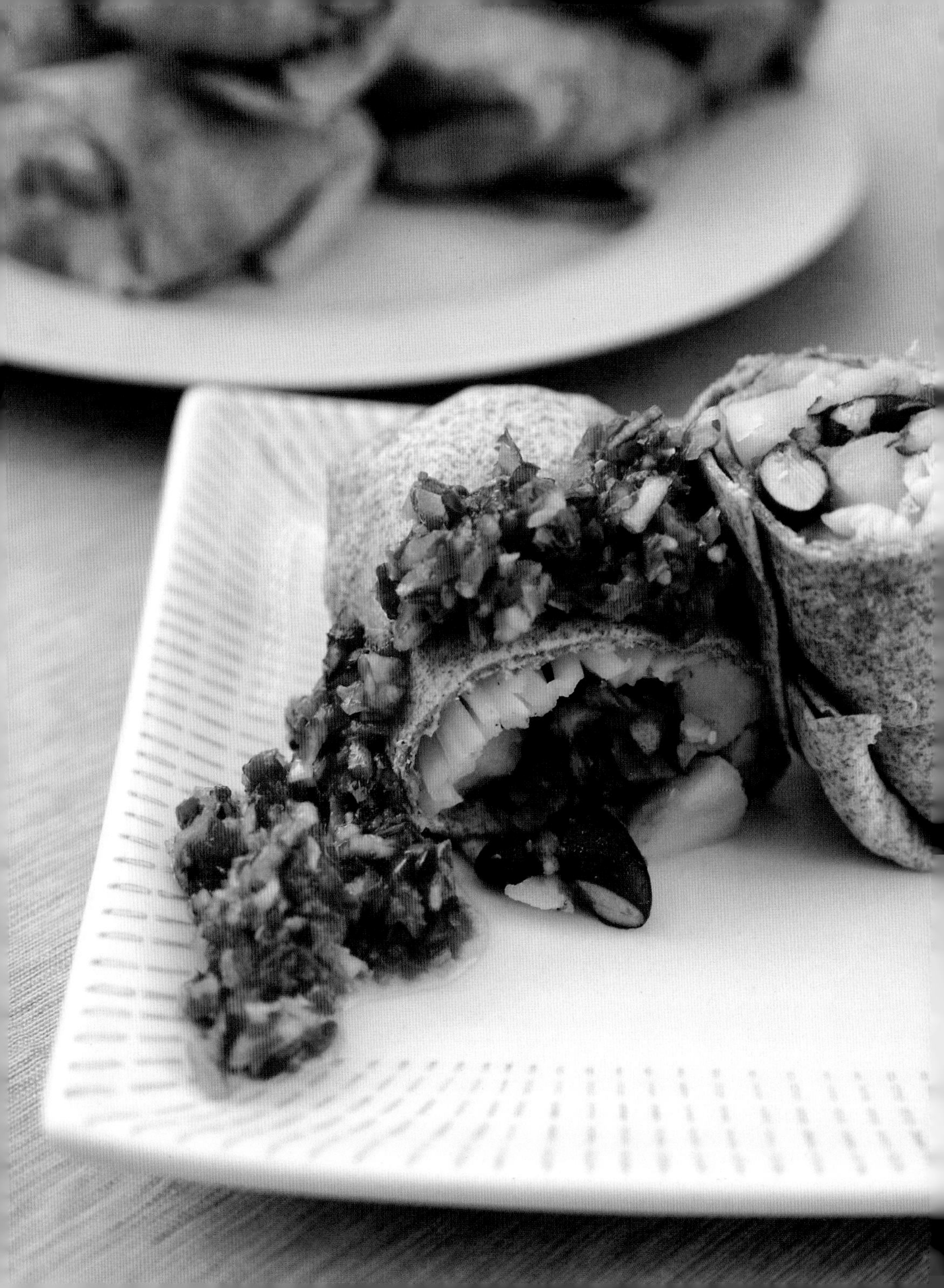

SERVINGS› 6
TIME› 10 minutes

Ham and Cheese Burritos

We keep burritos in the freezer for snacks, for post-ride meals, or even to stuff in our pockets and bring along. This simple version uses either cooked rice or potatoes as the base. Burritos are universally popular with athletes. It's just a matter of finding your favorite variety.

COOKED 3 cups cooked rice or cooked diced potatoes

1 cup diced ham

1 cup shredded cheddar cheese

½ cup prepared salsa

COOKED 1 cup cooked beans

4 scrambled eggs (optional)

6 large (10–12 inch) whole wheat tortillas

1. Combine all ingredients except tortillas, adding salt and pepper to taste. Scramble eggs over medium-high heat, if using.
2. Warm tortillas one at a time in a dry pan at medium-high heat, flipping after 1–2 minutes. Immediately stuff each with about 1 cup of the filling mixture. Roll tightly, being sure to fold in the short ends first.

Enjoy warm, or wrap and freeze for later use.

NOTE› For ready-to-serve burritos, combine all ingredients except cheese and tortillas in a sauté pan and heat thoroughly before stuffing tortillas.

TIP To reheat frozen burritos, place in the microwave for 1½ to 2 minutes.

PER SERVING (1 burrito)› **Energy** 445 cal • **Fat** 13 g • **Sodium** 688 mg • **Carbs** 64 g • **Fiber** 4 g • **Protein** 18 g
Nutrition for optional additions can be found in Appendix A.

SERVINGS> 2
TIME> 10 minutes

Honey Ginger Chicken Wraps

This simple recipe requires almost no equipment and not much time. It's perfect as an "on the road" item because you can easily find the ingredients and put it together in your hotel room. If you're doing this, mix the honey, ginger, and oil ahead of time and bring it along in a tightly sealed bottle.

- COOKED 2 cups cooked rice
- COOKED 2 cups cooked chicken, shredded
- 2 tablespoons honey
- 2 teaspoons freshly grated ginger
- 1 tablespoon olive oil
- juice of ½ a lemon or a splash of vinegar

OPTIONAL ADDITIONS

- a small handful of fresh greens or vegetables
- minced chiles or garlic
- red pepper flakes
- radishes

- 6 large (10–12-inch) whole wheat tortillas

1. Add a splash of water to the cooked rice and warm in a sauté pan over medium-high heat. Put rice aside.
2. Combine all ingredients (including optional additions, if using) and let sit for just a minute so that the chicken absorbs the flavors. Add salt and pepper to taste.
3. Warm tortillas one at a time in a dry pan at medium-high heat, flipping after 1–2 minutes. Immediately stuff each with about 1 cup of the filling mixture. Roll tightly, being sure to fold in the short ends first.

TIP Use grilled, sautéed, rotisserie, or baked chicken—all go great with steamed rice.

PER SERVING> **Energy** 500 cal • **Fat** 15 g • **Sodium** 228 mg • **Carbs** 19 g • **Fiber** 0 g • **Protein** 71 g

Nutrition for optional additions can be found in Appendix A.

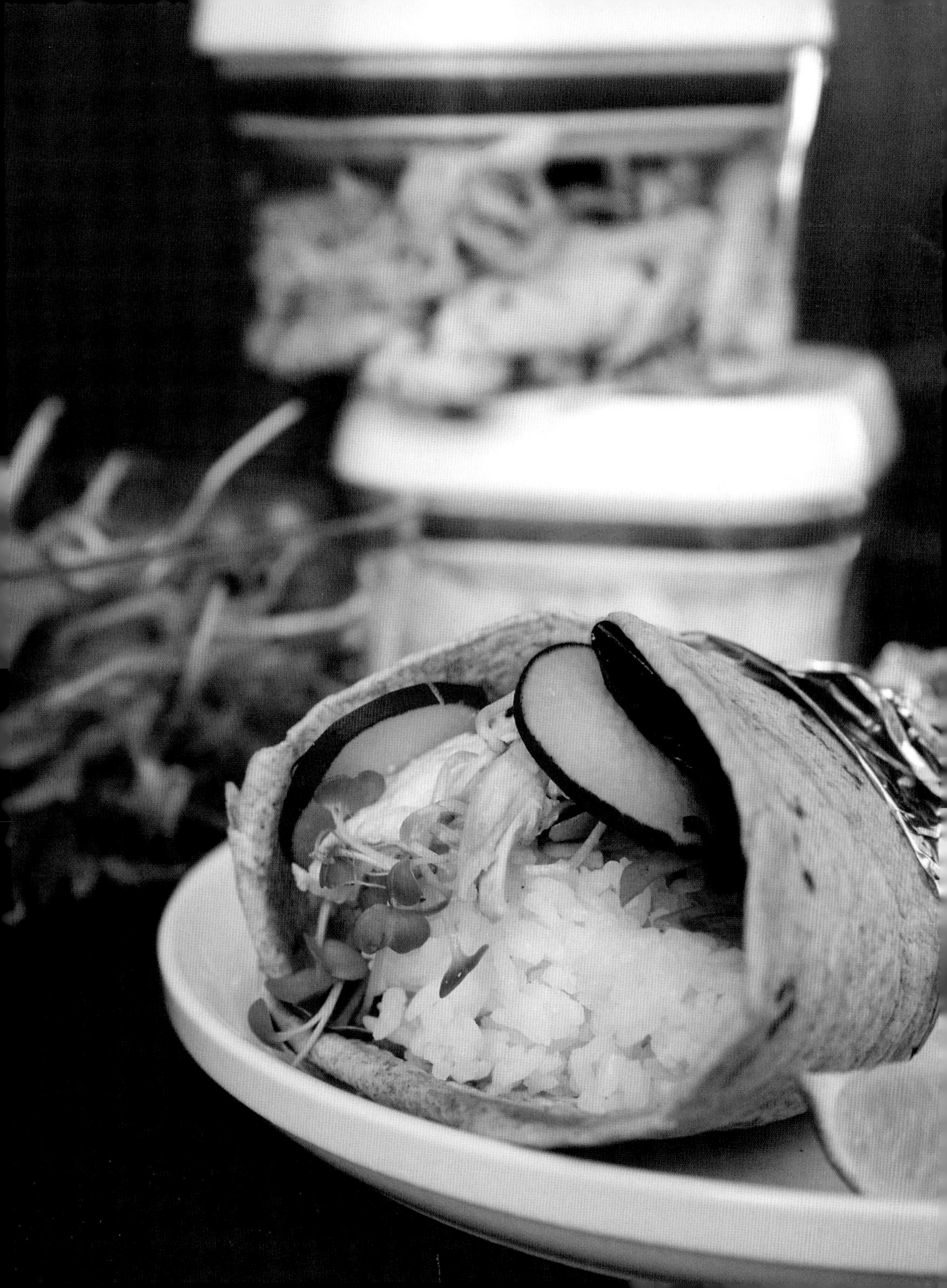

SERVINGS› 1
TIME› 10 minutes

Recovery Grilled Cheese

This is your basic grilled cheese sandwich with a whole lot of love added. Start with the basic recipe and then add whatever sounds interesting. Because this sandwich has more fat and dairy than most, save it for a mid- to late-season recovery meal when your body can use more calories.

1 tablespoon softened cream cheese

2 thick slices of bread

dash of ground nutmeg

4 thin slices Swiss cheese

2 ounces canned roasted red peppers or green chiles, drained

olive oil

OPTIONAL ADDITIONS

grilled asparagus

cooked bacon

sun-dried tomatoes

goat cheese

truffle oil

1. Spread cream cheese onto 2 slices of bread (these are the sides that will be matched together).
2. Sprinkle ground nutmeg on top of the cream cheese, then top with slices of Swiss cheese and a few pieces of roasted red pepper or green chiles.
3. Put sandwich together, brush olive oil on the outsides, and grill in a hot sauté pan until cheese is melted and bread is golden brown on both sides.

PER SERVING› **Energy** 686 cal • **Fat** 38 g • **Sodium** 1,033 mg • **Carbs** 58 g • **Fiber** 6 g • **Protein** 32 g

Nutrition for optional additions can be found in Appendix A.

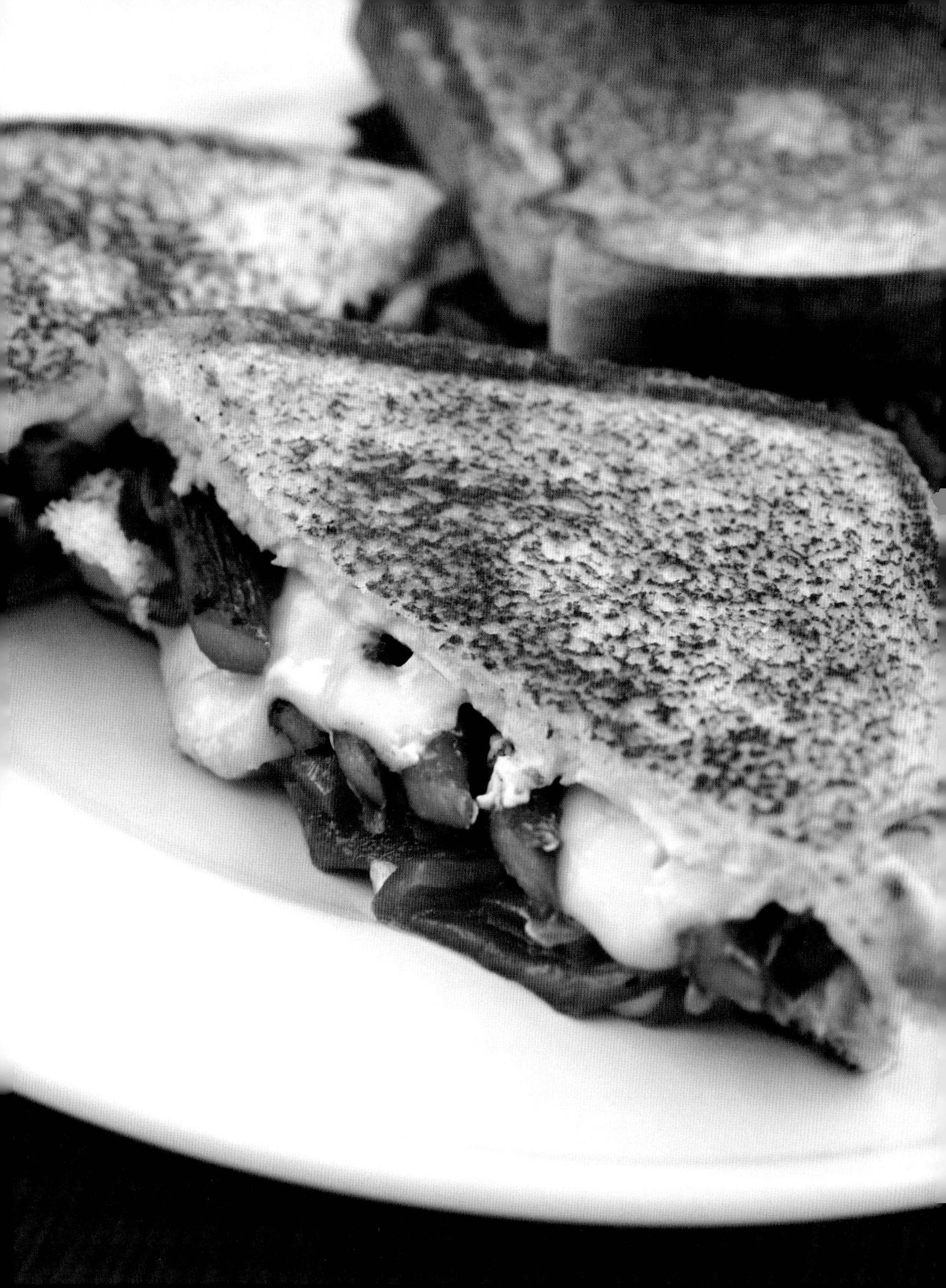

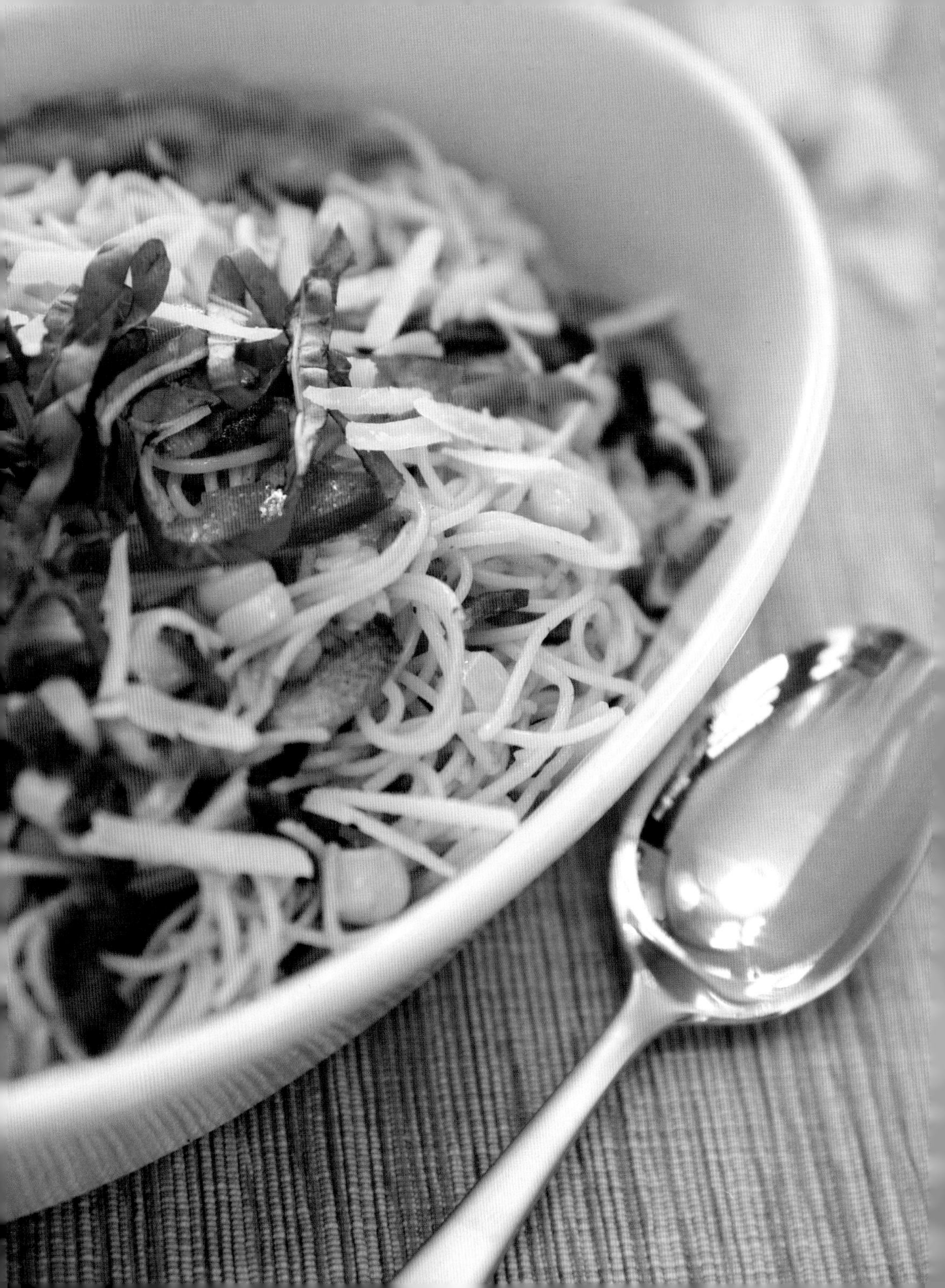

SERVINGS› 2
TIME› 15 minutes

Angel Hair with Bacon and Sweet Corn

This is a light-bodied, flavorful pasta that carries a bright burst of fresh uncooked corn. We typically prepare this dish fresh prior to a day of training or racing and put it in the cooler for immediately after the ride. Hot or cold, it's an excellent way to recover.

8 ounces angel hair pasta

8 ounces bacon, chopped

2 ears of uncooked sweet corn

1 tomato, diced

¼ cup fresh basil leaves, cut into strips

1½ tablespoons olive oil

1. Bring a large pot of water to a boil. Add the pasta and cook for 6–8 minutes, or until al dente.
2. While the pasta is boiling, fry the bacon in a medium sauté pan. When bacon gets crispy, drain off fat and wrap in paper towels to remove any excess fat.
3. Use a knife to carefully cut the kernels off the ears of corn.
4. Drain the pasta. Transfer pasta, bacon, and corn to a large bowl. Add tomato, basil, olive oil, and salt and pepper to taste. Fold everything together.

Top with grated parmesan and a squeeze of lemon juice.

TIP Use roasted chicken or eggs in place of the bacon to get more protein in this dish.

PER SERVING› **Energy** 679 cal • **Fat** 20 g • **Sodium** 969 mg • **Carbs** 108 g • **Fiber** 7 g • **Protein** 23 g

SERVINGS› 2
TIME› 10–15 minutes

Chicken Fried Rice

This recipe is exactly as Allen presented it to his class in the third grade and exactly as he serves it to athletes at training camps, races, or impromptu dinners at his place in Boulder, Colorado. At the 2010 Tour de France, this was Lance Armstrong's favorite post-race dish.

- 1 tablespoon minced garlic (about 2 cloves)
- 2–3 green onions, diced or thinly sliced
- 3 eggs
- 2 tablespoons low-sodium soy sauce
- COOKED 2 cups cooked rice
- COOKED 1 cup boneless chicken thighs (2–3 pieces)
- 1 cup frozen peas and corn

OPTIONAL ADDITIONS

- Sriracha sauce
- sesame oil

1. Bring a lightly oiled sauté pan to medium-high heat. Add the garlic and green onions and sauté for about 1 minute.
2. In a small bowl, beat the eggs and soy sauce vigorously and pour into the hot pan. The pan should be hot enough to cause the eggs to fluff. Stir the eggs to cook them quickly.
3. Add the rice and cooked chicken thighs and fry the mixture for 5–6 minutes.
4. Add the peas and corn and cook until the vegetables heat through and are vibrant in color.

Season to taste with salt, Sriracha sauce, and additional soy sauce or sesame oil.

PER SERVING› **Energy** 605 cal • **Fat** 17 g • **Sodium** 727 mg • **Carbs** 68 g • **Fiber** 4 g • **Protein** 39 g
Nutrition for optional additions can be found in Appendix A.

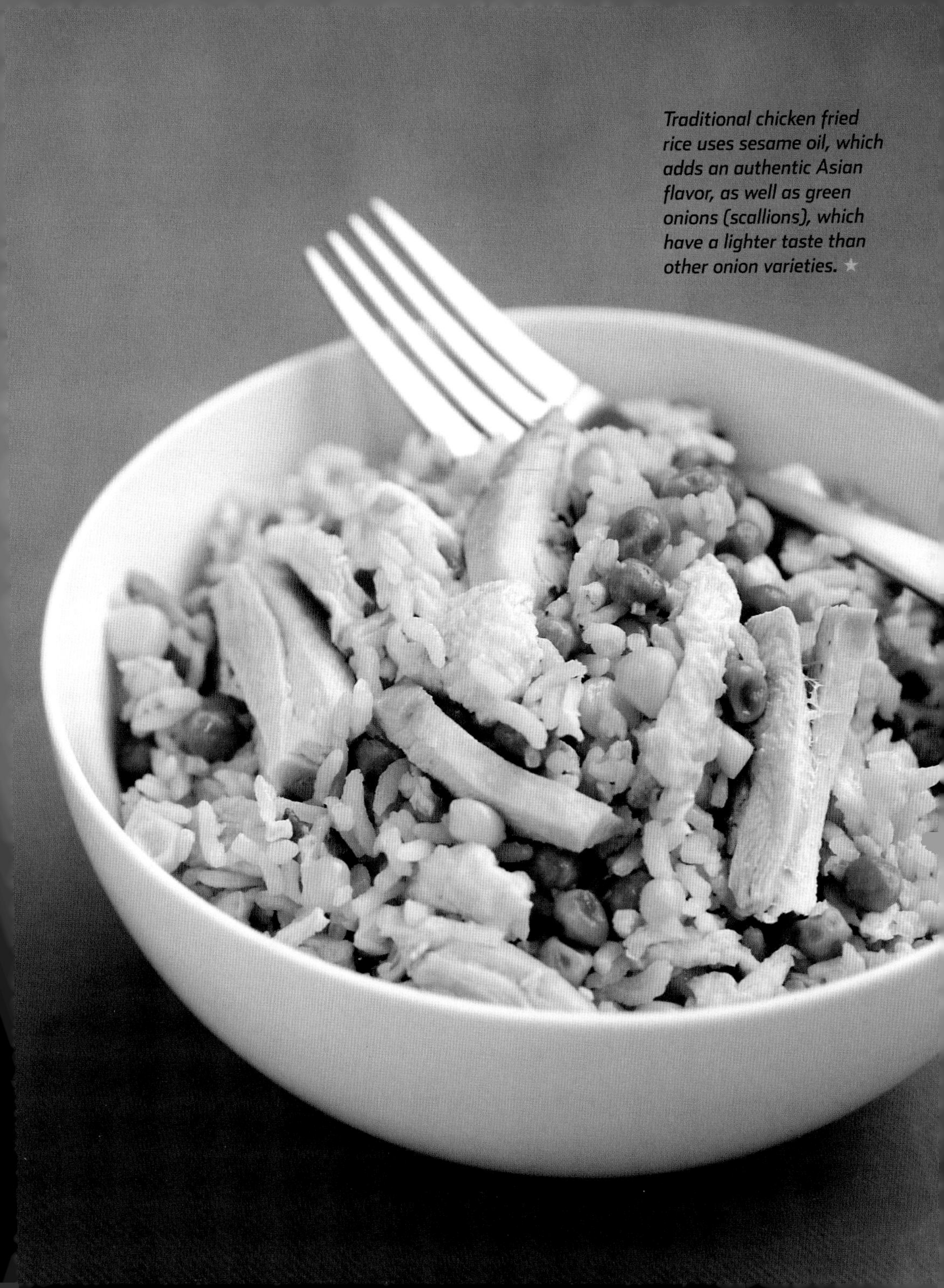

Traditional chicken fried rice uses sesame oil, which adds an authentic Asian flavor, as well as green onions (scallions), which have a lighter taste than other onion varieties. ★

SERVINGS› 2
TIME› 10 minutes

Pasta Salad with Olives and Beets

We don't like to boil and then drain vegetables since nutrients are lost that way. Instead, microwave the beets for this salad and then quickly sauté them, which imparts great flavor and sweetness.

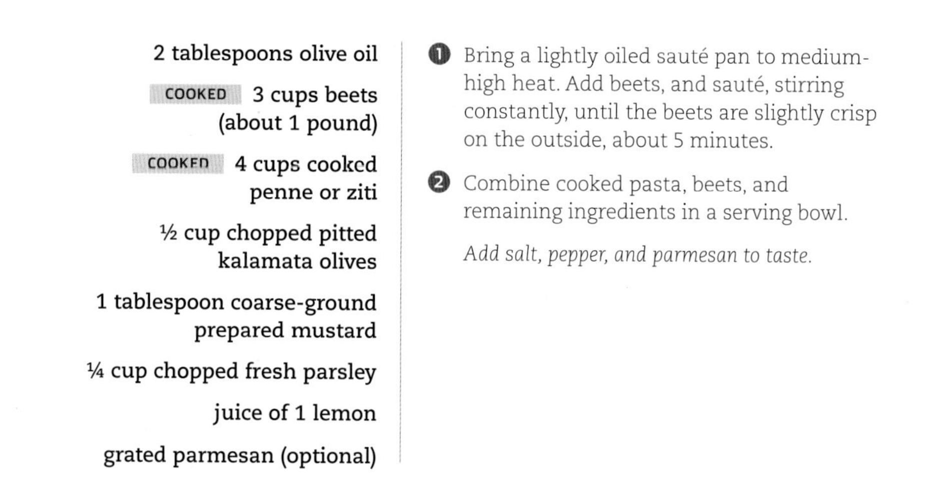

- 2 tablespoons olive oil
- COOKED 3 cups beets (about 1 pound)
- COOKED 4 cups cooked penne or ziti
- ½ cup chopped pitted kalamata olives
- 1 tablespoon coarse-ground prepared mustard
- ¼ cup chopped fresh parsley
- juice of 1 lemon
- grated parmesan (optional)

1. Bring a lightly oiled sauté pan to medium-high heat. Add beets, and sauté, stirring constantly, until the beets are slightly crisp on the outside, about 5 minutes.
2. Combine cooked pasta, beets, and remaining ingredients in a serving bowl.

Add salt, pepper, and parmesan to taste.

PER SERVING› **Energy** 607 cal • **Fat** 16 g • **Sodium** 551 mg • **Carbs** 112 g • **Fiber** 13 g • **Protein** 10 g

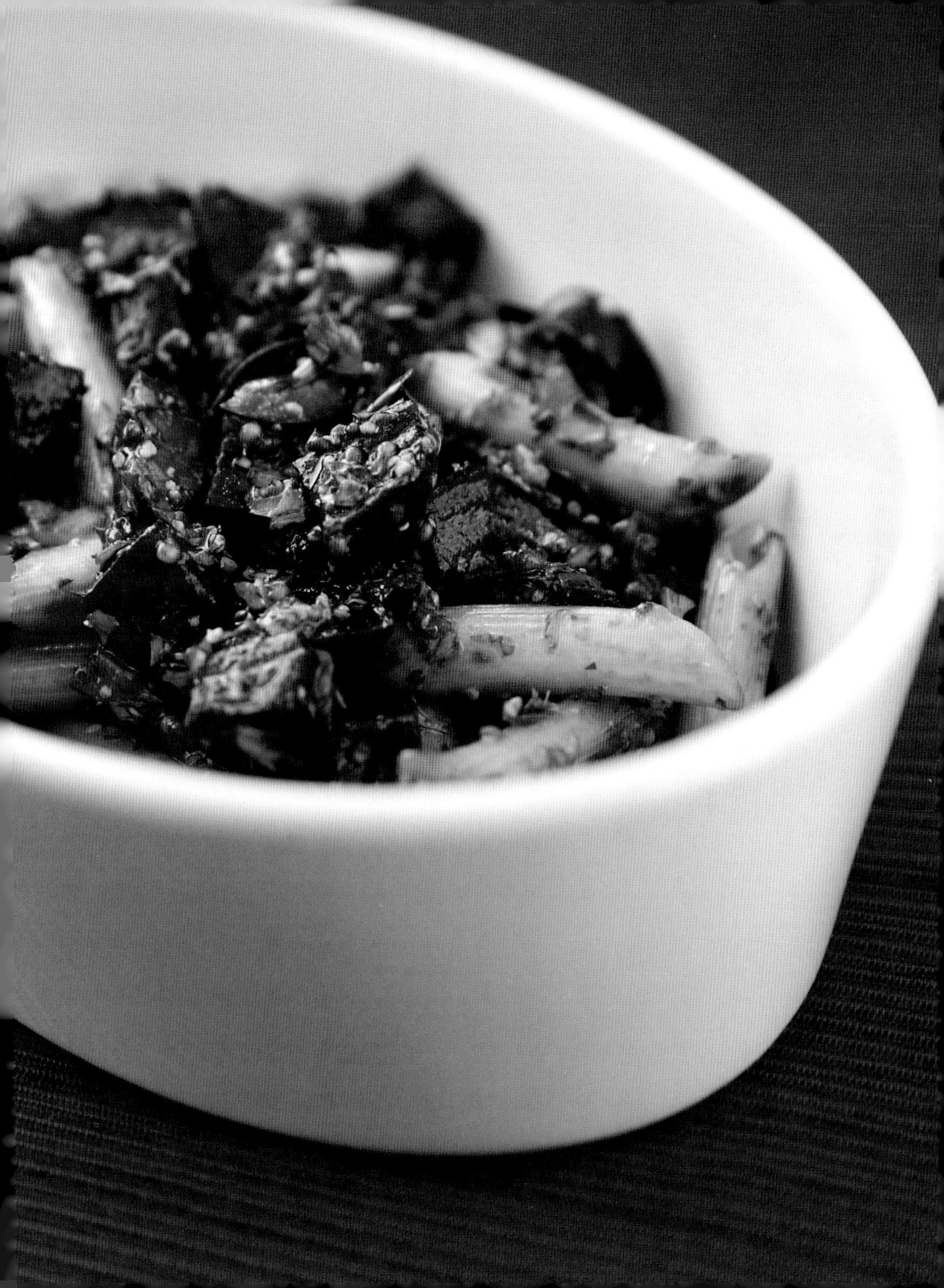

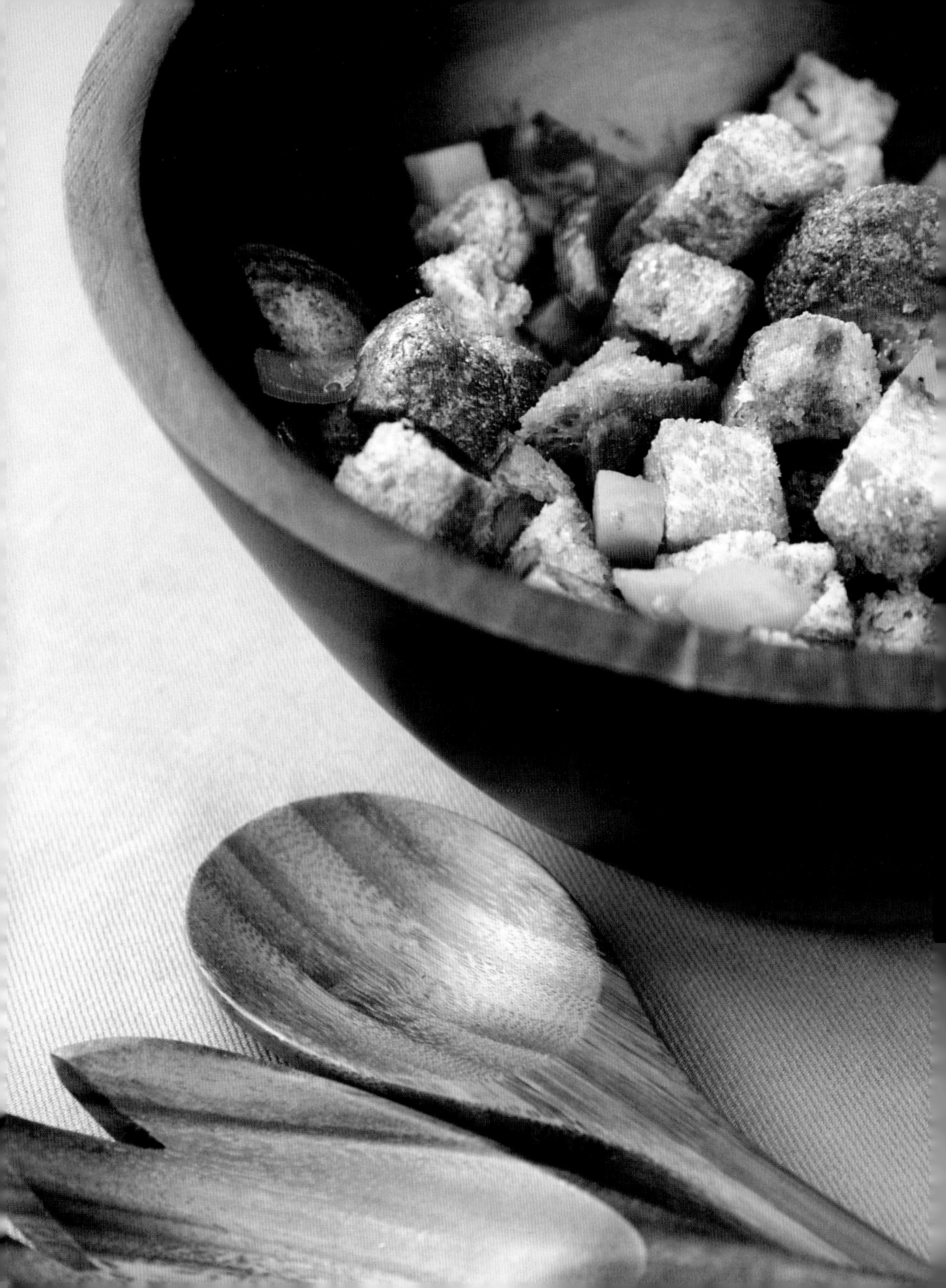

SERVINGS> 2
TIME> 15 minutes

Bread Salad

When you are ready for a break from rice and pasta, this salad is perfect. It's also practical because it can quickly transform stale bread into a delicious après dish. Be creative and change the flavors with the seasons: fresh herbs, sprouts, and hard-boiled eggs in spring; sweet corn and basil in summer; carmelized onions (in place of uncooked onions) and roasted beets in fall; and salmon, thyme, and bacon in winter.

4 cups cubed hearty bread (bite-size pieces)

4 tablespoons olive oil

1 tomato, diced

¼ small onion, thinly sliced

1 teaspoon red wine vinegar or balsamic vinegar

2 tablespoons grated parmesan

OPTIONAL ADDITIONS

See seasonal variations above

1. If the bread is very stale and hard, sprinkle some water over it. Let soak for a few minutes and then press out any excess water.
2. Warm the bread first by sautéing the cubes in a pan on the stove top or toasting them on a baking sheet in the oven.
3. In a large bowl, toss all ingredients together, adding salt, pepper, and parmesan to taste.

NOTE> To caramelize onions (see variation for fall as shown here), sauté in ½ cup water and ¼ cup brown sugar until golden brown.

TIP Use more olive oil and juice from diced tomatoes to wet the bread if it is super dry.

PER SERVING> Energy 663 cal • Fat 34 g • Sodium 856 mg • Carbs 75 g • Fiber 11 g • Protein 21 g

SERVINGS› 2
TIME› 20 minutes

Tuna and Broccoli with Noodles

This après dish is versatile in all the right ways. If you return from a workout well past hungry, use canned tuna and frozen broccoli to fix the problem fast. When you have more time, use an ahi tuna steak and fresh broccoli. Regardless of how you make it, this dish tastes even better on a base of egg noodles.

8 ounces ahi tuna

1 tablespoon olive oil

2 cups broccoli, cut into bite-size pieces

1 teaspoon minced garlic

½ a small onion, diced

1 tablespoon low-sodium soy sauce

COOKED **4 cups cooked pasta**

red pepper flakes (optional)

1. Lightly salt and pepper both sides of ahi tuna. Bring a lightly oiled sauté pan to a high heat; add tuna and sear both sides. Continue to cook until the flesh is almost white inside. Remove from heat; cool slightly, and chop. (If using canned tuna or beans, just proceed to next step.)
2. Add broccoli, garlic, and onion to pan. Sauté over high heat 3–5 minutes, until broccoli has a bright green color.
3. Add chopped tuna and soy sauce; stir gently to combine. Turn off heat. Add the cooked pasta and stir again.

Season with red pepper flakes or ground black pepper.

TIP If you don't have ahi tuna on hand, substitute a 5-ounce can of albacore or 1 cup of cooked beans.

PER SERVING› Energy 665 cal • Fat 13 g • Sodium 672 mg • Carbs 88 g • Fiber 7 g • Protein 48 g

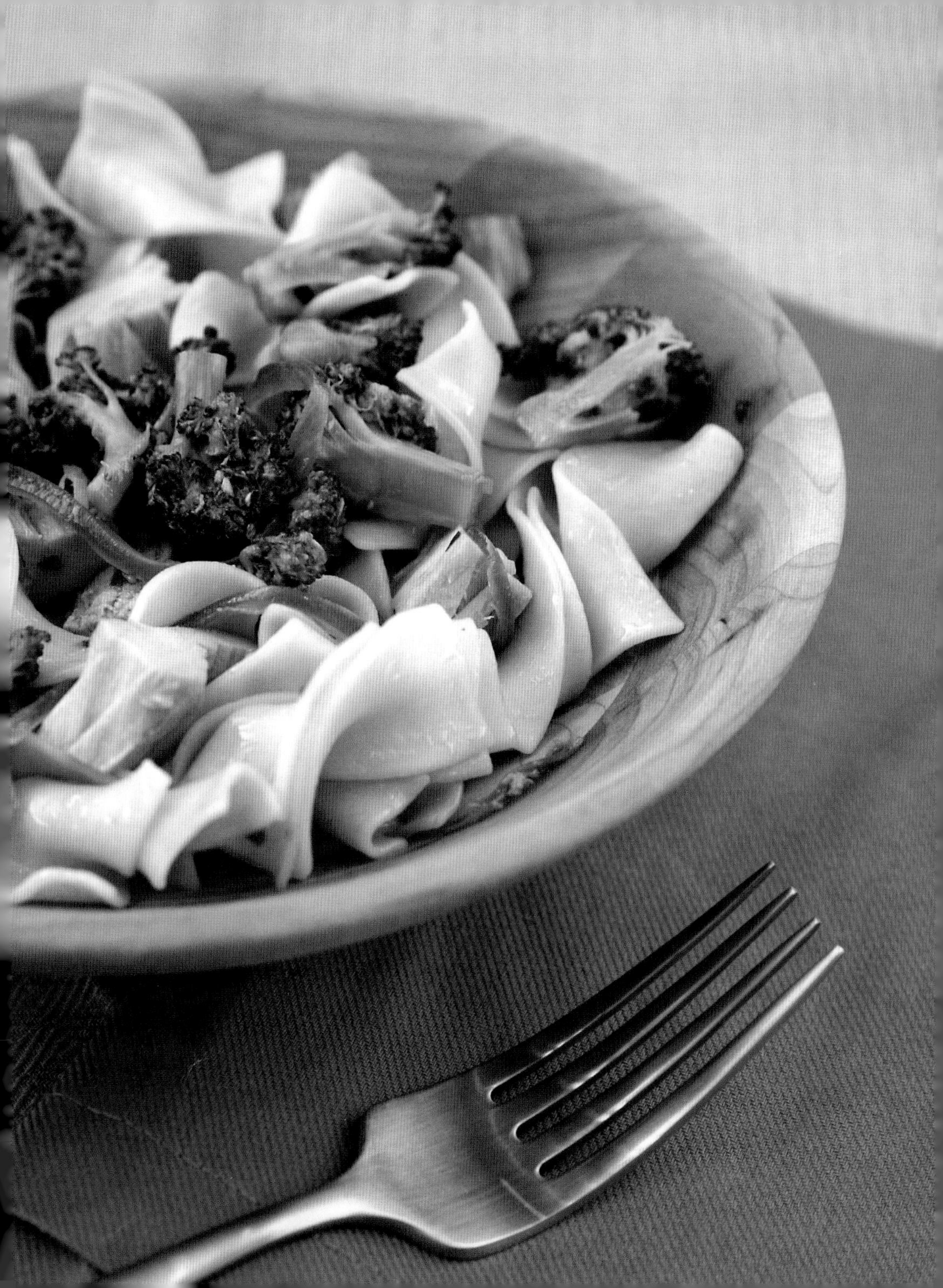

SERVINGS> 2
TIME> 10 minutes

Chicken Pasta Salad

This salad goes together quickly if you keep pre-portioned bags of cooked pasta in your fridge. If you're using gluten-free pasta, check the carb content and make sure you're getting enough.

- COOKED 2 cups cooked elbow pasta
- COOKED ½ cup cooked diced chicken
- ½ cup cherry tomatoes, cut in half, or ½ cup diced tomato
- handful of coarsely chopped fresh parsley
- 2 tablespoons olive oil
- juice of ½ a lemon
- 2 cups mixed salad greens
- grated parmesan

OPTIONAL ADDITIONS

- ¼ cup raisins
- ¼ cup toasted nuts (walnuts, pecans, or almonds)

1. Combine all ingredients except salad greens in a large bowl, adding salt and pepper to taste. Add greens and optional additions, if using; toss.

Top with grated parmesan and freshly ground salt and pepper.

PER SERVING> **Energy** 441 cal • **Fat** 17 g • **Sodium** 678 mg • **Carbs** 50 g • **Fiber** 5 g • **Protein** 24 g
Nutrition for optional additions can be found in Appendix A.

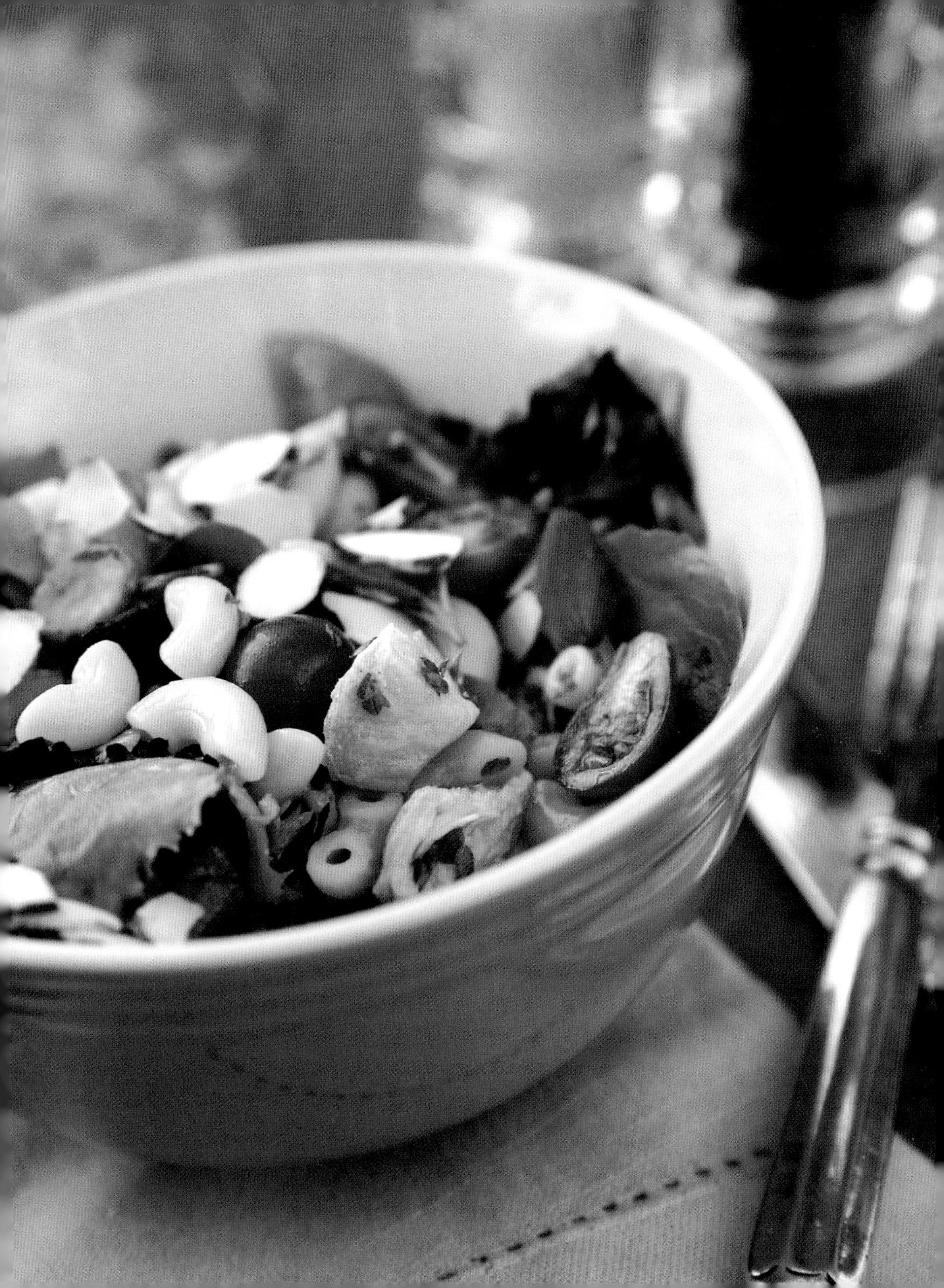

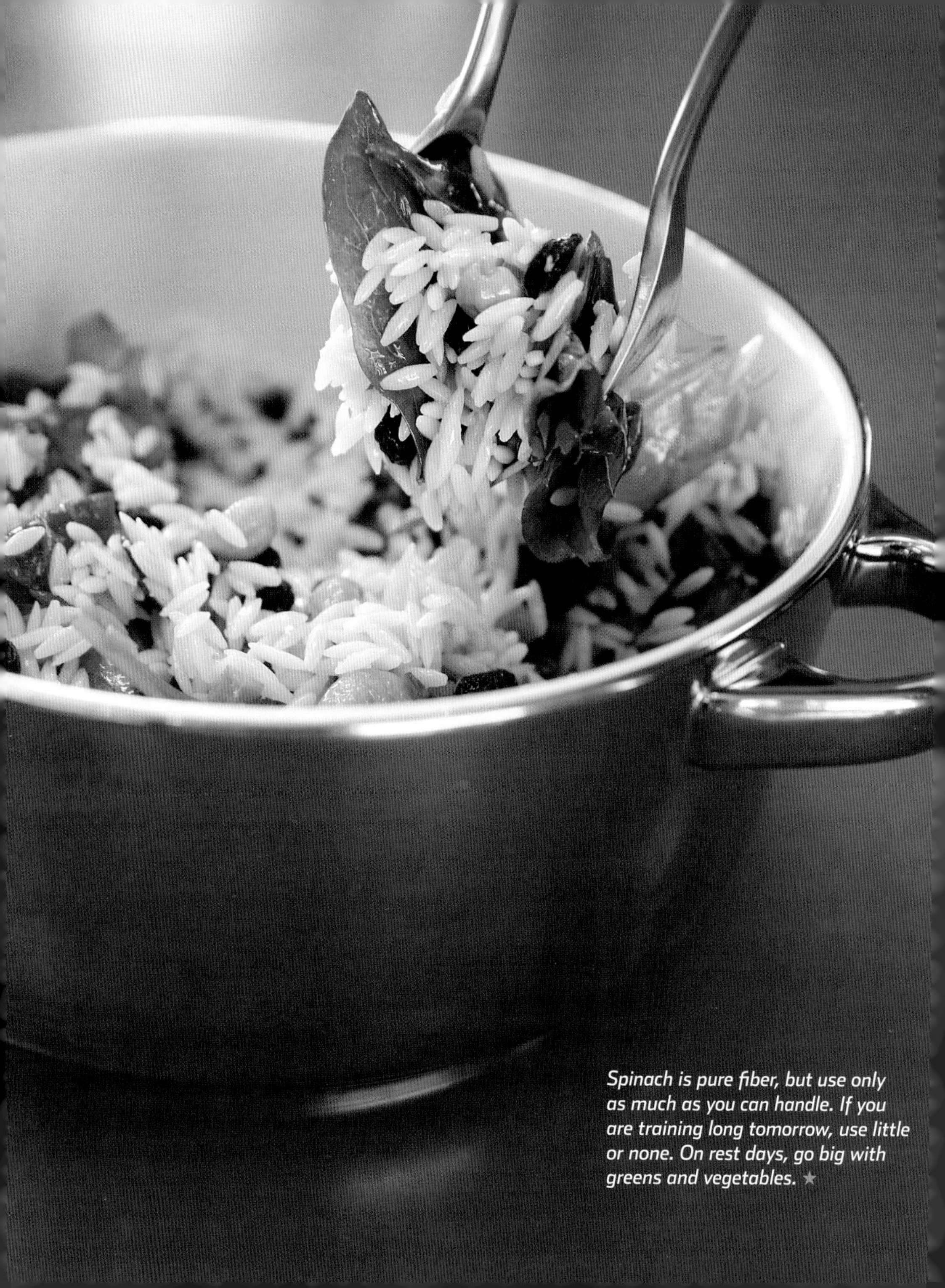

Spinach is pure fiber, but use only as much as you can handle. If you are training long tomorrow, use little or none. On rest days, go big with greens and vegetables. ★

SERVINGS› 4
TIME› 10 minutes

Orzo and Basil Salad

Orzo is one of our favorite pastas to store in the fridge for an "emergency" meal. Because of its compact size, orzo cooks fast and mixes well with smaller ingredients like the cashews and raisins in this recipe.

- COOKED 3 cups cooked orzo
- COOKED ½ cup cooked kidney beans, drained
- ¼ cup cashews or pine nuts
- ¼ cup raisins
- 2 tablespoons olive oil
- 4–5 fresh whole basil leaves

OPTIONAL ADDITIONS
(¼ cup of each or all)

- fresh spinach leaves
- crumbled feta cheese
- plain yogurt
- chopped carrot, apple, or bell pepper

1. Combine cooked orzo with other ingredients, including any desired optional additions, in a big bowl. Add salt and fresh lemon juice to taste.

PER SERVING› **Energy** 251 cal • **Fat** 12 g • **Sodium** 190 mg • **Carbs** 63 g • **Fiber** 3 g • **Protein** 12 g
Nutrition for optional additions can be found in Appendix A.

SERVINGS› 2
TIME› 5–15 minutes

Pasta Salad with Walnuts and Blue Cheese

Start with chilled cooked pasta, and this salad can come together in under five minutes. It makes a great entrée with the addition of cooked meat or grilled vegetables.

- 2 tablespoons olive oil
- ¼ cup chopped walnuts
- 2 tablespoons chopped fresh parsley
- 1 tablespoon coarse-ground prepared mustard
- 1 tablespoon crumbled blue cheese
- COOKED 3 cups cooked fettucini
- 2 cups mixed baby greens
- fresh lemon juice

OPTIONAL ADDITIONS

- roasted chicken
- grilled vegetables
- fresh basil

1. In a large bowl, combine olive oil, walnuts, parsley, mustard, and blue cheese. Fold in chilled pasta, along with any optional ingredients.

Serve greens with pasta on top. Add lemon juice and salt to taste.

TIP Toasting the walnuts makes this salad more flavorful and takes only a few extra minutes. You can do this in a small dry pan or in a 350-degree oven. Watch them closely so they do not burn!

PER SERVING› **Energy** 660 cal • **Fat** 28 g • **Sodium** 503 mg • **Carbs** 89 g • **Fiber** 6 g • **Protein** 20 g
Nutrition for optional additions can be found in Appendix A.

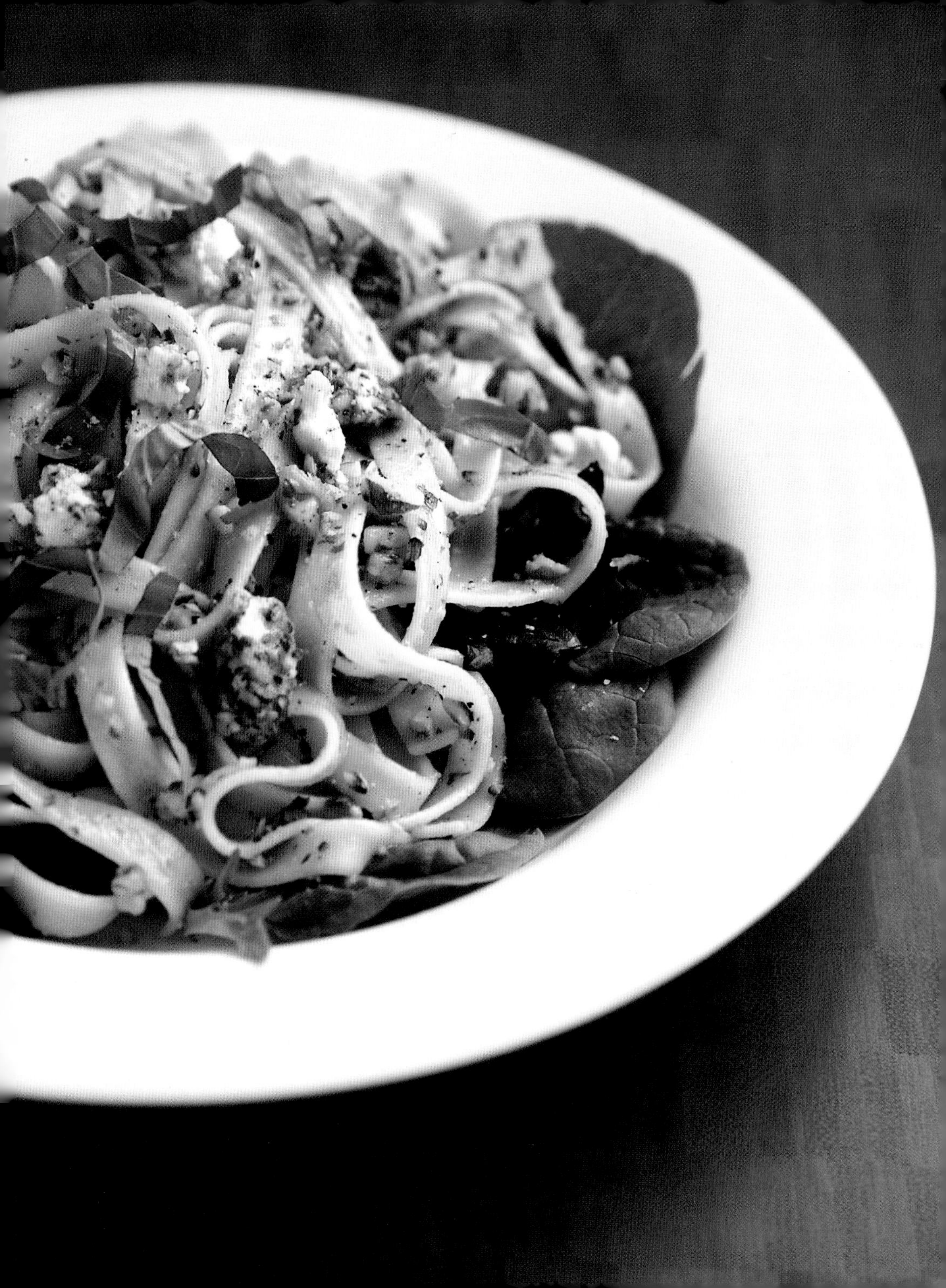

SERVINGS› 4
TIME› 20 minutes

Orange Chicken

The marmalade in this dish makes it delightfully sweet. Sugary sauces like this one are best after training rather than at dinner. Though it might take a few extra minutes, you'll find this version of orange chicken surprisingly simple.

2 cups uncooked calrose or medium-grain rice

1½ cups water

1 pound boneless, skinless chicken, cut into bite-size pieces

1 cup rice flour

½ cup red cabbage

¼ cup red onion, thinly sliced

1 jalapeno, thinly sliced

DRESSING

¼ cup orange marmalade

1 tablespoon soy sauce

1 teaspoon chili sauce (or to taste)

1. Combine rice and water in a rice cooker.
2. While rice is cooking, dust chicken pieces with rice flour in a bowl or large ziplock bag.
3. In a lightly oiled medium sauté pan, cook the chicken until lightly browned, about 5 minutes.
4. Add cabbage, onion, and jalapeno and sauté until all are softened, about 3–5 minutes. Remove pan from heat.
5. To make the dressing: In a small bowl, whisk together orange marmalade, soy sauce, and chili sauce.

Pour dressing over chicken and vegetable mixture and stir well to incorporate. Add salt and pepper to taste. Serve over rice.

PER SERVING› **Energy** 707 cal • **Fat** 17 g • **Sodium** 378 mg • **Carbs** 107 g • **Fiber** 7 g • **Protein** 32 g

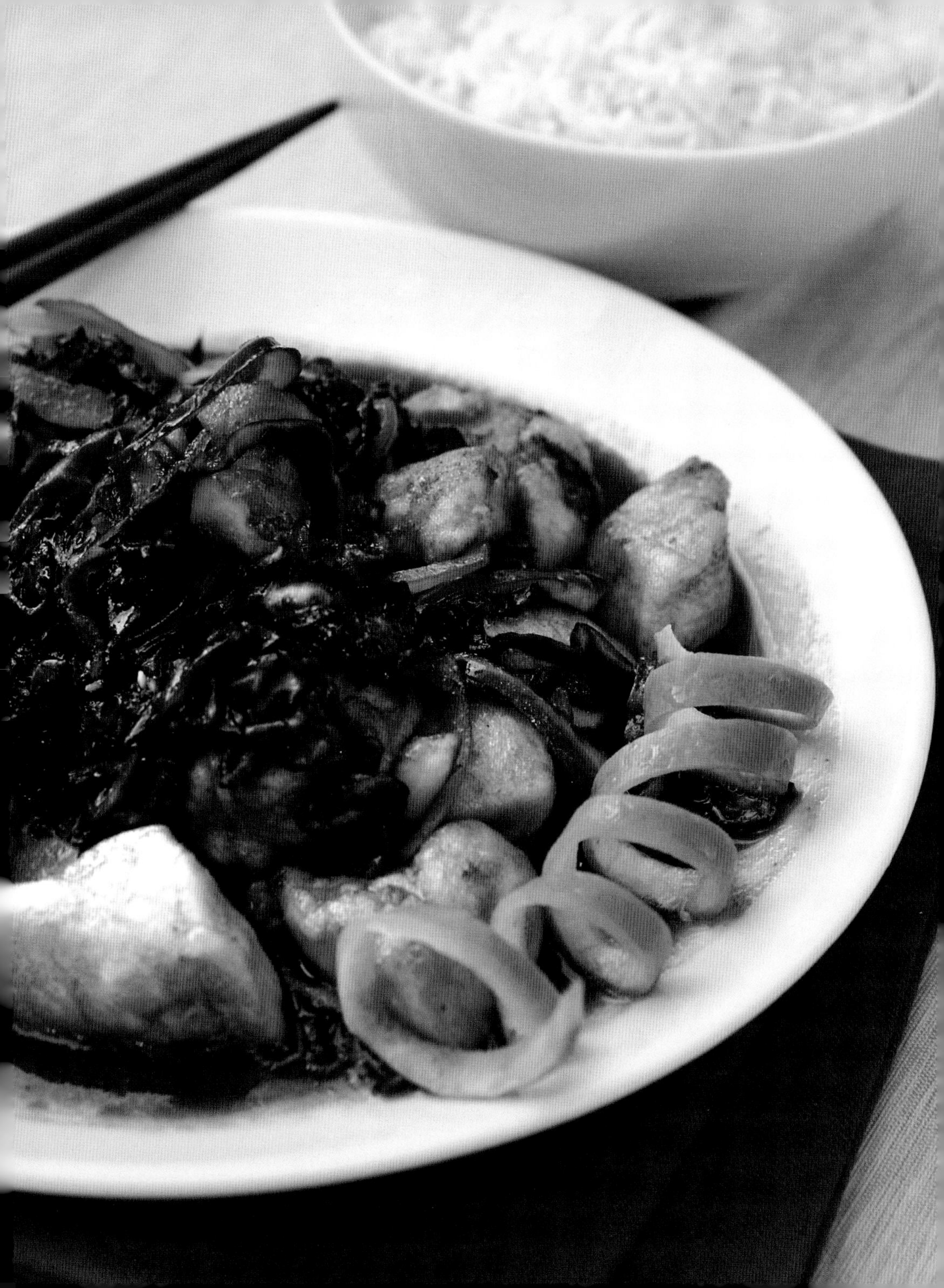

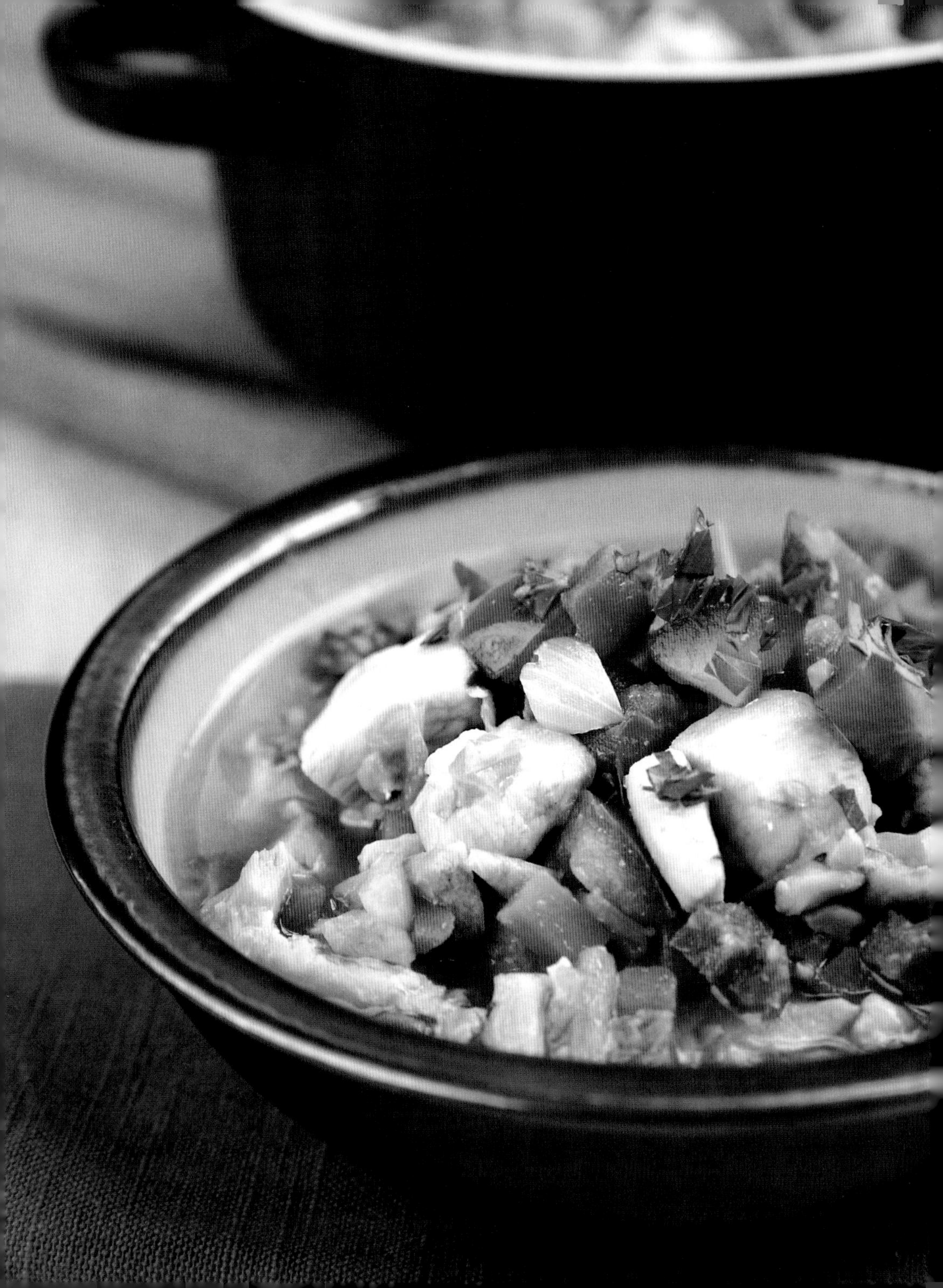

SERVINGS› 4
TIME› 1 hour

Spanish Chicken and Tomato Stew

Make this simple stew before your ride so that you can enjoy it afterward. The recipe calls for boneless and skinless chicken, but you can use bone-in meat.

1 tablespoon olive oil

2 pounds boneless, skinless chicken thighs, cut into cubes

1 cup chorizo or Italian sausage

1 cup carrots, chopped

1 cup tomatoes, diced

1 onion, chopped

2 mild green chile peppers, chopped, seeds left in

2–4 cups chicken stock or water (see note)

OPTIONAL ADDITIONS

½ cup apple cider vinegar

1 tablespoon brown sugar

1 cup cooked white beans, rinsed

1. Pour olive oil into a heavy pot and set over medium-high heat. While oil is heating, sprinkle salt and pepper over chicken.
2. Add sausage to pot and brown thoroughly. Add chicken and cook about 5–6 minutes, until browned.
3. Add vegetables and 2 cups chicken stock (including any desired optional ingredients), cover pot with lid, and bring to a rolling boil. Reduce heat to medium and let simmer for 45 minutes. Add salt and pepper to taste.

Add canned beans, if using, just before serving and garnish with parsley. Serve with warm polenta or steamed rice.

NOTE› To prepare in a slow cooker, first cook the meat as instructed in steps 1 and 2, but simply sear the meat until it is lightly browned on each side. The meat will not be cooked through. Transfer the meat and all of the ingredients, along with an additional 2 cups of chicken stock, to the slow cooker and cook on low for 3 to 4 hours.

PER SERVING› Energy 543 cal • Fat 31 g • Sodium 226 mg • Carbs 10 g • Fiber 2 g • Protein 53 g

Nutrition for optional additions can be found in Appendix A.

SERVINGS› 4
TIME› 1 hour

Dry-Spiced Chicken and Figs

The sugar of the figs and hints of cinnamon, cumin, nutmeg, and coriander make for a rich stew that restores the body after a tough training session. The hearty flavors are most suitable for fall or winter, atop a pile of wide noodles or steamed rice.

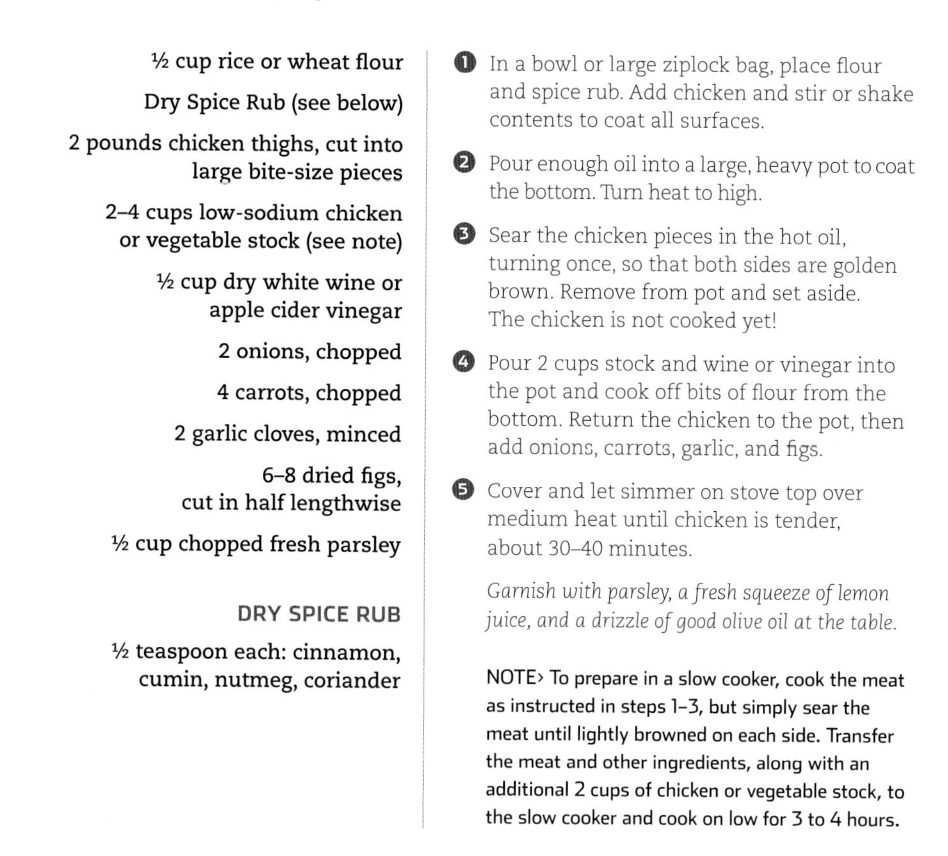

- ½ cup rice or wheat flour
- Dry Spice Rub (see below)
- 2 pounds chicken thighs, cut into large bite-size pieces
- 2–4 cups low-sodium chicken or vegetable stock (see note)
- ½ cup dry white wine or apple cider vinegar
- 2 onions, chopped
- 4 carrots, chopped
- 2 garlic cloves, minced
- 6–8 dried figs, cut in half lengthwise
- ½ cup chopped fresh parsley

DRY SPICE RUB

- ½ teaspoon each: cinnamon, cumin, nutmeg, coriander

1. In a bowl or large ziplock bag, place flour and spice rub. Add chicken and stir or shake contents to coat all surfaces.
2. Pour enough oil into a large, heavy pot to coat the bottom. Turn heat to high.
3. Sear the chicken pieces in the hot oil, turning once, so that both sides are golden brown. Remove from pot and set aside. The chicken is not cooked yet!
4. Pour 2 cups stock and wine or vinegar into the pot and cook off bits of flour from the bottom. Return the chicken to the pot, then add onions, carrots, garlic, and figs.
5. Cover and let simmer on stove top over medium heat until chicken is tender, about 30–40 minutes.

Garnish with parsley, a fresh squeeze of lemon juice, and a drizzle of good olive oil at the table.

NOTE› To prepare in a slow cooker, cook the meat as instructed in steps 1–3, but simply sear the meat until lightly browned on each side. Transfer the meat and other ingredients, along with an additional 2 cups of chicken or vegetable stock, to the slow cooker and cook on low for 3 to 4 hours.

PER SERVING› **Energy** 676 cal • **Fat** 28 g • **Sodium** 471 mg • **Carbs** 53 g • **Fiber** 9 g • **Protein** 50 g

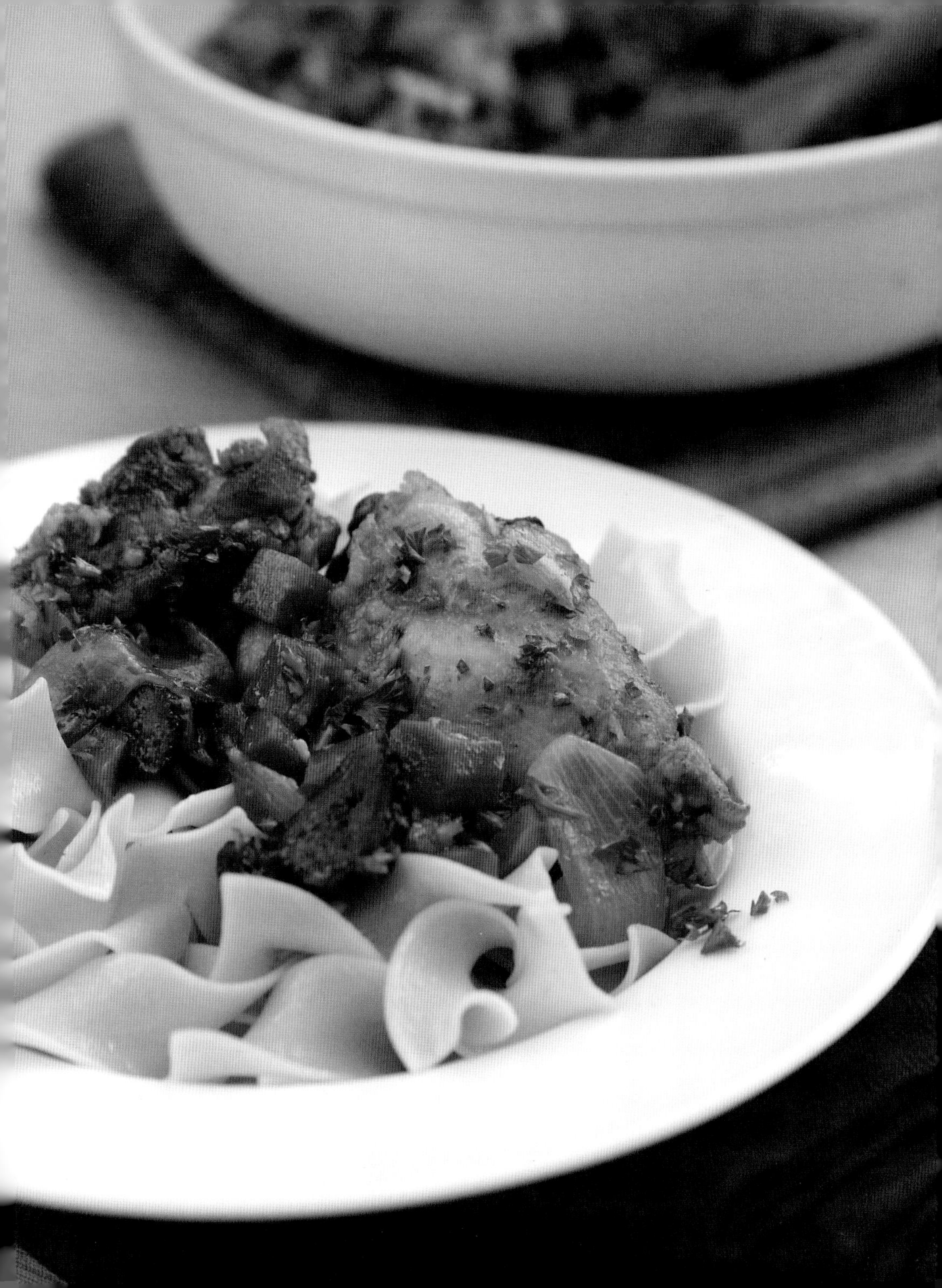

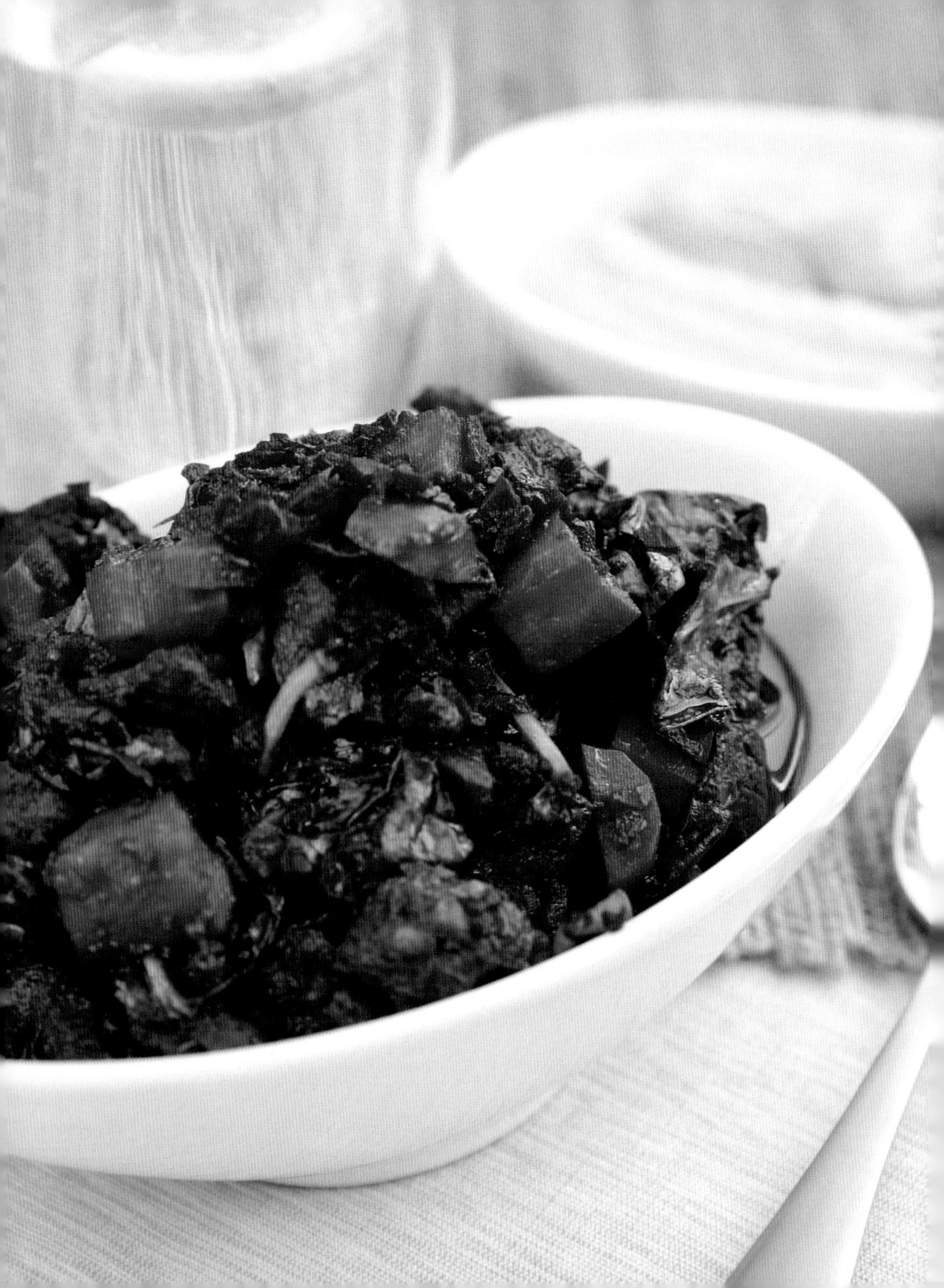

SERVINGS› 6
TIME› 15 minutes prep, cook 2 hours

Braised Beef and Vegetable Stew

This is a basic stew recipe adapted to make use of the veggie pulp that we generate when we serve up lots of beet juice. If you don't have veggie pulp on hand you can simply add some potatoes. In fact, any assortment of chopped vegetables or fresh herbs will do just fine.

STEW BASE

2 pounds stewing beef (such as chuck), cut into bite-size pieces

1 cup water

1 cup stock (see note)

½ cup red wine

¼ cup low-sodium soy sauce

¼ cup apple cider vinegar

1 teaspoon each coarse salt and black pepper

1 tablespoon brown sugar

½ cup carrots, chopped

½ of a small onion, chopped

2 cups chopped spinach

1 cup veggie pulp (from juicer)

COOKED 1 cup cooked red kidney beans (if using canned, add after meat is fully cooked)

1. Heat oven to 325 degrees.
2. Combine all stew base ingredients in a heavy covered pot. Cook in oven for 1 hour.
3. Add all vegetables, pulp, and beans to meat and stew base. Add more water or stock if needed to completely cover the beef and vegetables.
4. Return pot to oven and cook 1 hour. Check for tenderness. Adjust seasonings to taste.

This dish goes great with polenta, grilled breads, or rice.

NOTE› To prepare in a slow cooker, increase liquids to 2 cups stock and 2 cups water. Cook the meat and stew base on high for 1 hour. Add the vegetables, stirring to combine, and add water and stock to cover the beef and vegetables completely. Let simmer on low for 4–6 hours.

TIP Old Bay seasoning, a favorite of Biju's, can take a pot of beef stew to another level. Be sure to try your favorite seasoning or spice mix.

PER SERVING› Energy 404 cal • Fat 17 g • Sodium 936 mg • Carbs 12 g • Fiber 3 g • Protein 44 g

SERVINGS› 4
TIME› 15 minutes prep,
cook 2 hours

White Beans and Chicken

Here's an easy dish to put together before you head out on cold days. It will keep in the refrigerator for up to a week. You can use any cut of chicken. Dry beans soaked overnight are best, but canned will do. Just add them at the end after the chicken has cooked.

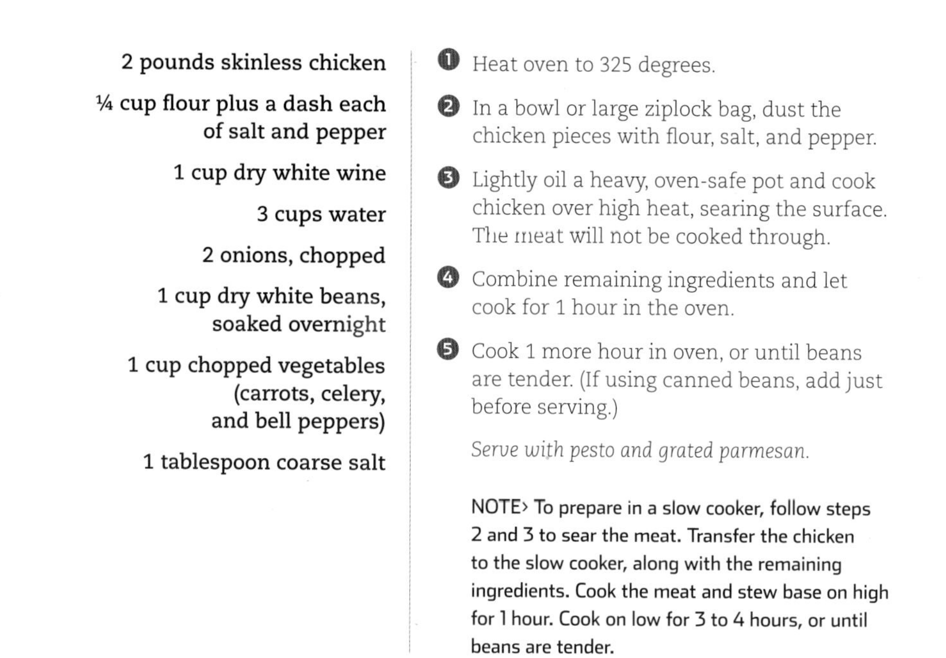

- 2 pounds skinless chicken
- ¼ cup flour plus a dash each of salt and pepper
- 1 cup dry white wine
- 3 cups water
- 2 onions, chopped
- 1 cup dry white beans, soaked overnight
- 1 cup chopped vegetables (carrots, celery, and bell peppers)
- 1 tablespoon coarse salt

1. Heat oven to 325 degrees.
2. In a bowl or large ziplock bag, dust the chicken pieces with flour, salt, and pepper.
3. Lightly oil a heavy, oven-safe pot and cook chicken over high heat, searing the surface. The meat will not be cooked through.
4. Combine remaining ingredients and let cook for 1 hour in the oven.
5. Cook 1 more hour in oven, or until beans are tender. (If using canned beans, add just before serving.)

Serve with pesto and grated parmesan.

NOTE› To prepare in a slow cooker, follow steps 2 and 3 to sear the meat. Transfer the chicken to the slow cooker, along with the remaining ingredients. Cook the meat and stew base on high for 1 hour. Cook on low for 3 to 4 hours, or until beans are tender.

PER SERVING› **Energy** 425 cal • **Fat** 4 g • **Sodium** 1,750 mg • **Carbs** 38 g • **Fiber** 7 g • **Protein** 39 g

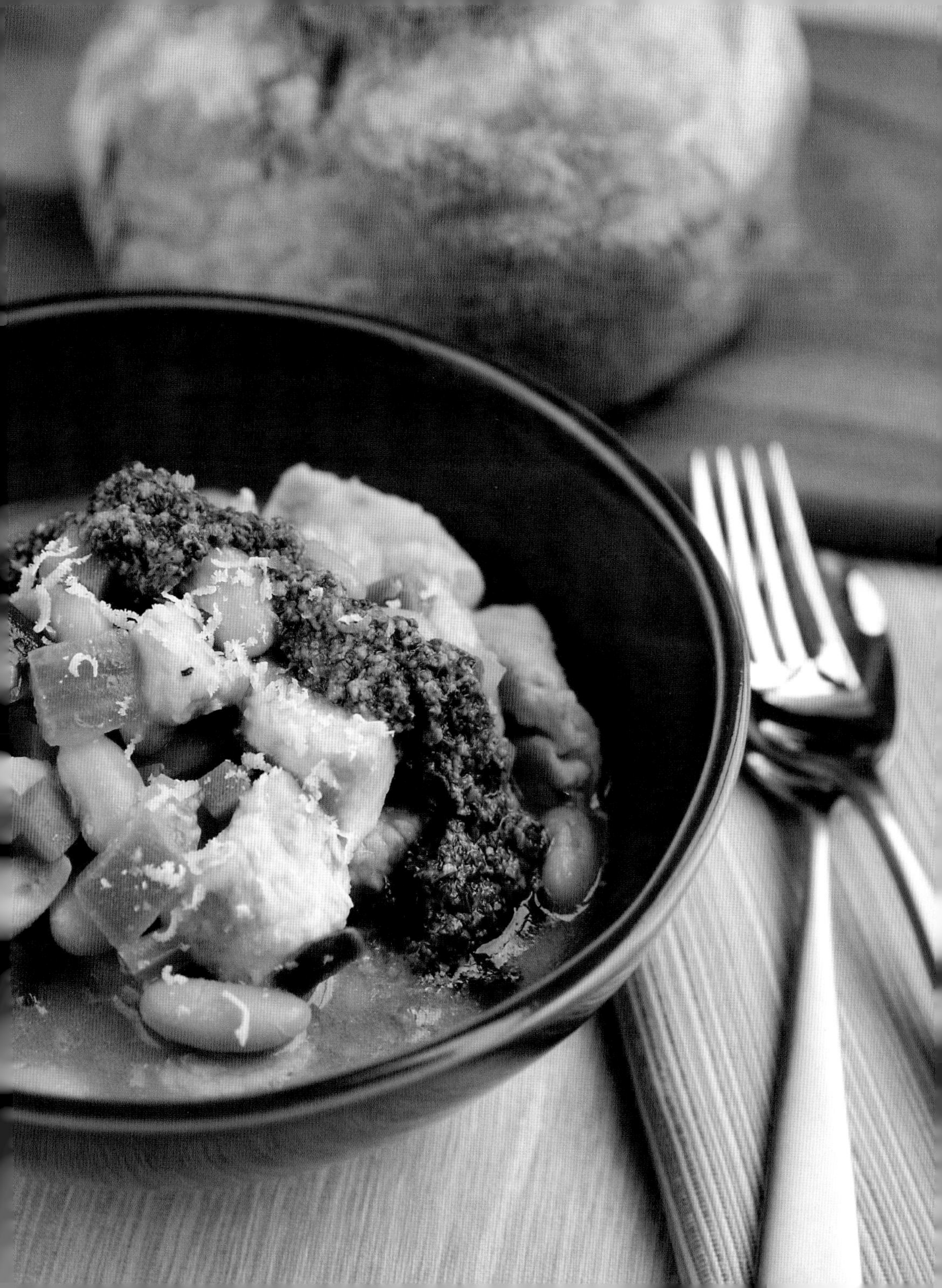

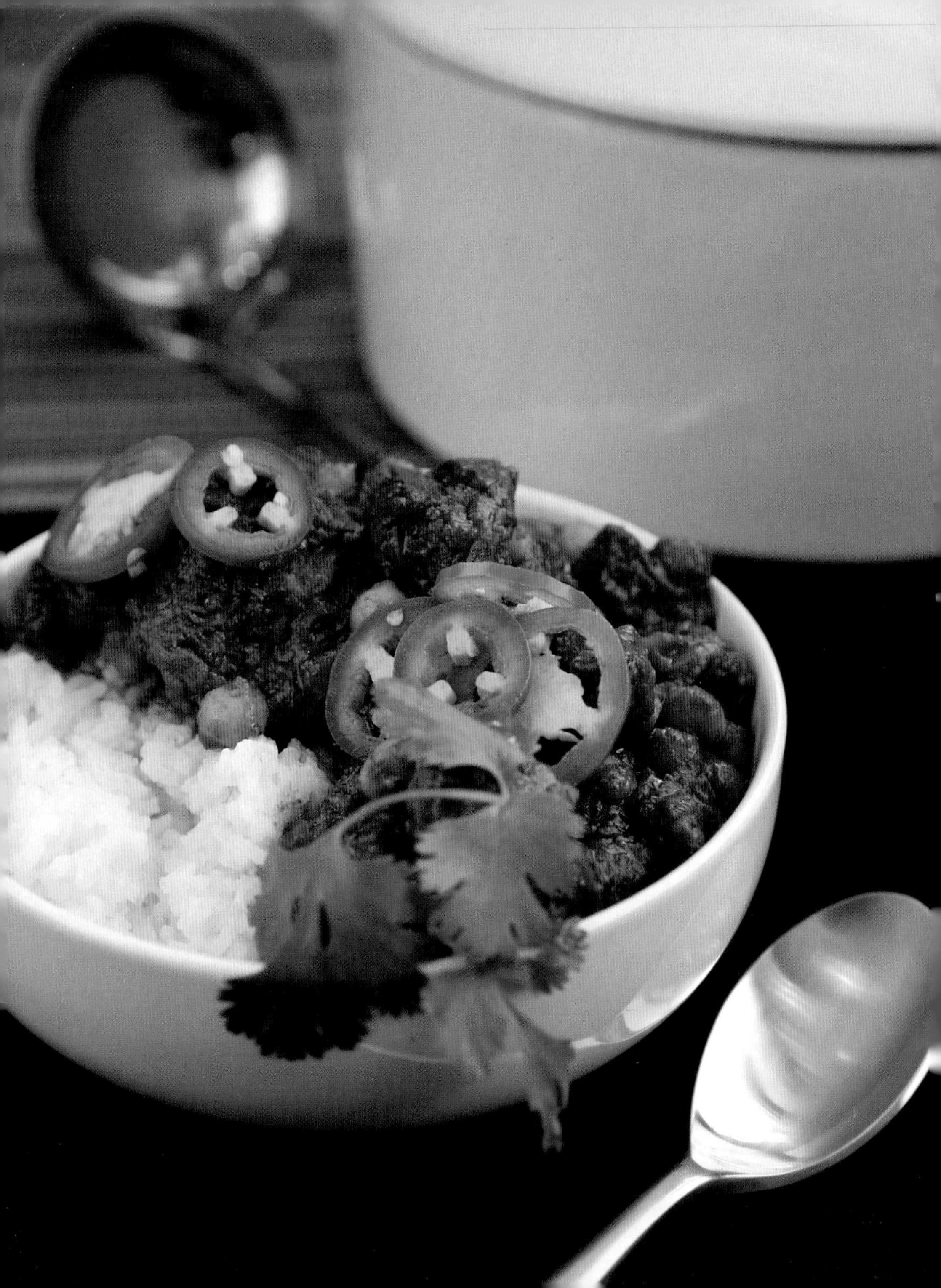

SERVINGS› 4
TIME› 15 minutes prep, cook 2 hours

Lamb and Chickpea Stew

This hearty stew is best for a post-ride dinner or on a rest day. Start the chickpeas (garbanzo beans) the night before, or use canned chickpeas. The stew can be finished on the stove top, in a crockpot, or in the oven and keeps in the fridge for up to a week.

olive oil or vegetable oil

2 pounds lamb, cut into cubes

2 onions, chopped

2–4 tablespoons curry powder (optional)

½ cup (small can) tomato paste

½ cup apple cider vinegar

3–6 cups water (see note)

2 cups dried chickpeas, rinsed and soaked in fridge overnight

2 garlic cloves, chopped (optional)

1. In large oven-safe pot, bring a few tablespoons of oil to a high heat, and then add lamb. Cook, turning to brown all sides. Add onions and stir for a few minutes until starting to soften.
2. Stir in curry powder, tomato paste, vinegar, and enough water to come just below the top of the lamb. Add soaked beans and garlic, if using. (If adding canned beans, wait until the meat has cooked and is tender.)
3. Stir well to combine. Cook on stove at a medium heat for roughly 2 hours or put in crockpot for about 4–5 hours. Check halfway; may need to stir or add additional water if lamb is looking dry. The stew is done when lamb is fork-tender.
4. Add salt and pepper to taste, and canned beans if using.

Garnish with chopped fresh green chiles and cilantro. Serve over steamed rice.

NOTE› If using canned beans, reduce water to 3 cups and add beans after stew is cooked.

PER SERVING› **Energy** 750 cal • **Fat** 35 g • **Sodium** 768 mg • **Carbs** 36 g • **Fiber** 10 g • **Protein** 71 g

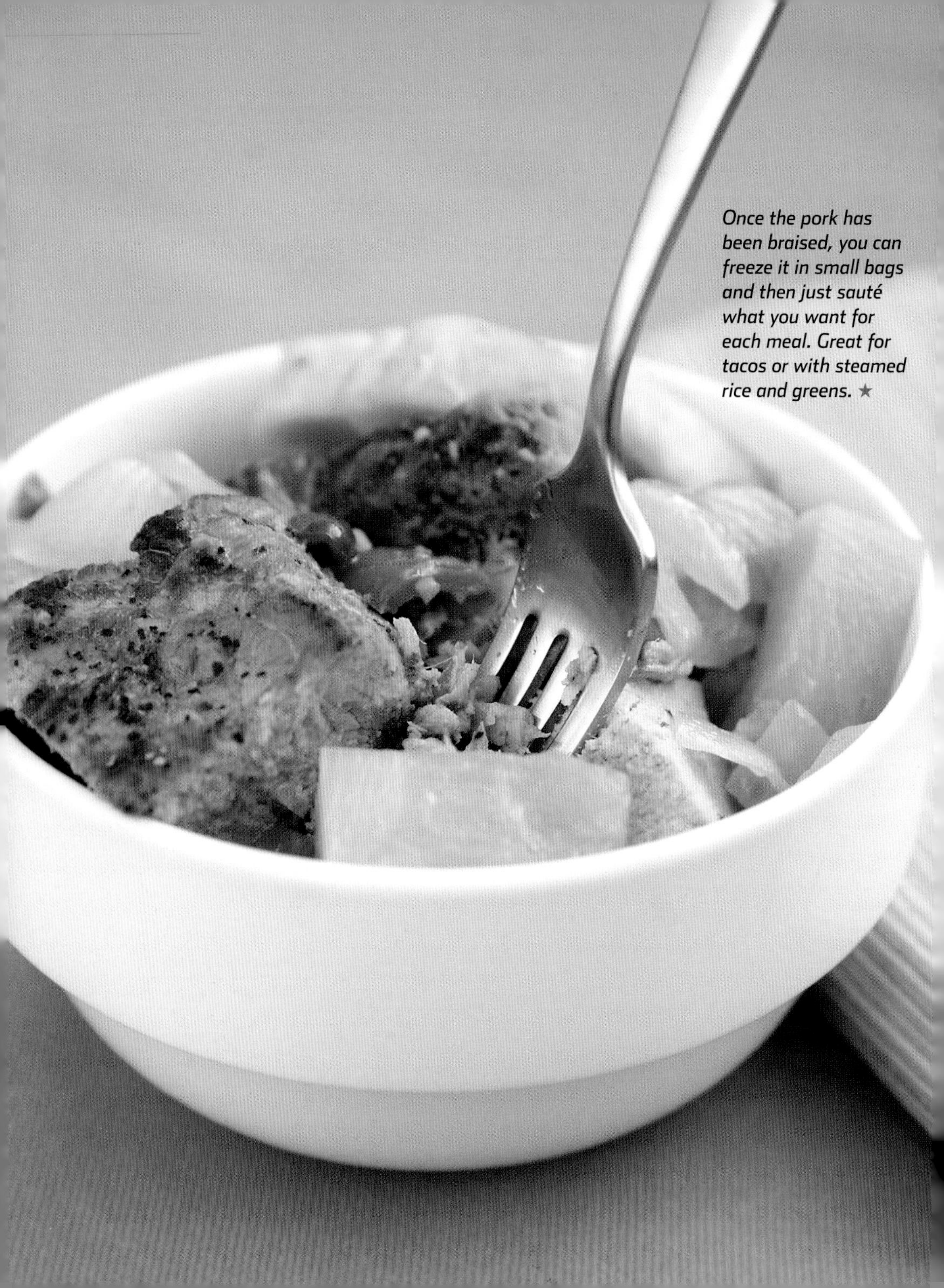

Once the pork has been braised, you can freeze it in small bags and then just sauté what you want for each meal. Great for tacos or with steamed rice and greens. ★

SERVINGS› 10
TIME› 20 minutes prep,
cook 2 hours

Fruit-Braised Pork

Here's a take on one of our all-time favorite things to make—you and your friends will love it. This is best as a post-ride or rest-day meal. The tropical fruits make the meat very tender and super easy to digest after a hard effort. The dry rub used on the pork is high in sodium, but timed right it will readily replace what you've lost in training.

4–6 pounds pork loin

1–2 cups fresh pineapple

2–3 medium onions, peeled, cut into large chunks

4 jalapenos, seeded and cut into chunks

1–2 cups apple and/or pineapple juice

1–2 cups white wine or light beer (see note)

DRY RUB

2 cups kosher salt

½ cup coarse raw sugar or brown sugar

¼ cup coarsely ground black pepper

1 tablespoon each: ground cinnamon, chili powder, and celery salt

1. Heat oven to 325 degrees.
2. To make the dry rub: Combine all ingredients in a bowl and mix thoroughly. Measure ½ cup and set aside. (Use leftover rub for any meats; it will keep in cupboard for several weeks.)
3. Cut pork into 3–4 large chunks and thoroughly coat with ½ cup of the dry rub. Bring a heavy, deep oven-safe pot to high heat on stove top. Add pork, and sear on all sides.
4. Add pineapple, onions, and jalapenos, stirring to combine.
5. Add fruit juice and beer or wine in equal parts until liquid covers the mixture completely. Cover tightly with lid or foil and transfer pot to the oven. Cook 2 hours.
6. Remove from oven, let cool, then cut pork into small pieces. Bag and store.

When ready to eat, sauté the braised pork in a hot pan with some fresh sliced onions if you like.

NOTE› In place of wine or beer, you may substitute 1½ cups chicken or vegetable stock and ½ cup vinegar.

PER SERVING› Energy 532 cal • Fat 27 g • Sodium 58 mg • Carbs 17 g • Fiber 1 g • Protein 49 g
SPICE RUB (½ cup)› Energy 40 cal • Fat 0 g • Sodium 1,000 mg • Carbs 12 g • Fiber 0 g • Protein 0 g
Nutritionals based on 4 pounds pork loin, 1½ cups pineapple, and 1 cup wine.

★★★

These meals are designed to be healthy, beautiful, and part of an experience, so they take a little more time and attention than some of our other menus and are meant to be shared with others. That said, we realize that sometimes dinner does need to accommodate our busy schedules, so we've also included a **handheld section** here.

The **bowls** are primarily nutrient-dense soups, a world away from the carbohydrate-packed sweet breakfast bowls. The **small plates** are primarily salads that you can eat before or after the main course or as a stand-alone meal if you're trying to watch your weight. Dinner's **big plates** are protein dishes that are meant to be served with carbohydrates. (See recipes for rice, pasta, couscous, quinoa, polenta, or potatoes in Basics.)

For an athlete, however, **dinner is also the one meal where being careful about portion size is critical.** We don't recommend that athletes skimp on what they eat before, during, or after training. So while we've designed these recipes as our largest and sometimes richest meals, this is the one place where you might have to occasionally pull the throttle back. Nonetheless, there's a lot to be enjoyed.

DINNER

BOWLS

SMALL PLATES

HANDHELDS

BIG PLATES

V **VEGETARIAN**
G **GLUTEN-FREE**

SERVINGS› 4
TIME› 20 minutes

Pasta and Herb Soup

I like soup any time of the year. It's easy to make and easy to digest, and soup's liquid form means that nutrients are easily absorbed—which becomes more important as you get further into your season.

½ onion, diced

1 tomato, chopped

4 cups chicken or vegetable stock

4 ounces uncooked small pasta

1 cup cut vegetables: carrots, peas, corn (frozen will work fine)

2–3 ounces shaved ham or prosciutto

1. In a large stock pot heat 1 tablespoon of olive oil to medium-high. Add the onions. Sauté until onions begin to sweat, 3–5 minutes.
2. Lower the heat, then add the tomato and stock. Bring to a low boil.
3. Add the pasta to the pot and stir. Check the pasta often; when it seems halfway cooked, add the cut vegetables. Add more water or stock if you like your soup thinner.
4. Bring the soup to a simmer and let the pasta cook to al dente. Turn off heat; add salt and pepper to taste.

Ladle soup into bowls and garnish with diced ham or prosciutto, along with grated parmesan, fresh herbs, and a splash of olive oil. Serve with chunks of crusty bread.

TIP Make sure to turn heat off before the pasta is cooked through, or the pasta will be mushy. Really small shapes of pasta, such as orzo and acini de pepe, take only a few minutes to fully cook.

PER SERVING› **Energy** 398 cal • **Fat** 12 g • **Sodium** 1,334 mg • **Carbs** 53 g • **Fiber** 7 g • **Protein** 21 g

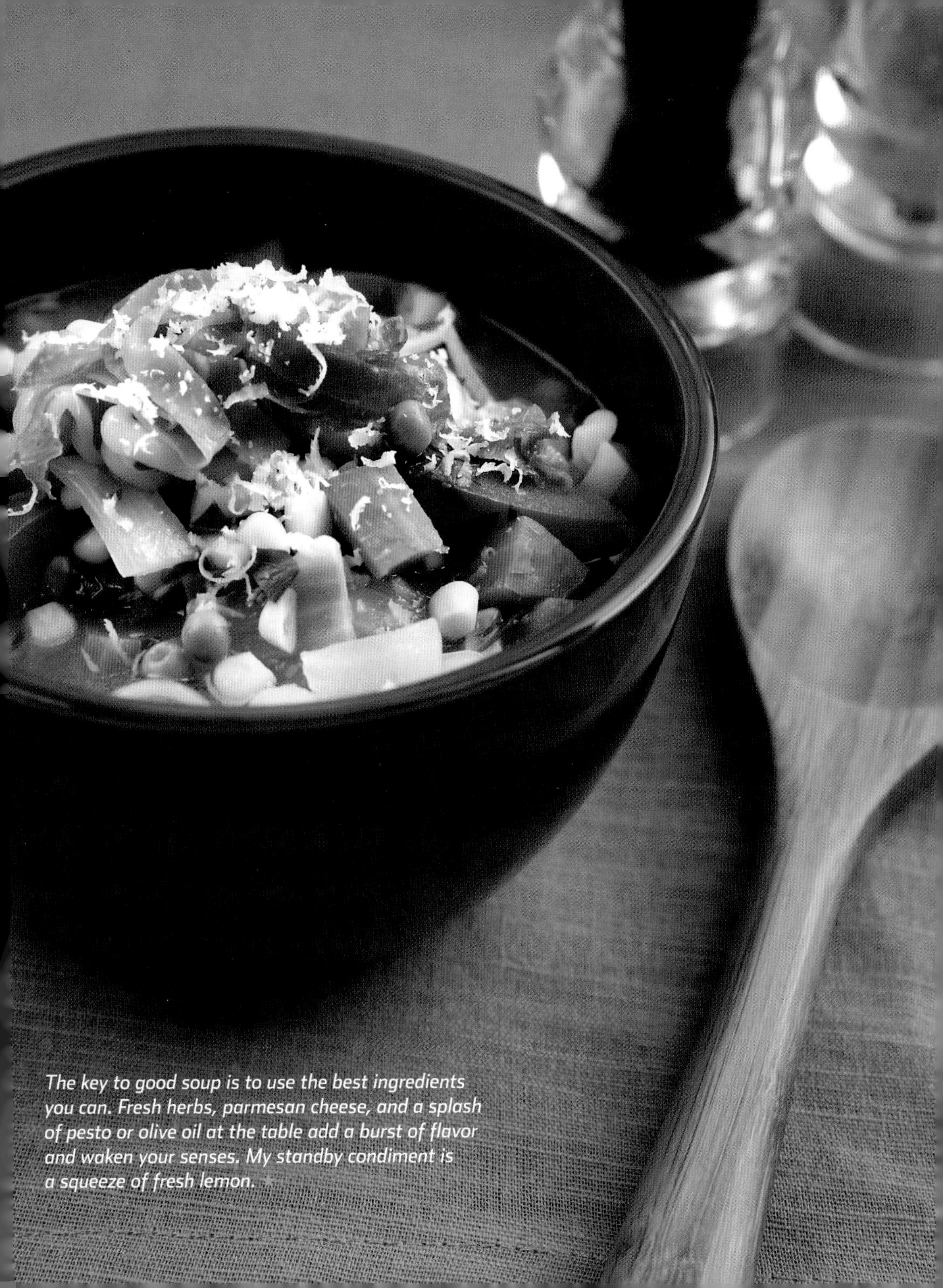

The key to good soup is to use the best ingredients you can. Fresh herbs, parmesan cheese, and a splash of pesto or olive oil at the table add a burst of flavor and waken your senses. My standby condiment is a squeeze of fresh lemon.

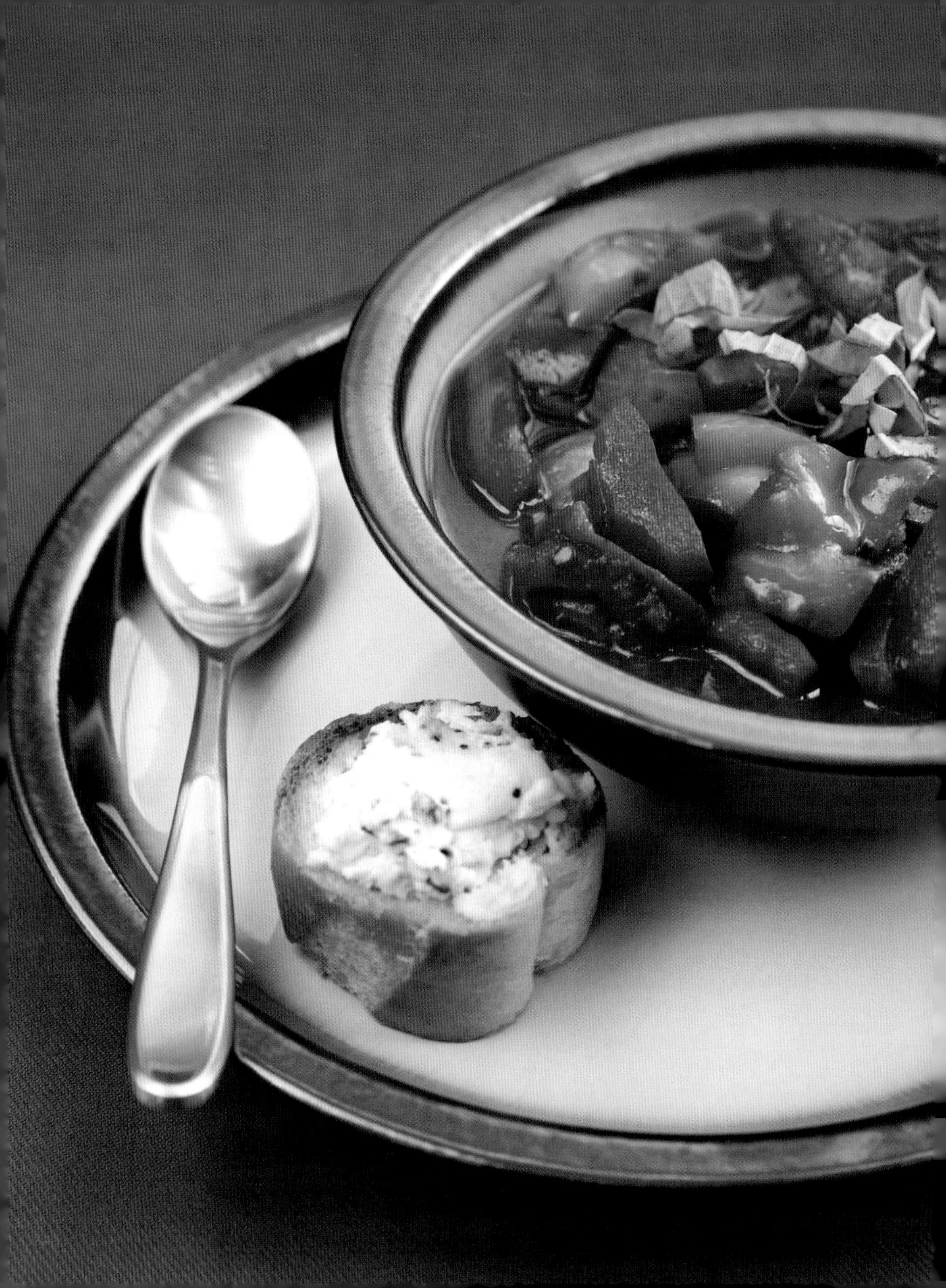

SERVINGS› 6
TIME› 45 minutes

Rustic Pepper and Tomato Soup

Our tasty croutons add a nice finish to this soup's complex tomato and pepper flavors. If you prefer a smooth consistency, you could opt to puree the soup in batches once it's cooked using a blender or a small food processor. Just be sure to reheat it afterward so it's good and hot when you bring it to the table.

1 cup chopped red bell peppers

1 cup chopped yellow bell peppers

1 cup chopped onions

2 cups chopped roma tomatoes

2 tablespoons brown sugar

1 teaspoon ground black pepper

¼ cup low-sodium soy sauce

1 cup red wine

1 cup water or stock (with extra to adjust for thickness)

CHEESE CROUTONS

6 thick slices of baguette (½ inch to 1 inch each)

olive oil

3 tablespoons soft goat cheese

3 tablespoons cream cheese

a few drops of truffle oil (optional)

1. In a large stock pot, add enough olive oil to cover the bottom and bring to medium-high heat.
2. Add the bell peppers and onions, and caramelize. Then add the tomatoes, brown sugar, and black pepper; sauté until the edges of the vegetables have begun to blacken.
3. Add the soy sauce, wine, and water. Turn heat down to medium and let cook for about 15 minutes, covered. Keep soup over low heat while you prepare the croutons.
4. To make the croutons: Brush baguette slices with olive oil and grill in a hot sauté pan or in the oven until brown and crusty. Blend together goat cheese, cream cheese, and a few drops of truffle oil. Spread cheese mixture onto one side of each slice of toast.

Ladle soup into bowls and place crouton on top or use for dipping. Garnish with fresh chopped parsley or basil.

PER SERVING› **Energy** 195 cal • **Fat** 9 g • **Sodium** 545 mg • **Carbs** 17 g • **Fiber** 2 g • **Protein** 6 g

Nutrition for optional addition can be found in Appendix A.

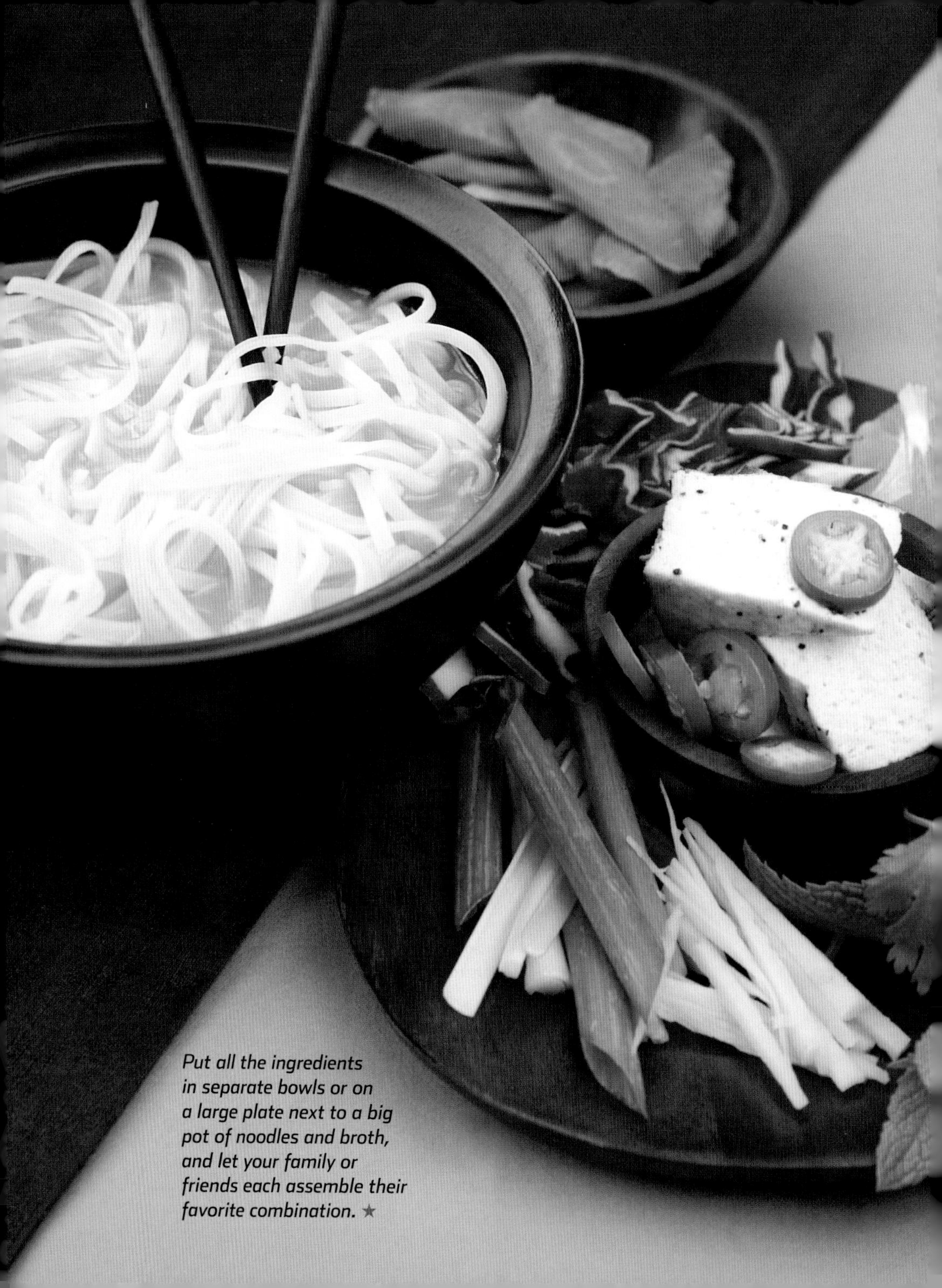

Put all the ingredients in separate bowls or on a large plate next to a big pot of noodles and broth, and let your family or friends each assemble their favorite combination. ★

SERVINGS› 4
TIME› 30 minutes

Spicy Asian Noodle Soup

This is our twist on the classic Vietnamese pho. It's traditionally made with beef bones and rice noodles, but we use readily available ingredients—things you probably have in your fridge and pantry.

8 ounces rice noodles

sesame or grapeseed oil

1 pound Italian bulk sausage (spicy or not) or 1 pound cubed firm tofu

¼ cup low-sodium soy sauce

4 cups chicken or vegetable broth

VEGETABLES/TOPPINGS

chopped green onions

chopped bell peppers

shredded or chopped carrots and/or radishes

shredded cabbage

chopped fresh ginger, garlic, and/or jalapeno

fresh mint, Thai basil leaves, and cilantro

soy sauce

Sriracha sauce

fresh limes

1. Bring a large stock pot filled with water to a boil. Cook the rice noodles as directed on the package. Drain water from noodles, tossing with a light sesame or grapeseed oil to prevent noodles from sticking. Set aside.
2. Brown the meat or tofu. Add a splash of oil once most of it is browned and then sauté until crisp. Add soy sauce and continue to mix. If using tofu, add some salt and pepper. Remove from heat.
3. While the meat or tofu is browning, bring the broth to a simmer in a large pot. Add an equal amount or more of water, depending on how strong you want the flavors to be.
4. Divide noodles among four bowls, add broth to each, and top with sausage or tofu.

Mix in the veggies and toppings as desired. Have ready bowls, chopsticks, and big spoons. Enjoy.

NOTE› If you don't separate the noodles before adding the broth, they may stick together and be harder to work with.

PER SERVING› **Energy** 419 cal • **Fat** 24 g • **Sodium** 2,139 mg • **Carbs** 25 g • **Fiber** 1 g • **Protein** 25 g

Nutrition includes Italian sausage and rice noodles. Nutrition for vegetables and toppings can be found in Appendix A.

SERVINGS› 4
TIME› 45 minutes

Red Lentil Soup

This is a super-easy way to make a last-minute soup that everyone will love. I use red lentils because they cook quickly and are available in the bulk food aisles of most natural food stores.

2 tablespoons vegetable oil

1–2 tablespoons curry powder (or substitute chili powder)

1 small onion, minced

2 cloves garlic, minced

1 tablespoon minced jalapeno

1 cup coconut milk

1 cup red lentils, rinsed

3 cups water or stock

OPTIONAL ADDITIONS

1 cup plain yogurt

¼ cup diced tomatoes

2 tablespoons chopped cilantro

1 teaspoon minced fresh ginger

1. In a large stock pot, heat oil over medium heat. Add the curry powder and toast for a few seconds, then add onion, garlic, jalapeno, and coconut milk. Stir together and let cook 5 minutes.
2. Add lentils and water or stock. Bring to a boil, then turn heat down and let simmer until lentils are tender, about 20–30 minutes.
3. If desired, add yogurt, tomatoes, cilantro, and ginger. Adjust flavor with salt.

Either serve as is, or puree in batches in a blender for a smooth consistency. The soup is fantastic with warm bread or tortillas and a little more yogurt and chopped jalapenos on top.

PER SERVING› **Energy** 360 cal • **Fat** 20 g • **Sodium** 304 mg • **Carbs** 31 g • **Fiber** 15 g • **Protein** 13 g

Nutrition for optional additions can be found in Appendix A.

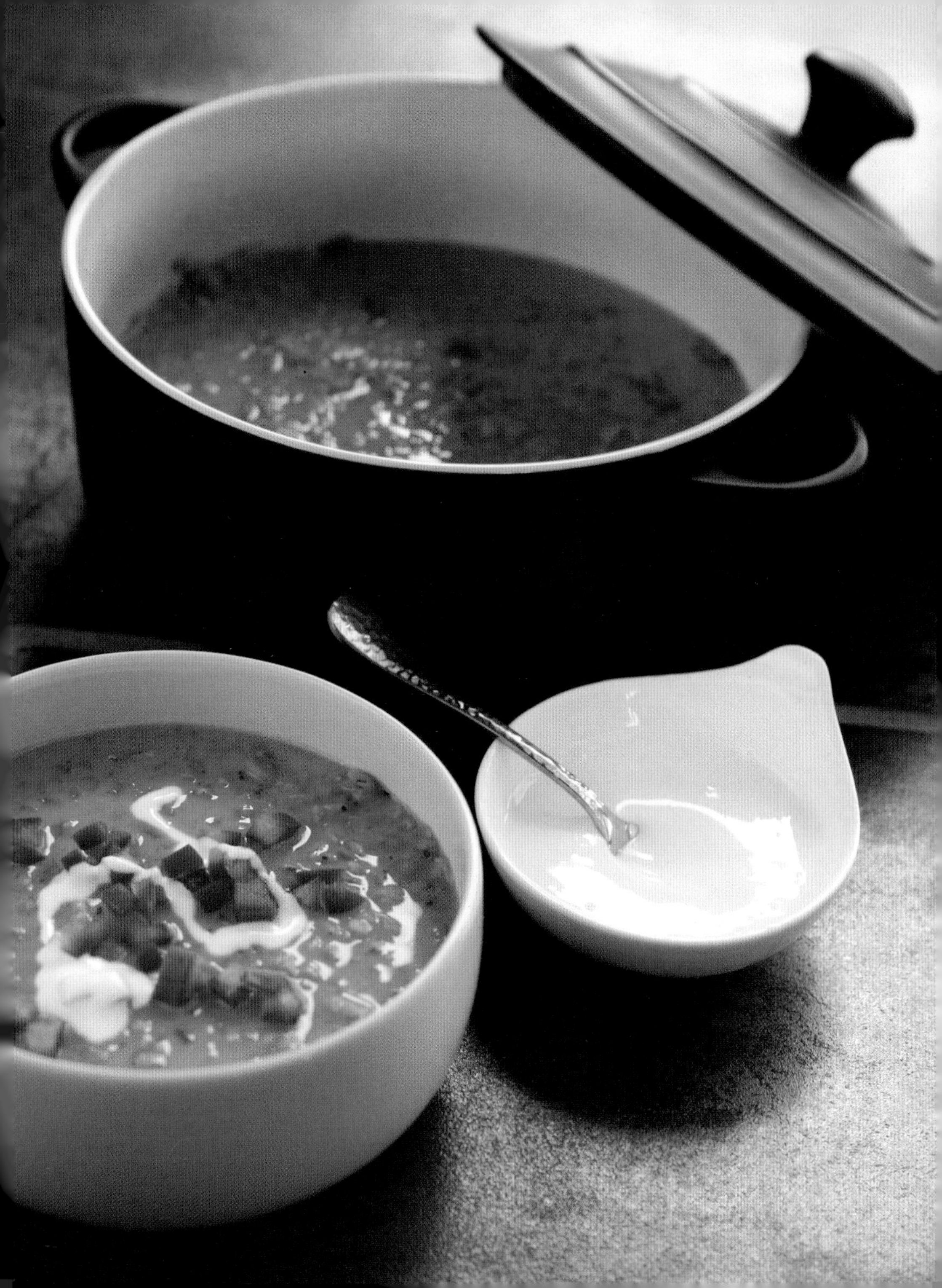

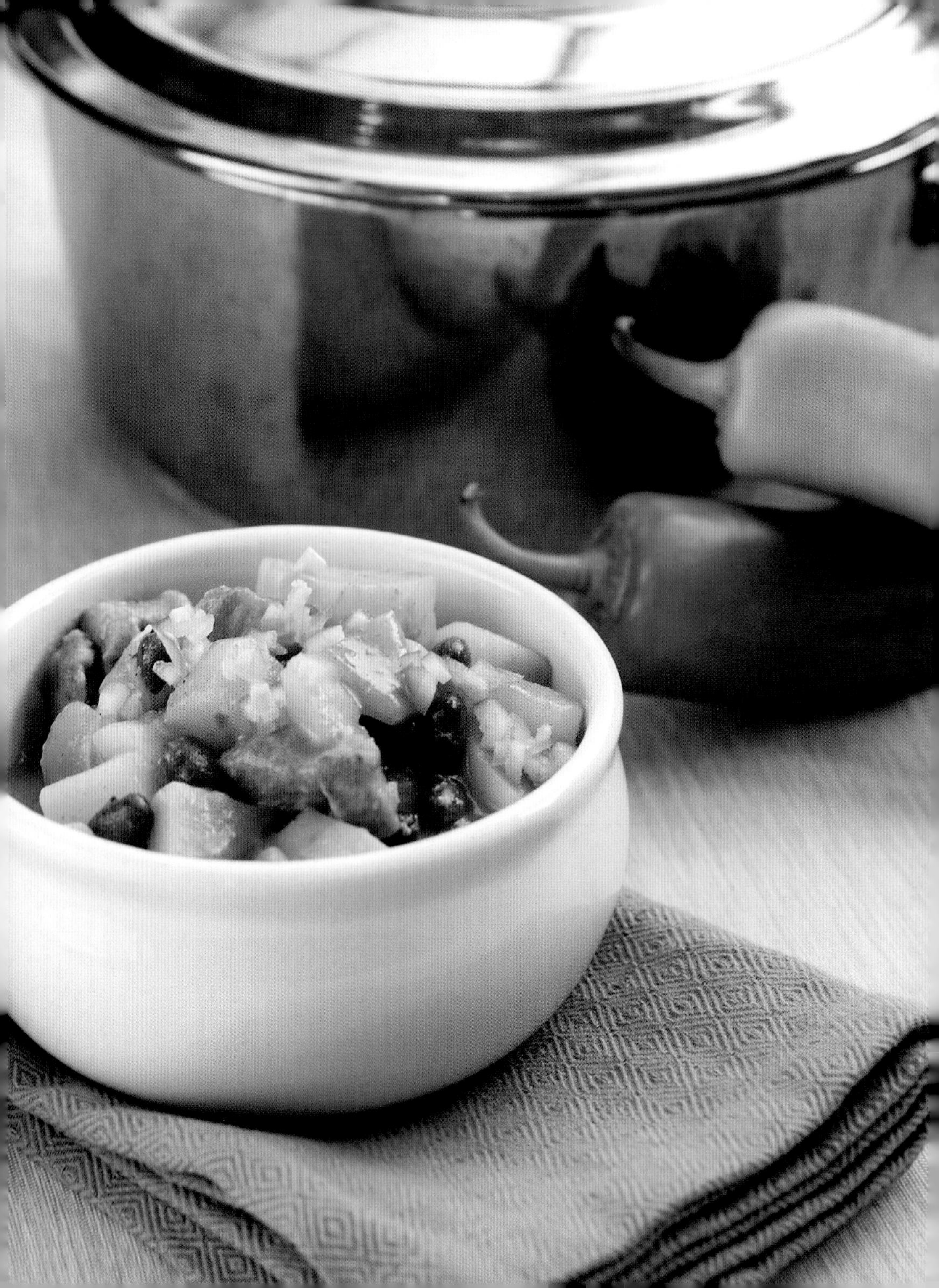

SERVINGS› 6
TIME› 40 minutes

Pork Green Chili

I like pork because it cooks very fast and remains tender. This green chili goes great with warm flatbreads or steamed rice. Best of all, tonight's dinner is tomorrow's hearty après meal.

¼ cup gluten-free flour (rice/potato/corn)

2 pounds pork, cut into bite-size cubes

1 onion, chopped

2–4 fresh chiles (such as anaheims or jalapenos), chopped

2 cups potatoes, cubed (skin left on if for post-ride)

2 tablespoons chili powder

stock or water

1 cup canned red beans, rinsed

OPTIONAL ADDITIONS

¼ cup apple cider vinegar

2 tablespoons low-sodium soy sauce

2 garlic cloves, chopped

1 tablespoon ground cumin

1. Heat a large stock pot to medium-high with enough oil to cover bottom. While the pot is heating, mix flour with a dash each of salt and pepper, then toss pork pieces in flour mixture, coating all sides.
2. Add pork to pot and stir gently to sear all sides. Add the onions, chiles, potatoes, and chili powder; stir. Pour enough water or stock in the pot to completely cover the vegetables and pork. Add any optional ingredients also at this point.
3. Bring to a boil, then turn heat down to a simmer. Cook at a simmer, stirring occasionally, until potatoes are tender and pork has cooked, about 20–30 minutes. Add beans, stir, and adjust flavor with salt and pepper.

Top with chopped cilantro, more chopped chiles, and plain yogurt.

PER SERVING› **Energy** 486 cal • **Fat** 15 g • **Sodium** 294 mg • **Carbs** 34 g • **Fiber** 5 g • **Protein** 52 g

Nutrition for optional additions can be found in Appendix A.

SERVINGS› 2
TIME› 10 minutes

Garden Fresh Tomato Soup

Summertime soups are a good prelude to dinner. If you have ripe tomatoes on hand you are just minutes away from enjoying this tomato soup. It's a perfect example of how a simple list of ingredients can be full of flavor. Just don't skimp on the basil.

4 medium vine-ripened tomatoes, peeled with stems removed

2 tablespoons red wine

2 tablespoons balsamic vinegar

juice of ½ a lemon

1 sprig of fresh basil, chopped

1 garlic clove, chopped

1. In a medium-sized saucepan, bring water to a boil. Use a knife to lightly score (or mark with an "x") the bottom of each tomato. Use a slotted spoon to place each tomato in the boiling water for about 5 seconds, or just long enough for the skin to loosen. Immediately transfer the tomato to a bowl of ice water while you finish up the other tomatoes. Then gently peel away the skin from the cooled tomatoes.
2. Combine all ingredients in blender or food processor. Add salt and pepper to taste.

Serve chilled or at room temperature. Garnish with minced onion, grated parmesan, and chopped fresh basil.

PER SERVING› **Energy** 66 cal • **Fat** 1 g • **Sodium** 163 mg • **Carbs** 13 g • **Fiber** 3 g • **Protein** 2 g

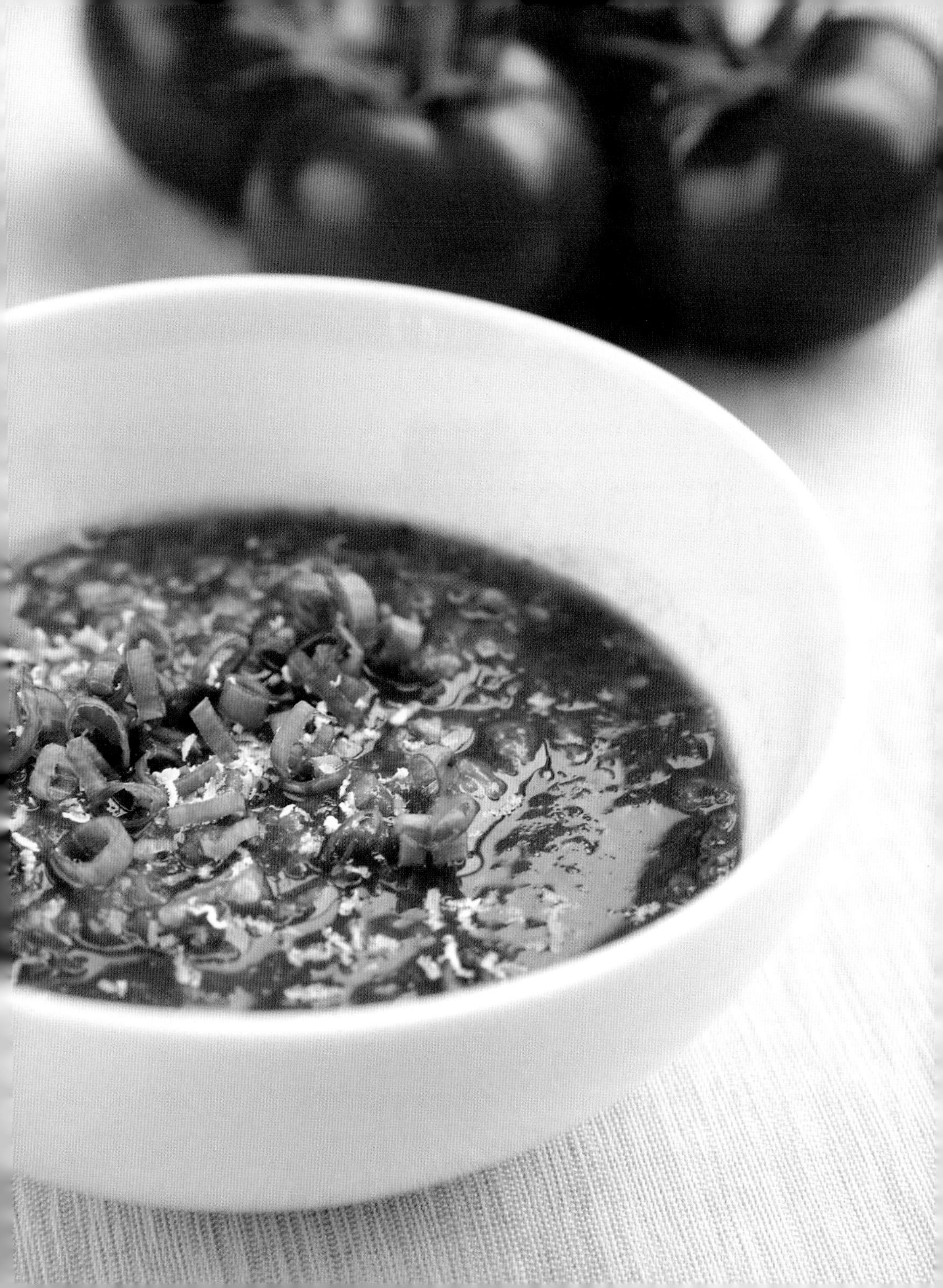

SERVINGS> 2
TIME> 10 minutes

Summer Melon Soup

Cantaloupe, honeydew, and seedless watermelon are but three of the types of melon that taste great in this refreshing soup. Experiment with your favorites—and be sure to keep this recipe in mind whenever you have overripe melon.

3 cups cubed watermelon (rind and seeds removed)

juice of ½ a lemon

½ cup apple juice

4–5 fresh mint leaves

½ cup plain or vanilla yogurt

honey or agave nectar to drizzle in as needed for sweetness

fresh mint or tarragon

1. Place melon, juice, and mint leaves in a blender or food processor (you may need to do this in two batches). Pulse, then add yogurt and honey in small amounts. You want the soup to be sweet without overpowering the delicate melon flavors and scents.

Serve chilled, within an hour or so of blending, garnished with fresh mint or tarragon, extra watermelon, and lime.

PER SERVING> **Energy** 87 cal • **Fat** 0 g • **Sodium** 53 mg • **Carbs** 19 g • **Fiber** 1 g • **Protein** 7 g

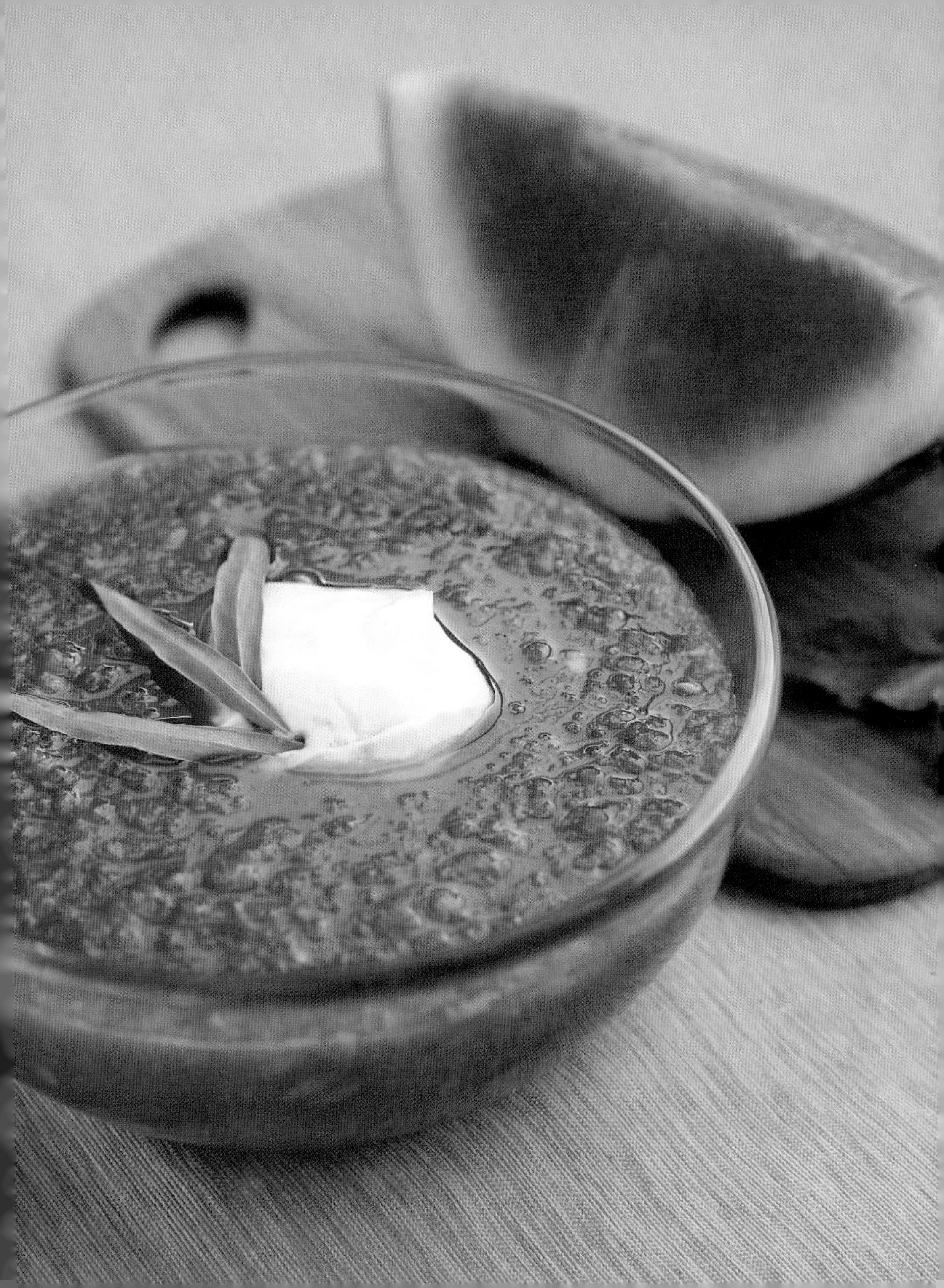

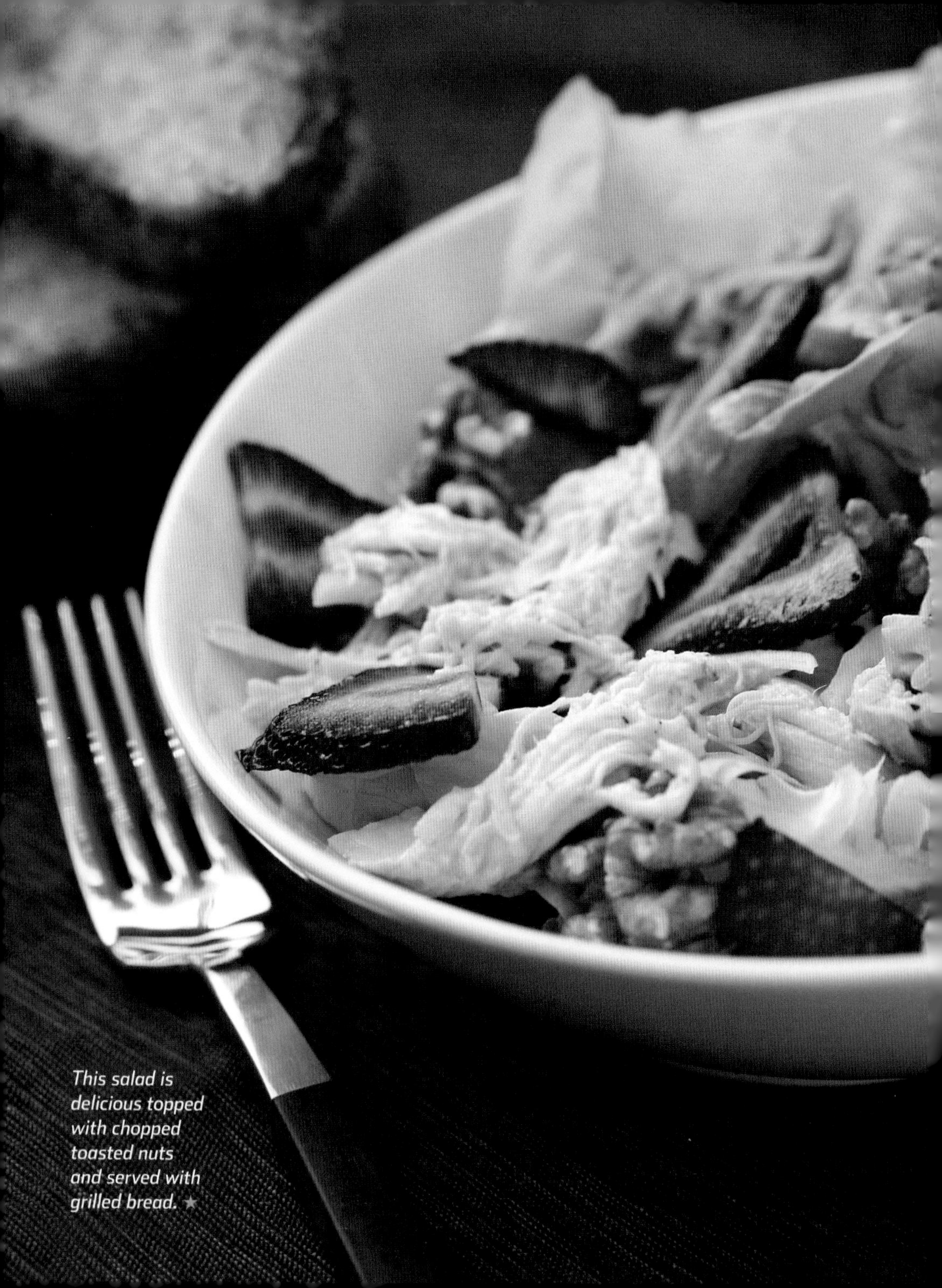

This salad is delicious topped with chopped toasted nuts and served with grilled bread. ★

SERVINGS› 2
TIME› 10 minutes

Strawberry Chicken Salad

This light and summery salad is incredibly easy to make. Either use chicken that you have cooked and ready or stop by the market for a rotisserie chicken. Let the chicken soak in the dressing while you put together the other ingredients so it can take on that sweet honey flavor that makes this salad so nice.

SALAD

COOKED 1 cup cooked and shredded chicken

2 cups loosely packed butter leaf lettuce, pulled into small pieces

¼ cup thinly sliced red onion

½ cup thinly sliced strawberries

grated parmesan

DRESSING

juice of 1 lemon

2 tablespoons honey or agave nectar

1 tablespoon white or apple cider vinegar

1 tablespoon light olive oil

a bit of fresh thyme

1. To make the dressing: In a bowl, combine the lemon juice, honey, and vinegar. While whisking, drizzle in oil; add salt and pepper to taste. Fresh thyme is a great finishing touch. Place the shredded chicken in the dressing while you prepare the salad, about 5 minutes.

2. Combine the lettuce, red onion, and strawberries in a medium-size serving bowl or individual plates. Place the chicken on top of the salad and drizzle with remaining dressing.

Add grated parmesan and salt and pepper to taste.

PER SERVING› Energy 304 cal • Fat 13 g • Sodium 403 mg • Carbs 25 g • Fiber 3 g • Protein 13 g

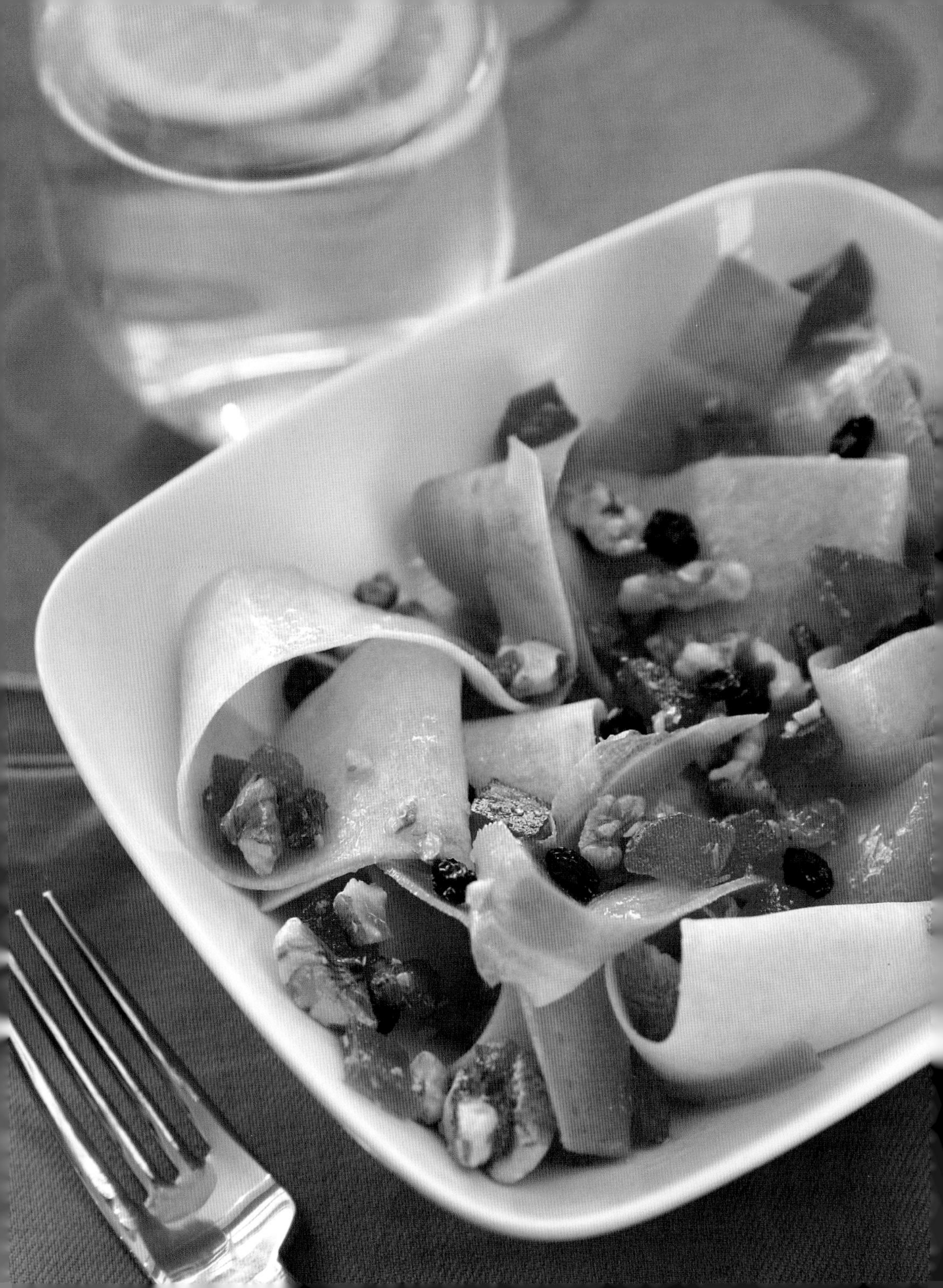

SERVINGS› 4
TIME› 30 minutes

Carrot and Butternut Squash Salad

This salad is delicious on its own or with wide pasta tossed in and topped with grated parmesan or goat cheese. When you can take the time, try peeling the vegetables into "ribbons" as shown for a beautiful dish that is sure to impress. On the nights when you don't have time for a grand presentation, just thinly slice the carrot and squash—the flavors will be equally great.

2 tablespoons olive oil

2 tablespoons chopped walnuts

2 tablespoons dried fruit (raisins, cranberries, diced mango, or peaches)

4 carrots, peeled

½ medium butternut squash (equal to the amount of carrots), cleaned and skinned

DRESSING

juice of ½ a lemon

juice of ½ an orange

2 tablespoons olive oil

1 tablespoon honey

1. Place a small sauté pan over medium heat. Add olive oil and let heat for a minute. Add walnuts and dried fruit and warm through, about 2–3 minutes, stirring continually. Set aside to cool slightly while you prepare the vegetables and dressing.
2. Using a vegetable peeler, peel long "ribbons" from the carrots and squash. Place in a serving bowl.
3. To make the dressing: Combine all dressing ingredients in a small bowl and whisk together, adding salt and pepper to taste.
4. Toss carrots and squash together, then fold in walnuts and fruit. Pour dressing over salad and mix together well.

Garnish with fresh parsley, if desired.

TIP Zucchini or yellow squash can be substituted for the butternut squash.

PER SERVING› **Energy** 291 cal • **Fat** 16 g • **Sodium** 302 mg • **Carbs** 38 g • **Fiber** 3 g • **Protein** 4 g

SERVINGS› 4
TIME› 25 minutes

Cobb Salad

Instead of the usual avocado, tomato, and blue cheese, my favorite cobb salad contains fruit. When you have the time, this simple dressing can be made with almost any jam or preserves you have in the house. As an alternative, use your favorite prepared dressing with a sweet and tangy taste.

SALAD

4 eggs

4 cups mixed greens

sliced meats and cheeses, a slice or two of each per serving: ham, turkey, Swiss, cheddar, etc.

2 bananas, sliced lengthwise

8–12 strawberries, sliced

juice of ½ a lemon

DRESSING

2 tablespoons orange marmalade or cherry jam, or other jam/preserves

1 tablespoon chopped onion

1 teaspoon chopped garlic

1 teaspoon chopped jalapeno

1 tablespoon chopped fresh parsley

½ cup white or apple cider vinegar

½ cup canola oil

1. To hard-boil eggs: Put whole eggs in a small pot and cover with water. Bring to a boil, cover with a lid, and let cook approximately 10 minutes. Remove eggs and rinse in cold water before peeling. If you are not using the eggs immediately, wait to peel them and cut into halves.

2. To make the dressing: Place all ingredients except oil in a blender. Turn on motor to a low speed and carefully drizzle in oil until a nice thick consistency is reached. Adjust seasoning with salt, pepper, and a bit of sugar. (Makes enough for at least 8 servings. Keep leftover dressing in the fridge for up to 4 days.)

3. Toss greens in a bowl with a squeeze of lemon juice and a sprinkle of salt.

Place about 1 cup of greens in center of each plate. Arrange an equal amount of meat and cheese, egg, and sliced fruit onto each plate of greens. Top with dressing.

PER SERVING› **Energy** 272 cal • **Fat** 14 g • **Sodium** 550 mg • **Carbs** 20 g • **Fiber** 3 g • **Protein** 19 g
DRESSING (2 tbsp.)› **Energy** 94 cal • **Fat** 9 g • **Sodium** 0 mg • **Carbs** 3 g • **Fiber** 0 g • **Protein** 0 g

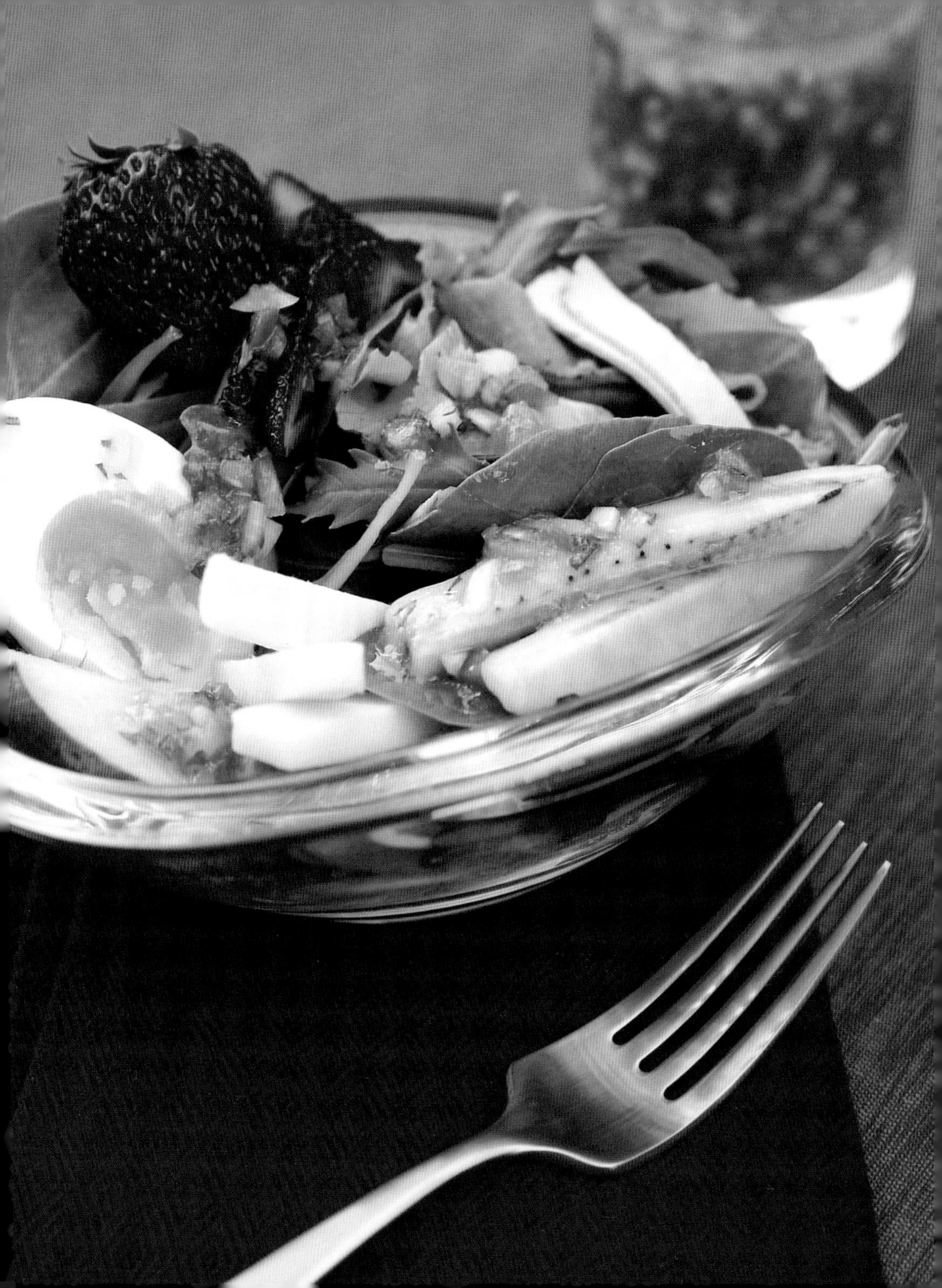

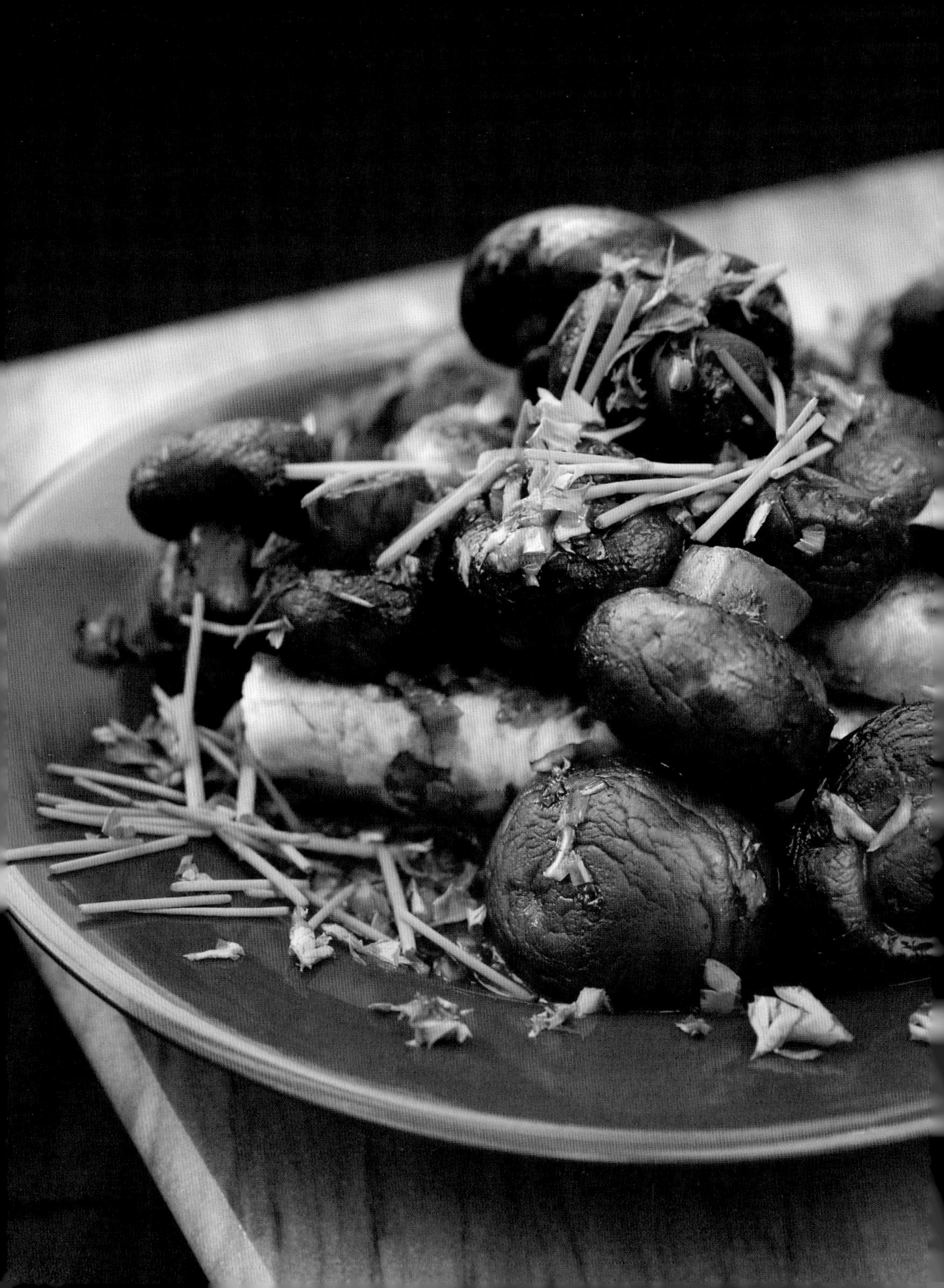

SERVINGS› 4
TIME› 15 minutes

Wine and Soy Mushrooms

Dry white wine is typically less expensive and more accessible than sake, which is traditionally used in recipes like this one. What's more, in a pinch you can cook the mushrooms in a light beer.

4 slices of Texas toast or baguette

2 tablespoons olive oil

1 pound small fresh mushrooms, washed and trimmed

1 teaspoon minced garlic

¼ cup dry white wine or beer

2 tablespoons low-sodium soy sauce

2 tablespoons fresh parsley or chives

½ cup low-sodium stock (any kind) or water

1. Lightly brush bread with olive oil and toast in a hot pan or under the broiler for just a few minutes. Keep a close eye so as not to burn the bread. Set aside.
2. Bring a lightly oiled sauté pan to medium-high heat. Add the mushrooms and garlic and sauté until the mushrooms get just a touch of crispness on the edges, 8–10 minutes.
3. Turn the heat down to medium-low. Add the wine and soy sauce.
4. Add the parsley or chives and half the stock; stir. Add remaining stock if you want more sauce. Add salt and pepper to taste.

Place two slices of toasted bread on each plate, then add a generous scoop of mushrooms. Top with grated parmesan or more fresh chopped herbs.

TIP Replace the bread with white rice to make this a gluten-free dish.

PER SERVING› **Energy** 317 cal • **Fat** 12 g • **Sodium** 733 mg • **Carbs** 39 g • **Fiber** 3 g • **Protein** 9 g

SERVINGS› 4
TIME› 30 minutes

Steak and Eggplant Salad

This is a delicious dish that you'll want to master. If you don't have cooked noodles on hand, put water on to boil before you start the other steps.

- 1 pound flank or skirt steak
- 2 tablespoons Spice Rub (page 295; see note)
- 1 medium eggplant, cut into ½-inch-thick disks
- 2 tablespoons olive oil
- 1 cup rice or wheat flour, seasoned with salt and pepper
- 2–3 garlic cloves, chopped
- 1 tomato, diced
- COOKED 1 cup cooked flat, wide noodles
- grated parmesan
- 4 cups fresh mixed greens

1. Heat oven to 350 degrees. Rub both sides of the steak with the spice rub; set aside.
2. Lay eggplant slices flat on a baking sheet. Brush both sides with olive oil.
3. In a large ziplock bag lightly dust each piece of eggplant with seasoned flour.
4. Bring a lightly oiled sauté pan to medium-high heat. Add eggplant. Cook on both sides, about 5–6 minutes or until golden brown, then transfer to an oven-safe dish and keep warm in the oven while you prepare the steak.
5. Place steak in the same pan you used for the eggplant. Let cook for about 3 minutes, then flip. Add garlic and diced tomatoes to the pan, stirring occasionally. Let cook 3–5 minutes or until steak is done as you like it. Remove from heat and let rest before cutting into strips.

Cut eggplant into chunks and combine with cooked pasta. Add grated parmesan and olive oil to taste. Next combine steak with mixed greens. Add lemon juice, salt, and pepper to taste. Load up plates with greens and steak, then top with eggplant and pasta.

NOTE› If you don't have Spice Rub on hand, use 1½ tablespoons of brown sugar mixed with 1 teaspoon each salt and pepper.

PER SERVING› **Energy** 453 cal • **Fat** 11 g • **Sodium** 296 mg • **Carbs** 48 g • **Fiber** 5 g • **Protein** 40 g

★ See page 295 for the handy Spice Rub which may be used on beef, pork, or lamb.

★ Serve warm with Chimichurri sauce (page 287).

SERVINGS› 8
TIME› 45 minutes

Jalapeno and Potato Empanadas

We will be the first to admit that empanadas are a labor-intensive food, but they are a tradition in the peloton that everyone should experience. Wrap up a few of these empanadas for a ride and you'll understand—that is, if you can manage to have any left over. (Remember to go light on the jalapeno for rides.)

FILLING

¼ cup minced onion

COOKED 2 cups cooked potatoes, cut into small cubes

1 tablespoon chopped jalapeno

¼ cup shredded or crumbled cheese: jack, cheddar, or queso fresco

1 tablespoon chopped fresh cilantro

EMPANADAS

1 recipe Pie Crust (page 276) or ready-made dough

1. To make the filling: Bring a lightly oiled sauté pan to medium-high heat. Add the onions and sauté until softened, about 3–5 minutes. Add the potatoes and jalapenos, mix thoroughly, and turn off heat.
2. Add cheese, cilantro, and a bit of salt and pepper. Taste; adjust seasonings. Set in fridge to let cool before making empanadas.
3. To make the empanadas: Heat oven to 375 degrees.
4. On a lightly floured surface, roll out small balls of the prepared pie crust dough, forming 6-inch rounds. You should have enough for 6–8 rounds.
5. Place a large spoonful of cooked filling on one side of each circle, then fold over to make a half-moon. Crimp sides together using a fork (you may need to wet the edges first with a bit of water to encourage them to adhere).
6. Transfer to a greased or nonstick baking sheet and bake until golden brown, about 15–20 minutes.

PER SERVING› **Energy** 429 cal • **Fat** 17 g • **Sodium** 248 mg • **Carbs** 62 g • **Fiber** 3 g • **Protein** 6 g

SERVINGS› 8
TIME› 45 minutes

Buffalo Curry Empanadas

I like to make these empanadas when having friends or family over for dinner. This particular variety is in celebration of those who like spicy food. To balance all that heat, serve up some Tomato Jam (page 289). It's a lovely blend of spicy and sweet that might entice you to make these handheld snacks more often.

FILLING

- 1 pound ground buffalo or grass-fed beef
- ¼ cup minced onions
- 1 tablespoon minced garlic
- 1 tablespoon minced jalapeno
- 2 tablespoons curry powder
- 1 teaspoon salt
- 1 cup peas
- 2 small tomatoes, chopped (optional)
- 2 tablespoons molasses
- 2 tablespoons low-sodium soy sauce

EMPANADAS

- 1 recipe Pie Crust (page 276) or ready-made dough

1. To make the filling: In a lightly oiled sauté pan, brown the meat and onions. Add the garlic, jalapeno, curry powder, and salt. Continue cooking, stirring, until all pink is gone from the meat.
2. Add peas (and tomatoes, if using), along with molasses and soy sauce. Cook 15 minutes. Adjust flavor with salt, then let cool before making empanadas.
3. To make the empanadas: Heat oven to 375 degrees.
4. On a lightly floured surface, roll out small balls of the prepared pie crust dough, forming 6-inch rounds. You should have enough for 6–8 rounds.
5. Place a large spoonful of cooked filling on one side of each circle, then fold over to make a half-moon. Crimp sides together using a fork (you may need to wet the edges first with a bit of water to encourage them to adhere).
6. Transfer to a greased or nonstick baking sheet and bake until golden brown, about 15–20 minutes.

PER SERVING› **Energy** 454 cal • **Fat** 24 g • **Sodium** 624 mg • **Carbs** 41 g • **Fiber** 2 g • **Protein** 18 g
Nutrition for optional additions can be found in Appendix A.

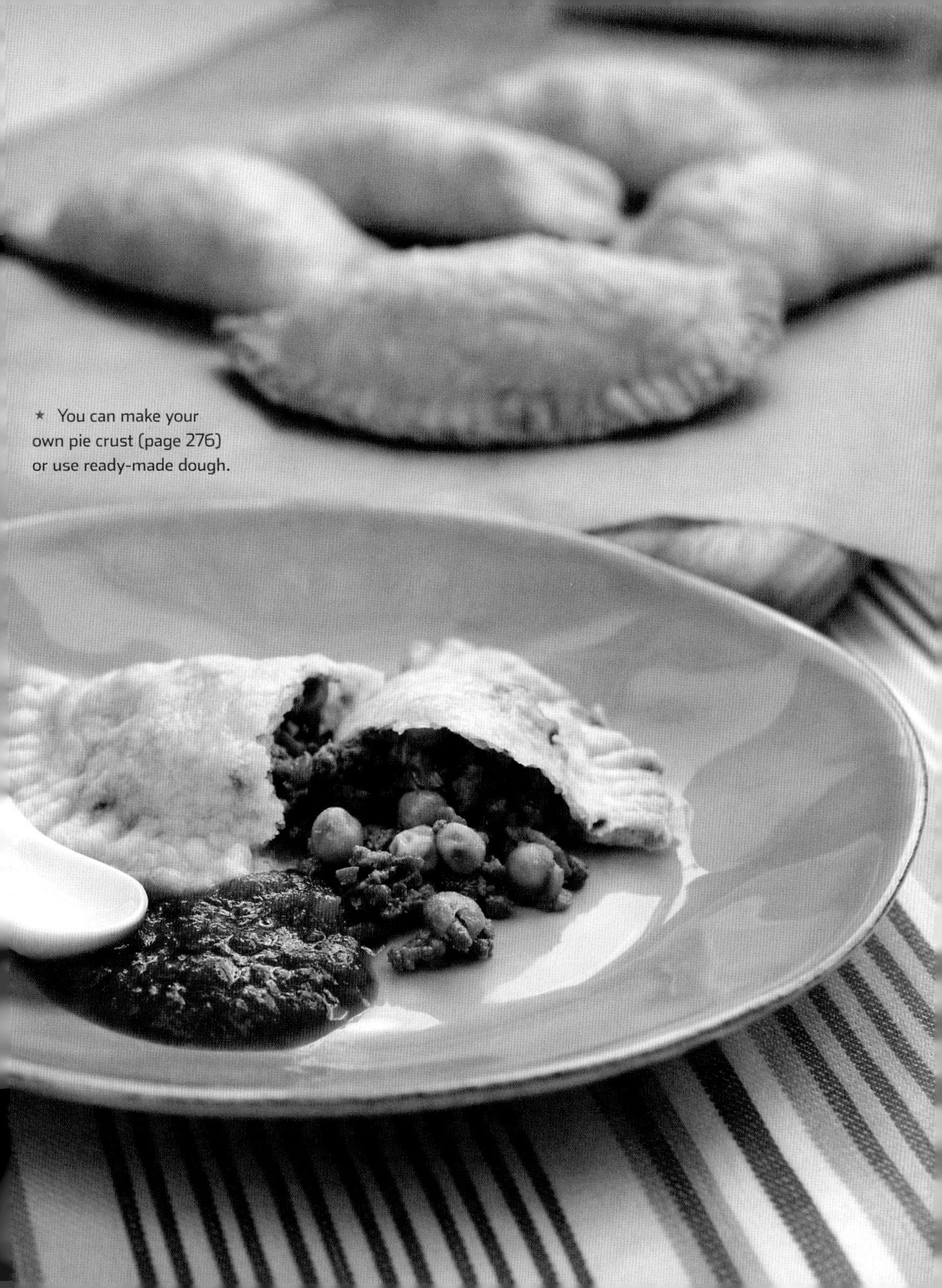

* You can make your own pie crust (page 276) or use ready-made dough.

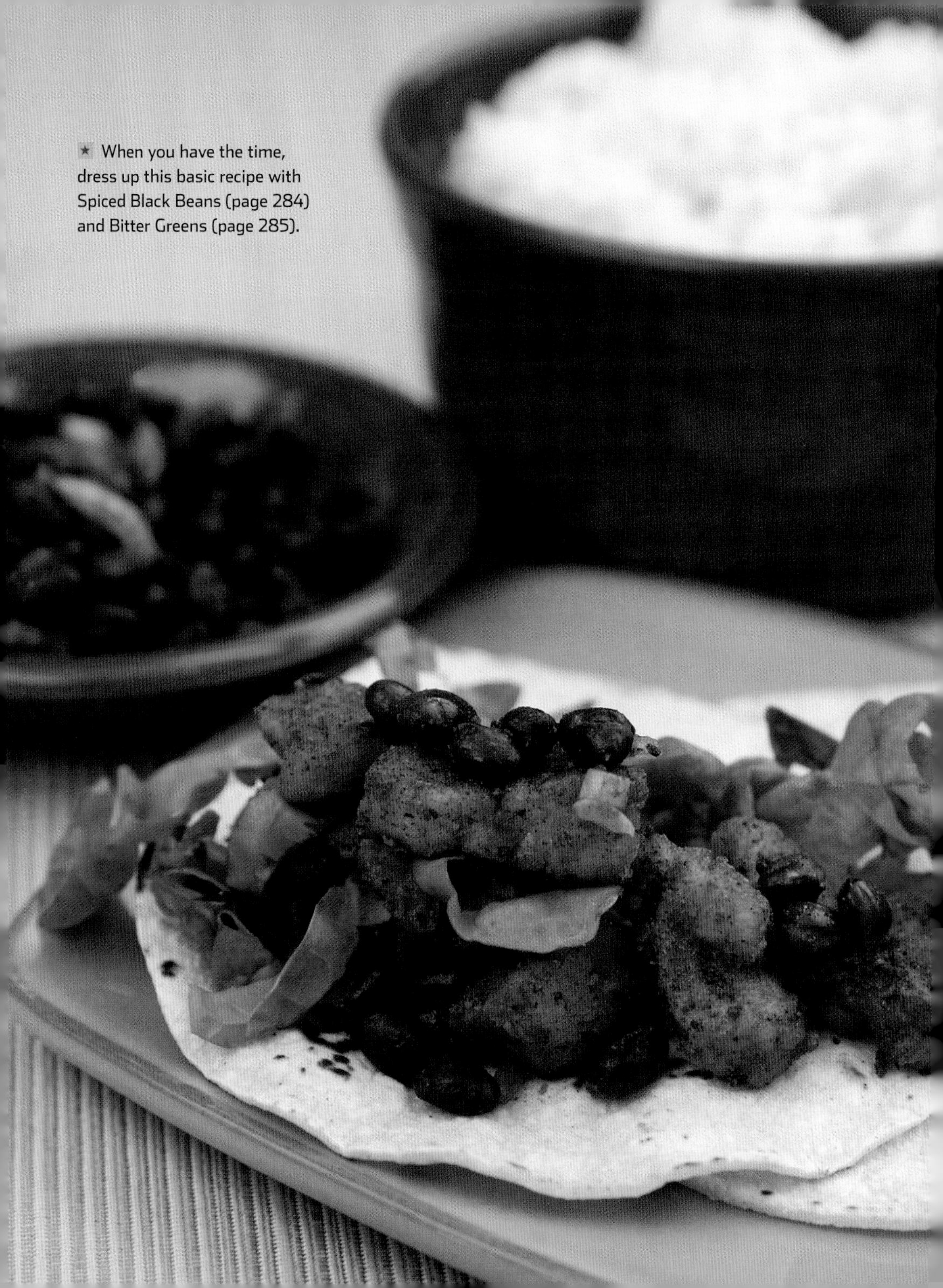

★ When you have the time, dress up this basic recipe with Spiced Black Beans (page 284) and Bitter Greens (page 285).

SERVINGS› 6
TIME› 25 minutes

Fish Tacos

Fish tacos are excellent year-round. Stock your freezer with frozen filets, which are affordable and readily available. Thin, firm filets like tilapia, snapper, or sole work especially well. Allow 12–24 hours to thaw the fish in the fridge and pat it dry with a paper towel prior to cooking. This allows the breading to cook up crispy and delicious.

RICE

- 1 cup basmati rice
- 1½ cups water
- 1 tablespoon white vinegar

FISH

- ½ cup flour
- 1 tablespoon taco seasoning
- 1 teaspoon ground black pepper
- 1 pound firm white fish filets
- 1 tablespoon grapeseed oil

- 12 corn tortillas
- 1 can (16 ounces) black beans, drained and rinsed
- 2 cups loosely packed greens
- lime wedges

1. To make the rice: Put rice, water, and vinegar in a medium pot. Bring to a boil; turn down to a simmer and cover with a lid. Let simmer until all the moisture is cooked away, about 15 minutes. Turn heat off and let sit with lid on.
2. To make the fish: Combine flour, taco seasoning, and pepper in a wide bowl or deep plate. Dredge fish in flour.
3. Pour the oil into a sauté pan and turn heat to medium-high. Add fish; fry about 3–5 minutes per side or until light golden brown. Set aside.
4. Warm the tortillas in a hot, dry pan, one at a time, flipping after 1–2 minutes.

Pile rice, beans, and fish on each warmed tortilla. Top with pico de gallo and greens, and garnish with lime wedges.

TIP Grapeseed oil is great for cooking fish because it doesn't overpower or alter the flavor. If you don't have it on hand, canola oil makes a good substitute.

PER SERVING› **Energy** 424 cal • **Fat** 8 g • **Sodium** 967 mg • **Carbs** 62 g • **Fiber** 5 g • **Protein** 27 g

SERVINGS› 4
TIME› 30 minutes

Buffalo and Sweet Potato Tacos

Both of these fillings are very easy to make and cook quickly. You can ratchet up the heat by using more jalapenos or adding some ground cayenne. Also, I like the dish to have a bit of sweetness to contrast with the rustic buffalo flavor.

BUFFALO FILLING

1 pound ground buffalo/bison
2 teaspoons taco seasoning
2 teaspoons chili powder
1 teaspoon brown sugar
¼ cup peas
1 lime

SWEET POTATO FILLING

COOKED 1 cup cooked sweet potato, cut into large cubes
1 onion, thinly sliced
1 bell pepper, thinly sliced

8 corn tortillas, warmed
plain yogurt
cilantro sprigs

1. To make the buffalo filling: Pour enough oil into a large sauté pan to thinly coat the bottom. Place pan over high heat and add the ground buffalo, stirring often to keep meat from sticking. Let the meat brown.
2. Add the dry spices and sugar, and cook for a minute. Turn the heat to medium and continue cooking until it's all a nice dark color and most of the liquid has cooked off.
3. Add peas. Season with fresh lime juice and salt to taste. Remove pan from heat while peas are still bright green.
4. To make the sweet potato filling: Pour enough oil into a medium nonstick sauté pan to thinly coat the bottom. Add sweet potatoes, onions, and peppers, and sauté until edges of the potatoes begin to crisp, about 5 minutes.
5. Add chili powder and salt to taste. Stir well; turn off heat.

Pile a good amount of buffalo and sweet potato fillings on each warmed tortilla. Top with yogurt and a few sprigs of cilantro. Makes 8 tacos.

PER SERVING› **Energy** 540 cal • **Fat** 25 g • **Sodium** 628 mg • **Carbs** 45 g • **Fiber** 6 g • **Protein** 35 g

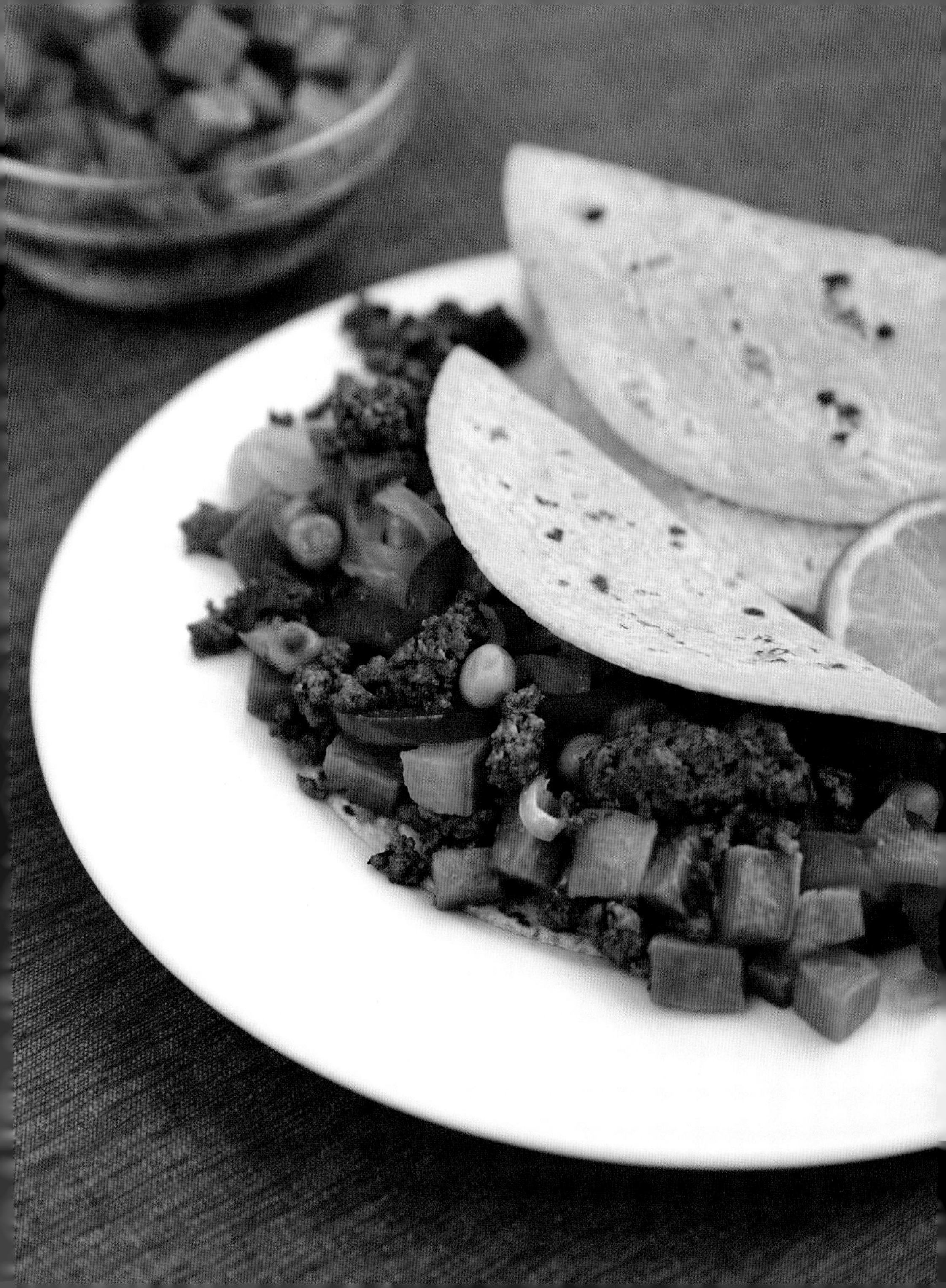

SERVINGS› 4
TIME› 30 minutes

Turkey Lettuce Wraps

Lettuce wraps are great when you want a lighter dinner that is still full of fantastic flavor. With the help of a big bowl of rice, you can get the right balance of carbs and protein to satisfy your hunger.

FILLING

1 pound ground turkey

2 tablespoons favorite spice mix (Asian, Mexican, or Indian curry blend)

¼ cup raisins

¼ onion, minced

1–2 fresh chiles, chopped

PEANUT SAUCE

½ cup peanut butter

1 tablespoon fresh lemon or lime juice

2 tablespoons olive oil

1 tablespoon apple cider or white vinegar

1 teaspoon red pepper flakes (optional)

WRAPS

1 large head of lettuce, leaves pulled apart, washed and dried

1. To make the filling: Pour enough oil into a large sauté pan to thinly coat the bottom. On medium-high heat, brown the turkey.
2. Add spice mix and remaining ingredients. Combine thoroughly, cover, and let cook 10 minutes. Mix again, adding salt and pepper to taste.
3. While the filling is cooking, make the peanut sauce: In a small bowl, combine the peanut butter, lemon or lime juice, olive oil, and vinegar. Adjust ingredients to achieve a pourable consistency, adding salt and red pepper flakes if desired.

Let filling cool a bit, then scoop it into lettuce leaves and top with peanut sauce. Roll up or fold over the leaves and eat the wraps with your hands.

TIP Most recipes call for iceberg lettuce, but I prefer to use other varieties for their nutritional value.

PER SERVING› **Energy** 157 cal • **Fat** 1 g • **Sodium** 148 mg • **Carbs** 11 g • **Fiber** 2 g • **Protein** 27 g
PEANUT SAUCE (2 tbsp.)› **Energy** 170 cal • **Fat** 15 g • **Sodium** 99 mg • **Carbs** 7 g • **Fiber** 1 g • **Protein** 5 g

If you need carbs with your meal, add cooked rice, pasta, or potatoes to the filling. ★

★ For a quick and easy Pizza Dough recipe, see page 275.

SERVINGS› 4
TIME› 50 minutes

Pizza with Tomatoes and Basil

This pizza is topped with just three ingredients. You can of course add any number of toppings, but if your ingredients are at the peak of summer freshness, why bother?

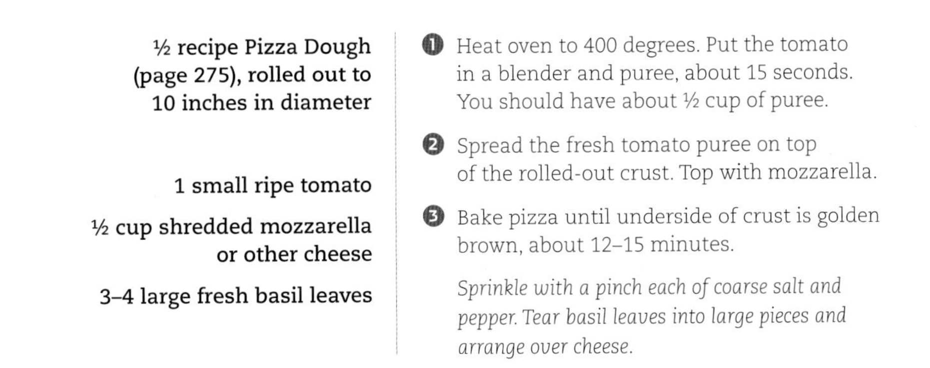

½ recipe Pizza Dough (page 275), rolled out to 10 inches in diameter

1 small ripe tomato

½ cup shredded mozzarella or other cheese

3–4 large fresh basil leaves

1. Heat oven to 400 degrees. Put the tomato in a blender and puree, about 15 seconds. You should have about ½ cup of puree.
2. Spread the fresh tomato puree on top of the rolled-out crust. Top with mozzarella.
3. Bake pizza until underside of crust is golden brown, about 12–15 minutes.

Sprinkle with a pinch each of coarse salt and pepper. Tear basil leaves into large pieces and arrange over cheese.

PER SERVING› **Energy** 444 cal • **Fat** 10 g • **Sodium** 653 mg • **Carbs** 73 g • **Fiber** 3 g • **Protein** 14 g

SERVINGS› 4
TIME› 1 hour

Pizza with Potatoes

Pizza is a big morale booster for a professional cycling team in the middle of a tough race season. This particular pizza is wonderfully mild so you could eat it before a race if the opportunity presented itself. Or you can add a flourish of your own choosing.

- ½ recipe Pizza Dough (page 275), rolled out to 10 inches in diameter
- olive oil
- ¼ cup onion, thinly sliced
- COOKED 1 cup cooked potatoes, thinly sliced
- 3 tablespoons grated parmesan
- fresh thyme or other herbs

OPTIONAL ADDITIONS

- chopped garlic
- shredded mozzarella
- fresh chopped tomatoes

1. Heat oven to 400 degrees. In a small or medium sauté pan over medium-high heat, sauté the onions in a bit of olive oil until lightly brown. Remove from heat.
2. Brush uncooked pizza crust with olive oil. Top with potatoes, onions, grated parmesan, and herbs. (If using optional additions, add them here.)
3. Bake in oven until underside of crust is golden brown, about 12–15 minutes. Sprinkle with salt and pepper to taste.

TIP This pizza has a light, flaky crust. It's a great starter or snack.

PER SERVING› Energy 492 cal • Fat 11 g • Sodium 658 mg • Carbs 85 g • Fiber 4 g • Protein 13 g
Nutrition for optional additions can be found in Appendix A.

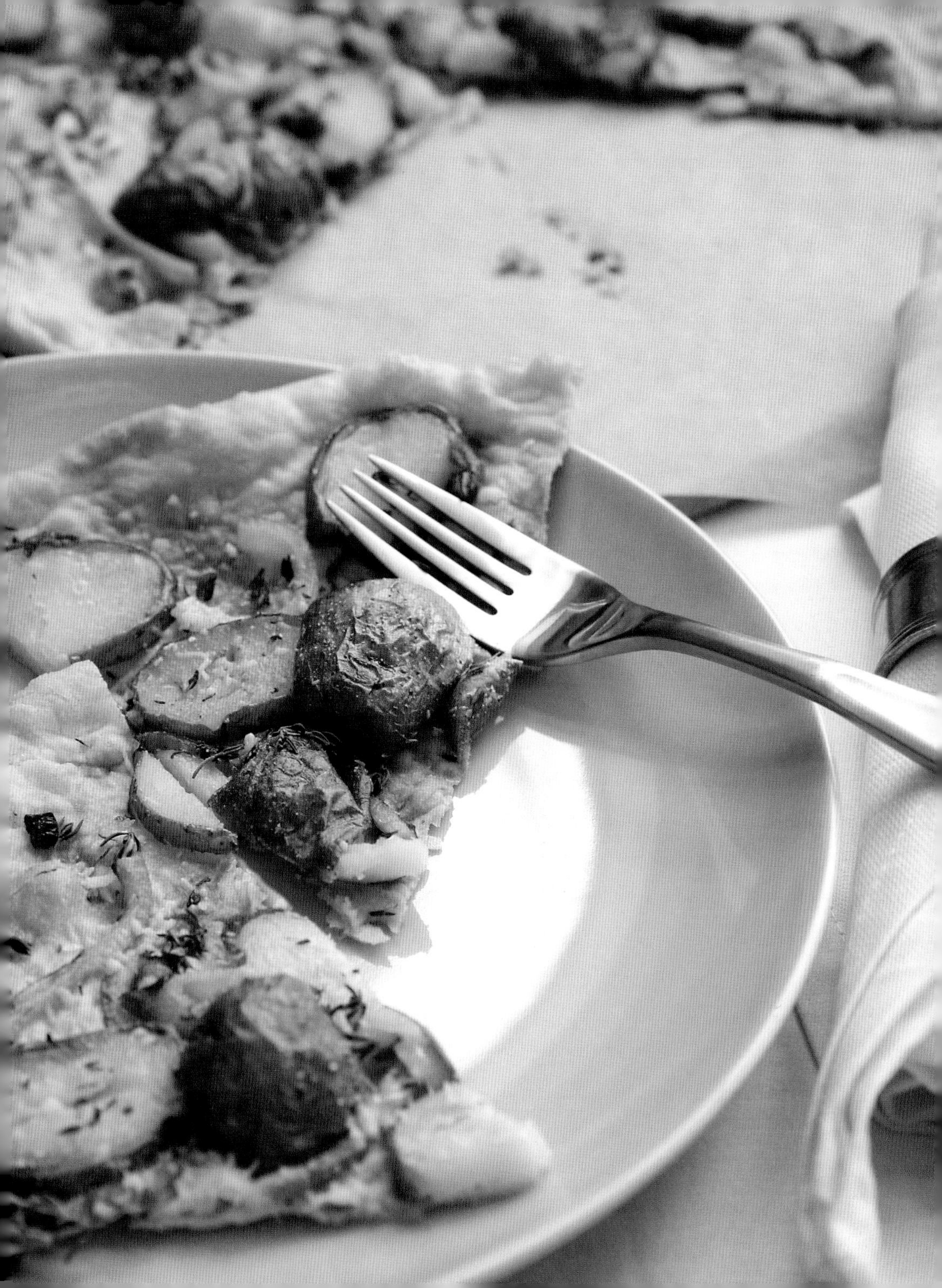

SERVINGS › 4
TIME › 50 minutes

Pizza with Spinach, Eggs, and Anchovies

Most athletes crave salt and tart flavors after hard efforts, especially on hot summer days. With anchovy and lemon juice among the ingredients, this nutritious starter satisfies both cravings. Cook the crust by itself, remove from oven, brush with olive oil, and top with fresh ingredients. It's simple!

½ recipe Pizza Dough (page 275), rolled out to 10 inches in diameter

1 cup fresh spinach leaves, washed and dried

1 teaspoon minced garlic

1 tablespoon olive oil, plus extra to brush on crust

1 tablespoon grated parmesan

6–8 thin slices of anchovy

COOKED 2 hard-boiled eggs, quartered

lemon juice

OPTIONAL ADDITIONS

toasted pine nuts or walnuts

fresh basil, torn or cut into slivers

1. Heat oven to 400 degrees. Cook pizza crust until it is golden brown, 8–12 minutes. Remove from oven and immediately brush lightly with olive oil.
2. While the crust is baking, combine the spinach, garlic, 1 tablespoon of olive oil, and parmesan (and any optional ingredients).
3. Top the hot crust with the spinach and parmesan mixture. Add anchovy slices and eggs, alternating. Finish with a fresh squeeze of lemon juice, and a sprinkle of coarse salt.

PER SERVING › Energy 515 cal • Fat 15 g • Sodium 1,210 mg • Carbs 72 g • Fiber 3 g • Protein 18 g
Nutrition for optional additions can be found in Appendix A.

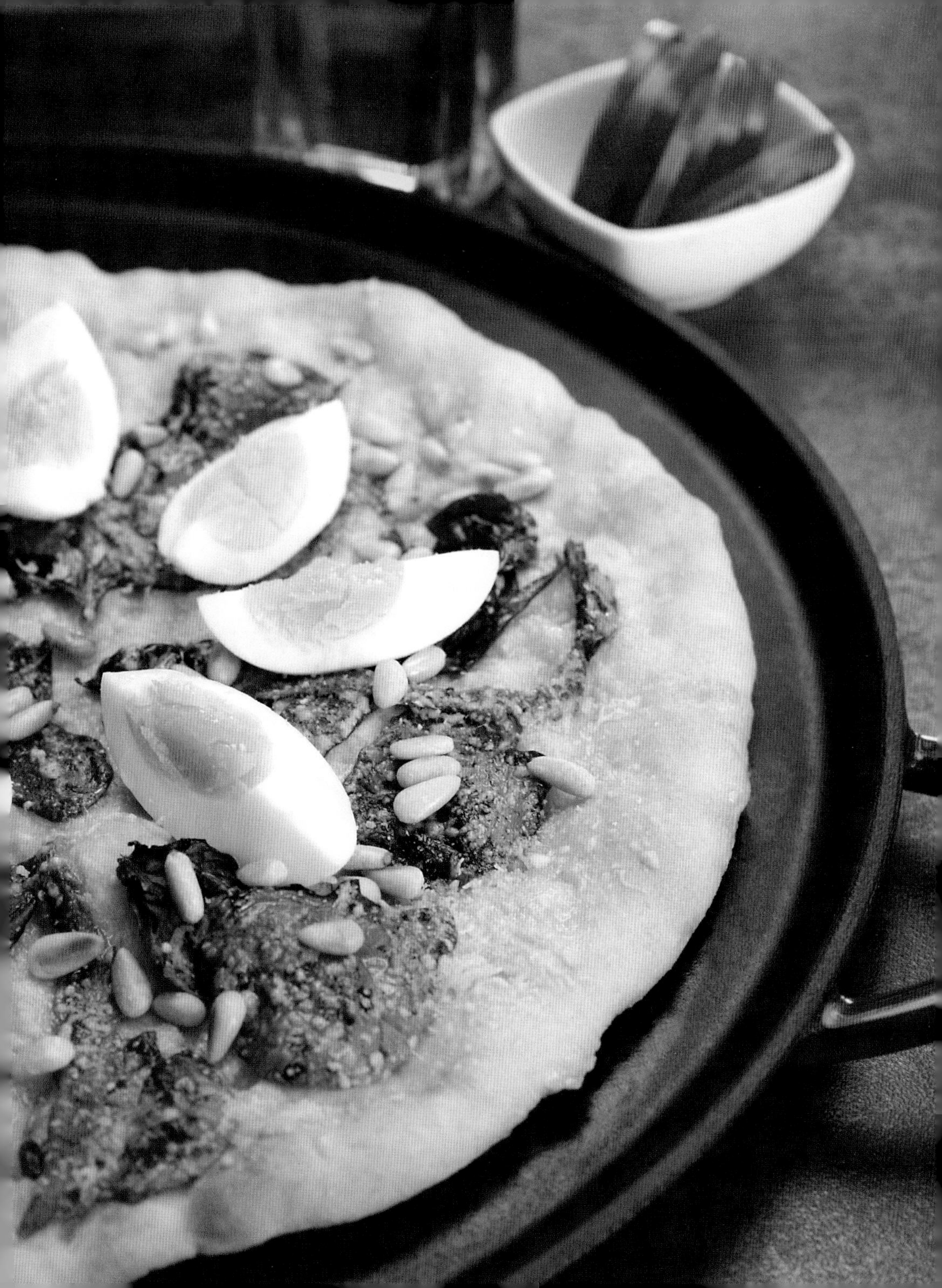

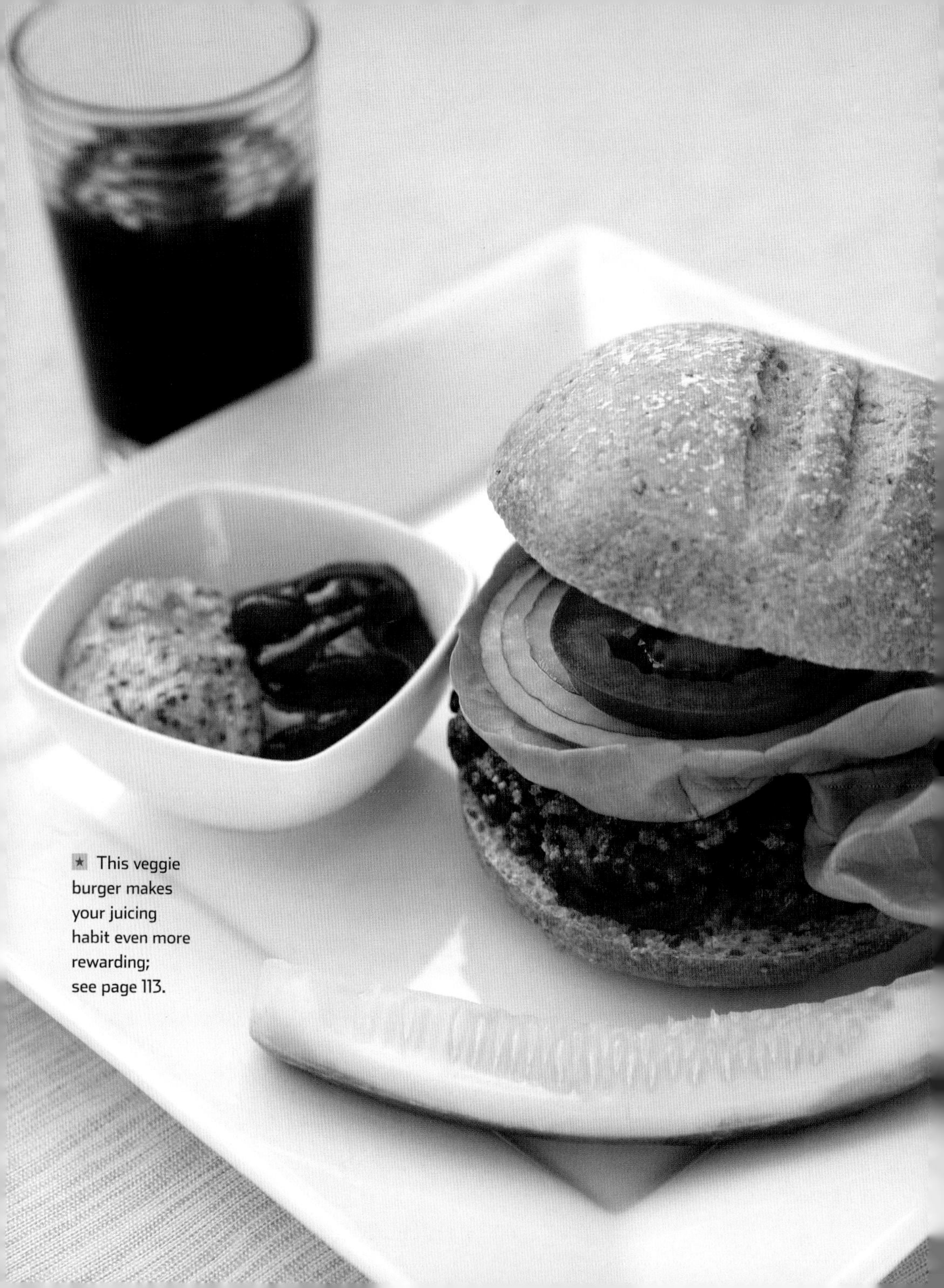

★ This veggie burger makes your juicing habit even more rewarding; see page 113.

SERVINGS> 8
TIME> 20 minutes

Veggie Burgers

My vegetarian friends are constantly trying to figure out a solid veggie burger recipe. To form a patty that doesn't fall apart, most recipes add flour or egg—and any number of things that don't really work well together. This loose recipe has just three ingredients plus whatever sounds good to you. It is free of dairy and gluten and has no added oils, eggs, or binders.

1 cup mixed veggie pulp (see note)

COOKED **4 cups cooked sticky rice**

COOKED **1 cup cooked or canned beans**

whole wheat buns

OPTIONAL ADDITIONS

mixed spices: up to 2 teaspoons total of ground coriander, cumin, chili powder, and celery salt

up to 1 cup of chopped mushrooms, carrots, and/or broccoli, lightly sautéed

1. Combine the pulp, rice, and beans. Taste; adjust for flavor with salt, brown sugar, any spices you like, and chopped cooked veggies, if using.
2. Once you are happy with the flavor, form into large balls, then press down to form patties. You should have enough for 8 patties.
3. Heat a lightly oiled sauté pan to medium-high. Add as many patties as will comfortably fit in the pan. When bottom sides are golden brown, flip patties and cook until golden brown on second side.

Let seared patties cool before wrapping and storing in the freezer, where they will keep for up to a month.

NOTE> You will need a juicer to make these burgers. Try beets, carrots, apples, and your favorite greens for the pulp.

TIP The mix ratio will vary depending on the moisture in the veggie pulp and also the rice. If your rice is really dry, try adding a splash of water to it and heating it over the stove or in the microwave.

PER SERVING> **Energy** 288 cal • **Fat** 2 g • **Sodium** 311 mg • **Carbs** 57 g • **Fiber** 8 g • **Protein** 3 g
Nutrition for optional additions can be found in Appendix A.

★ Cilantro-Mint Yogurt may be used on a variety of dishes for extra flavor; see page 291.

SERVINGS› 12
TIME› 45 minutes

Meatball Sliders

Like classic meatballs but with the addition of raisins and made a bit smaller, these are perfect for summer picnics or when unexpected guests arrive—you can freeze the cooked meatballs by themselves or with the sauce.

- 1 pound ground beef or lean ground turkey
- 1 pound spicy Italian bulk sausage
- ¼ cup golden raisins
- 1 cup cubed fresh bread
- 2 eggs, beaten

- 1 jar of your favorite prepared tomato sauce
- ½ cup of water
- 1 dozen dinner rolls, split
- Cilantro-Mint Yogurt (page 291)
- toppings of your choice: cheese, onions, chopped veggies, etc.

1. In a medium bowl, combine beef or turkey, sausage, raisins, cubed bread, and eggs. Let sit for a few minutes so the bread soaks up the egg.
2. Using your hands, form 12 meatballs. Adjust size to fit inside dinner rolls after they are fried.
3. Add oil to cover the bottom of a large heavy pot and turn heat to medium-high. Add meatballs as space allows (don't crowd them) and turn often to brown all sides. Remove meatballs from the pot after they brown and place on a paper towel.
4. After all the meatballs have been browned, return them to the pot, add tomato sauce and water, cover with a lid, and let cook over medium-high heat for 20 minutes, stirring occasionally to prevent sauce from scorching.

Place one meatball and a bit of sauce inside each split dinner roll. Top with Cilantro-Mint Yogurt and any other desired toppings.

PER SERVING (1 slider)› **Energy** 453 cal • **Fat** 20 g • **Sodium** 983 mg • **Carbs** 52 g • **Fiber** 5 g • **Protein** 25 g
Nutrition uses ground turkey. Nutrition for toppings can be found in Appendix A.

SERVINGS› 4
TIME› 30 minutes

Frittata with Red Pepper Oil

There are countless versions of a good frittata; here's a basic one of sliced vegetables and cheese. As you get more comfortable making this recipe, change up the cheeses and add cooked meats and fresh herbs. A frittata is great with a big chunk of crusty bread and a lemony salad.

FRITTATA

- 2–3 tablespoons olive oil (depending on size of pan)
- 1 onion, thinly sliced
- 2 bell peppers, thinly sliced
- 6–8 eggs, lightly beaten
- ½ cup shredded Swiss cheese
- 1 tablespoon total chopped fresh herbs: basil, thyme, parsley, tarragon
- dash of salt and pepper
- dash of ground nutmeg (optional)

RED PEPPER OIL

- ½ cup olive oil
- 2 tablespoons diced fresh red bell pepper or marinated red pepper
- dash of salt
- lemon juice

1. To make the frittata: In a large nonstick sauté pan, heat enough oil to coat bottom evenly. Over medium heat, sauté onions and peppers until tender, about 4–5 minutes.
2. Meanwhile, combine eggs, cheese, herbs, and a dash each of salt and pepper (and nutmeg, if using) in a medium bowl. Pour over the cooked vegetables and gently even out pan. Cook at medium heat, pushing eggs around until almost cooked through. Cover for a few minutes and let sit until eggs firm. Let rest in pan before serving.
3. To make the red pepper oil: Put oil, peppers, and salt in a blender. Blend until smooth. Add lemon juice to taste, along with more salt if needed to balance the flavors. Will keep stored in fridge for about a week.

Either flip frittata upside-down onto serving plate or cut in pan. Serve with a drizzle of red pepper oil.

PER SERVING› **Energy** 270 cal • **Fat** 20 g • **Sodium** 208 mg • **Carbs** 8 g • **Fiber** 2 g • **Protein** 14 g
RED PEPPER OIL (1 tbsp.)› **Energy** 97 cal • **Fat** 11 g • **Sodium** 28 mg • **Carbs** 2 g • **Fiber** 0 g • **Protein** 0 g

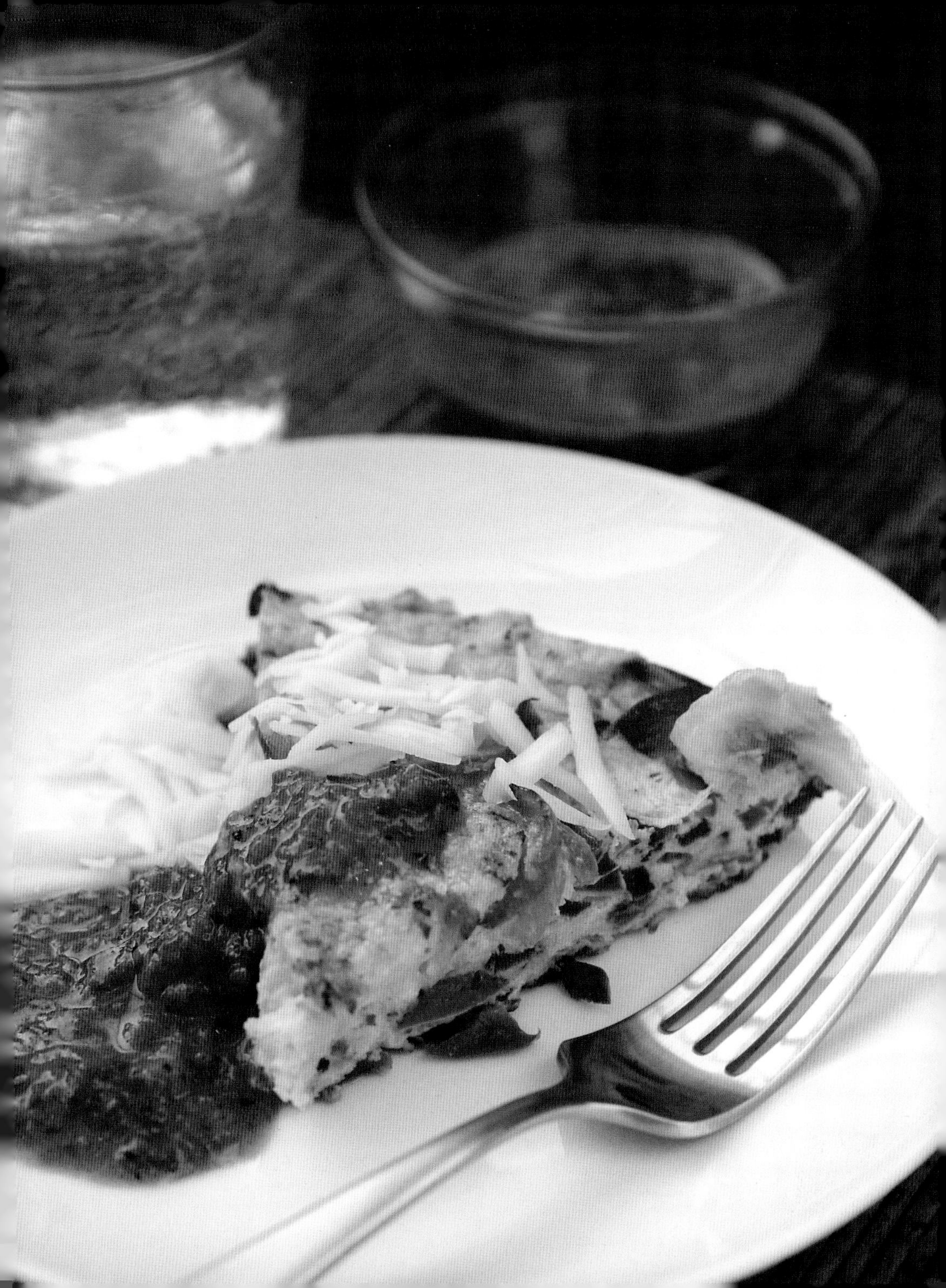

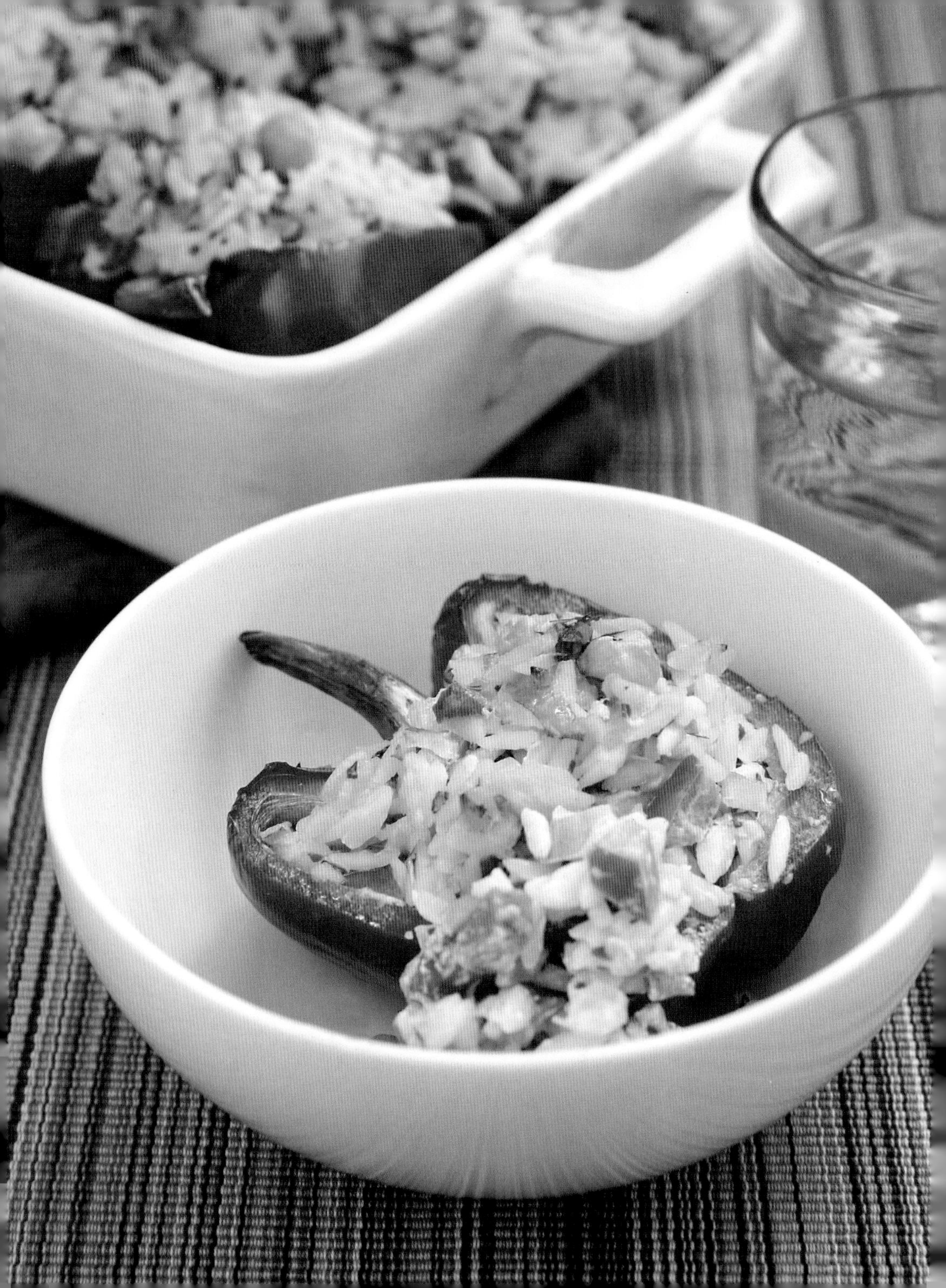

SERVINGS› 4
TIME› 45 minutes

Orzo-Stuffed Peppers

Stuffed peppers are not everyday fare for most athletes, but they use ingredients that we typically have on hand. It only takes about 15 minutes to prep the stuffing, but if you plan your week so as to have some leftover Orzo and Basil Salad (page 153) around, you can make some quick additions and have a delicious reincarnation on your plate.

- 8 ounces orzo
- 1 cup shredded sharp cheddar or mozzarella cheese
- 1 tomato, diced
- 1 small onion, chopped
- ¼ cup total of fresh chopped herbs: parsley, basil, chives
- ½ cup plain yogurt or low-sodium stock
- 2 tablespoons olive oil
- 4 medium–large bell peppers, washed, and halved

OPTIONAL ADDITIONS

- 2 ounces goat cheese or low-fat cream cheese
- 5 ounces canned tuna or salmon, drained
- COOKED 1 cup cooked garbanzo beans

1. Heat oven to 375 degrees. Cook the orzo according to package directions. Drain; toss with a bit of olive oil.
2. Combine orzo and remaining ingredients except peppers, adding salt and pepper to taste (plus any optional additions). Stuff each pepper with the orzo mixture and top with a little extra cheese or fresh herbs.
3. Set peppers upright on an oiled oven-safe dish. Cover with foil and bake for 30 minutes. Remove foil and let bake 5–10 minutes more, until the tops are slightly browned and the peppers are tender.

If you're in a hurry, microwave the stuffed peppers 3–4 minutes, then bake them in the oven for 15–20 minutes.

TIP You can substitute rice for orzo, but make sure to use "almost cooked" rice—fully cooked rice will become too soft when baked.

PER SERVING› **Energy** 386 cal • **Fat** 18 g • **Sodium** 220 mg • **Carbs** 44 g • **Fiber** 3 g • **Protein** 15 g

Nutrition for optional additions can be found in Appendix A.

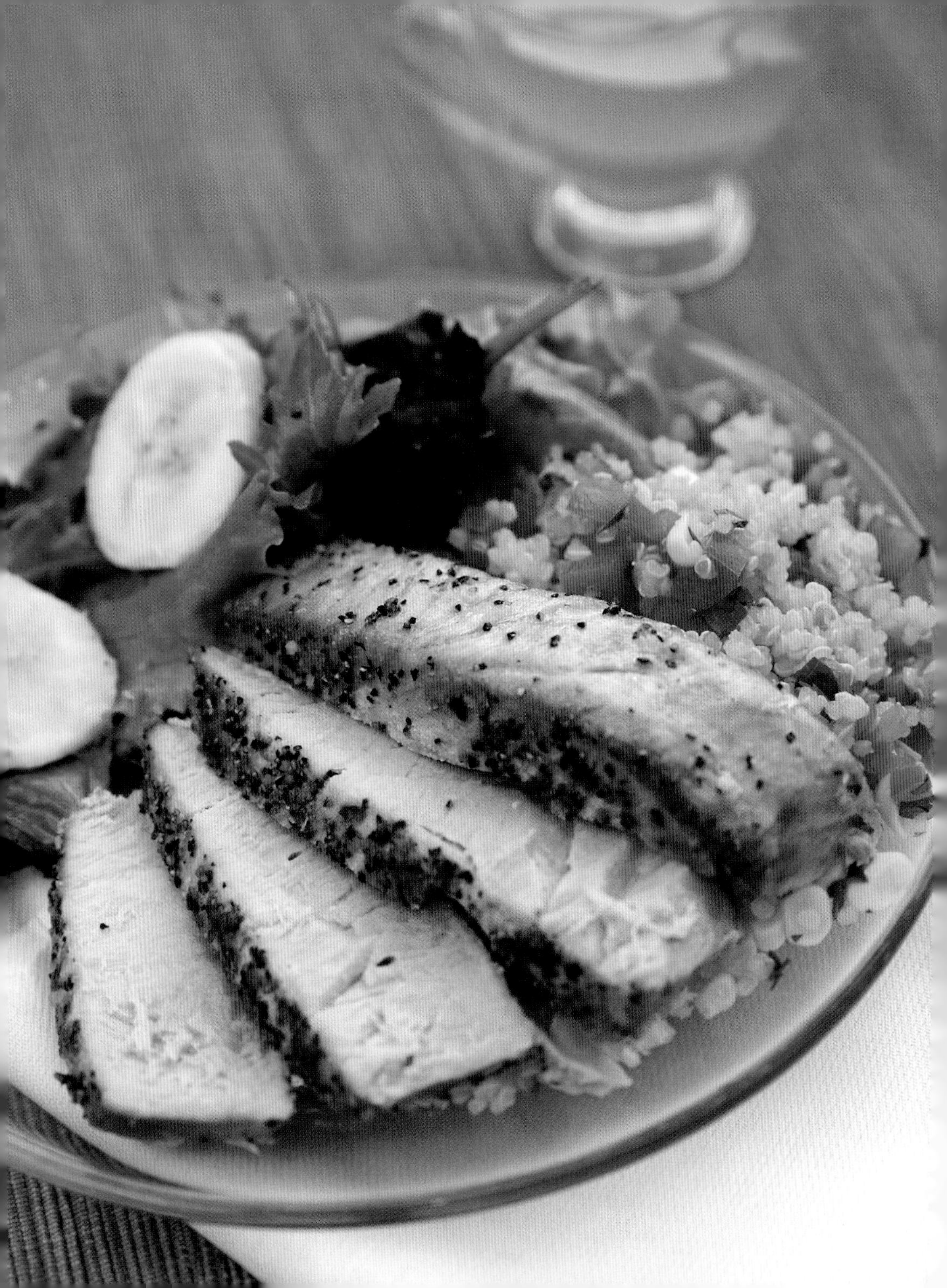

SERVINGS› 2
TIME› 15 minutes

Seared Ahi

Ahi (also known as yellowfin tuna) is a versatile and substantial fish—it's easy to work with and has great texture. I keep a few steaks on hand in the freezer and serve this dish with steamed rice, potatoes, or quinoa.

2 ahi steaks (3–4 ounces each), sprinkled with salt and coarse pepper on both sides

LEMON OIL

1 lemon

¼ cup olive oil

3 cups loosely packed mixed salad greens

1 banana, sliced

2 tablespoons honey

1. Bring a lightly oiled nonstick sauté pan to medium-high heat. Add ahi. Sear on one side, then flip over and sear the other side. (Each side should take about 3 minutes, depending on the thickness of the steaks.) Remove before the fish has completely cooked through; it should still be a bit pink in the center. Cut into thick strips.
2. To make the lemon oil: In a small bowl, combine olive oil and juice from one lemon with a pinch of salt and whisk together.

Toss greens with half the lemon oil dressing. Place ahi strips on individual plates beside mixed greens and banana slices. Drizzle with remaining lemon oil and honey. Finish with salt and pepper to taste.

TIP The safest method to thaw fish or meat is to place it in a dish in the refrigerator overnight. Do not leave out at room temperature!

PER SERVING› **Energy** 470 cal • **Fat** 29 g • **Sodium** 360 mg • **Carbs** 25 g • **Fiber** 3 g • **Protein** 32 g

SERVINGS› 4
TIME› 25 minutes

Pan-Seared Sole

Any mild-flavored white fish works well in this recipe. We've chosen sole because it's easy to find at the market and even easier to prepare. The mango and avocado in the salsa are sweet and buttery without overpowering the delicate flavor of the fish. This recipe works well with any thin, mild-flavored fish. It cooks quickly, so make it just before you're ready to serve.

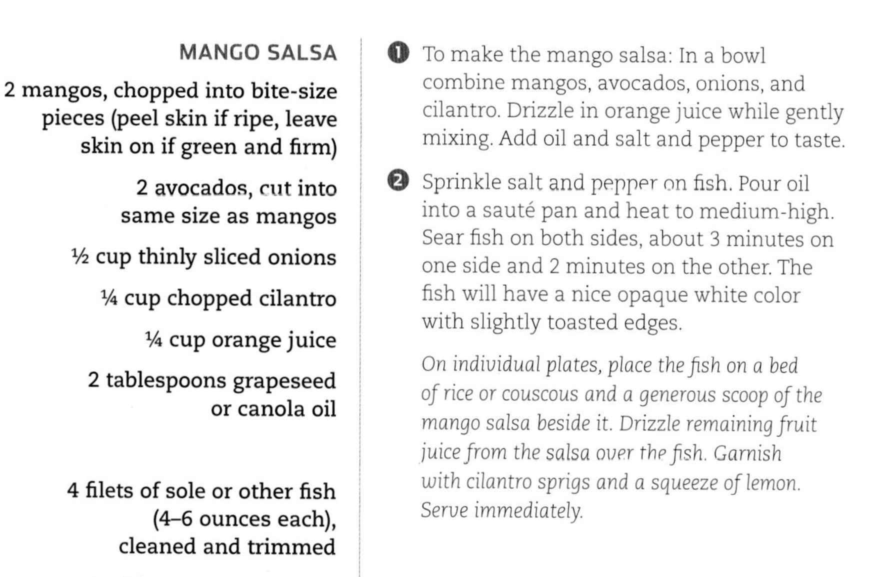

MANGO SALSA

2 mangos, chopped into bite-size pieces (peel skin if ripe, leave skin on if green and firm)

2 avocados, cut into same size as mangos

½ cup thinly sliced onions

¼ cup chopped cilantro

¼ cup orange juice

2 tablespoons grapeseed or canola oil

4 filets of sole or other fish (4–6 ounces each), cleaned and trimmed

2 tablespoons grapeseed or canola oil

1. To make the mango salsa: In a bowl combine mangos, avocados, onions, and cilantro. Drizzle in orange juice while gently mixing. Add oil and salt and pepper to taste.
2. Sprinkle salt and pepper on fish. Pour oil into a sauté pan and heat to medium-high. Sear fish on both sides, about 3 minutes on one side and 2 minutes on the other. The fish will have a nice opaque white color with slightly toasted edges.

On individual plates, place the fish on a bed of rice or couscous and a generous scoop of the mango salsa beside it. Drizzle remaining fruit juice from the salsa over the fish. Garnish with cilantro sprigs and a squeeze of lemon. Serve immediately.

PER SERVING› **Energy** 380 cal • **Fat** 21 g • **Sodium** 210 mg • **Carbs** 27 g • **Fiber** 7 g • **Protein** 1 g

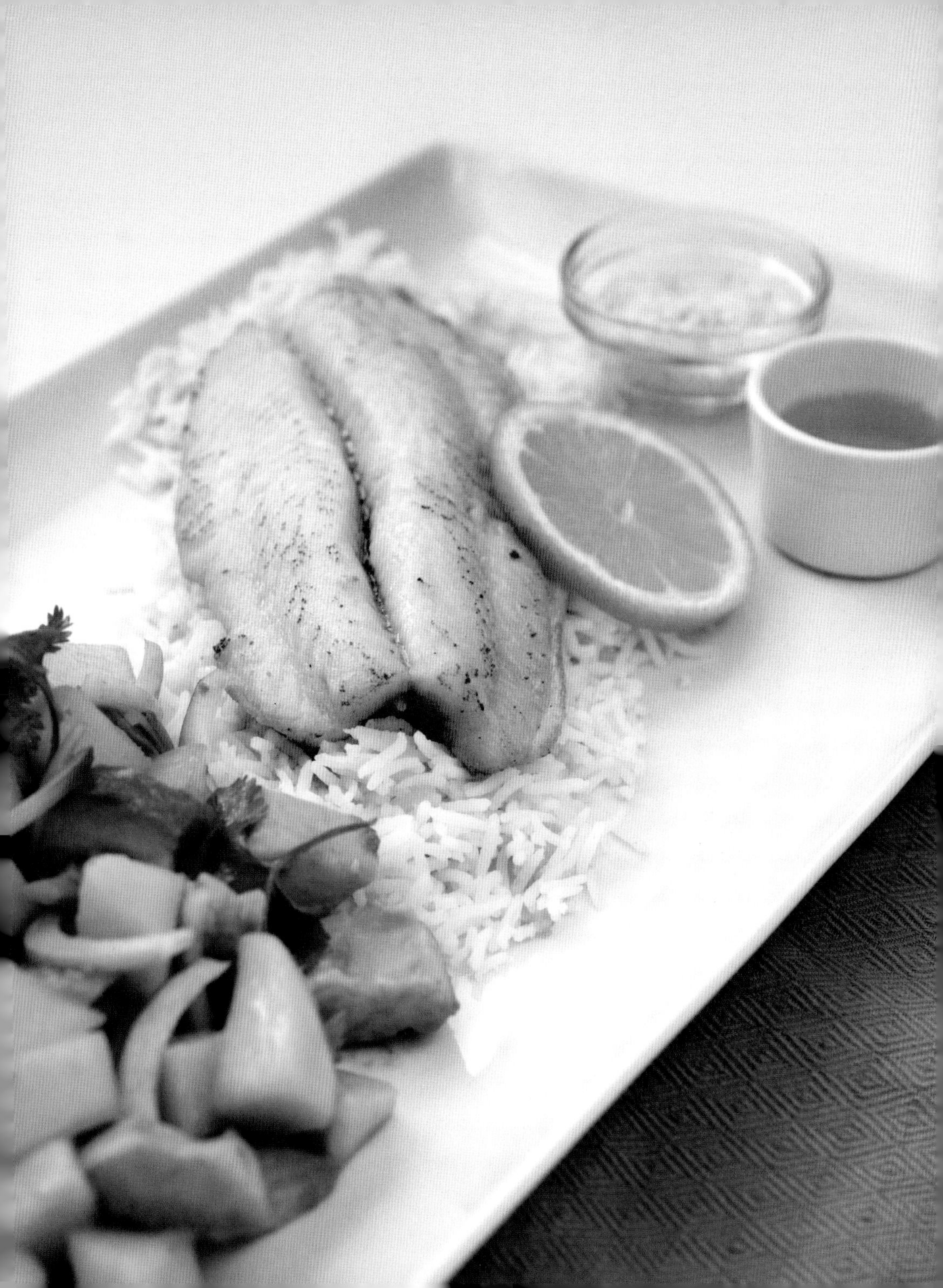

SERVINGS› 4
TIME› 20 minutes

Simple Biryani

Biryani is a classic South Indian dish that comes together in a hurry. Thanks to the fresh vegetables and the protein found in the cashews, biryani is a complete meal in itself.

2 cups rice (see note)

3½ cups water

2 tablespoons light olive oil

2 cups chopped vegetables (carrots, broccoli, yellow squash, zucchini, etc.)

1 onion, sliced into strips

¼ cup cashews or peanuts

¼ cup raisins

1 tablespoon curry powder (add more if you like)

1. Combine rice and water in a rice cooker.
2. While the rice is cooking, in a large deep pan, bring oil to medium-high heat. Add the other ingredients; sauté until raisins are plump and curry powder is fully incorporated, about 3–5 minutes.
3. Add rice; stir and cook until rice is evenly distributed among the vegetables and the color is uniform, about 8–10 minutes. Add salt to taste.

Serve with plain yogurt or just a squeeze of lemon juice.

NOTE› Jasmine rice works well in this dish.

TIP As you become more comfortable with the dish, add chopped fresh ginger, cilantro, or diced cooked potatoes. Chicken or garbanzo beans are great additions also.

PER SERVING› **Energy** 451 cal • **Fat** 15 g • **Sodium** 196 mg • **Carbs** 72 g • **Fiber** 9 g • **Protein** 11 g

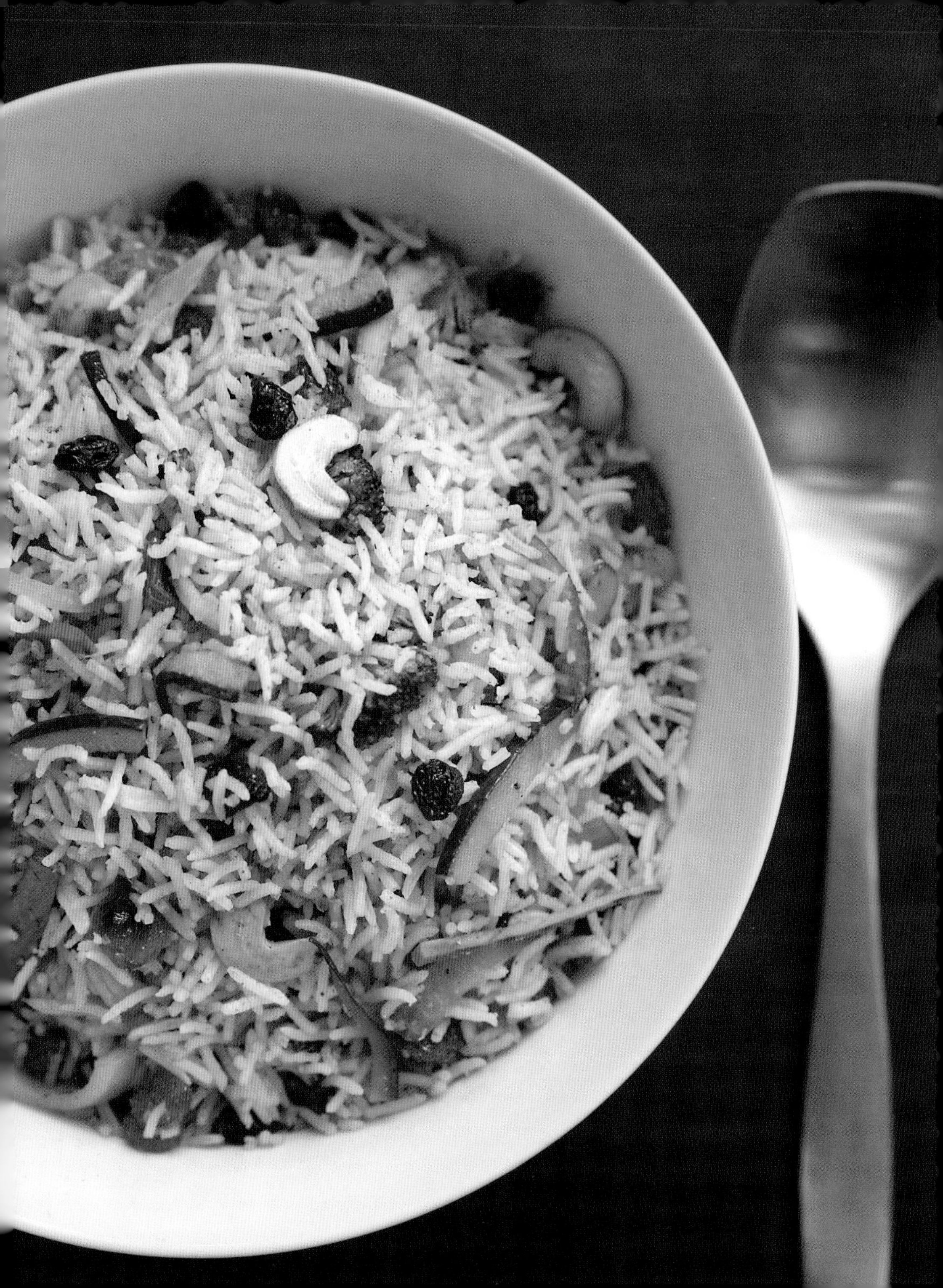

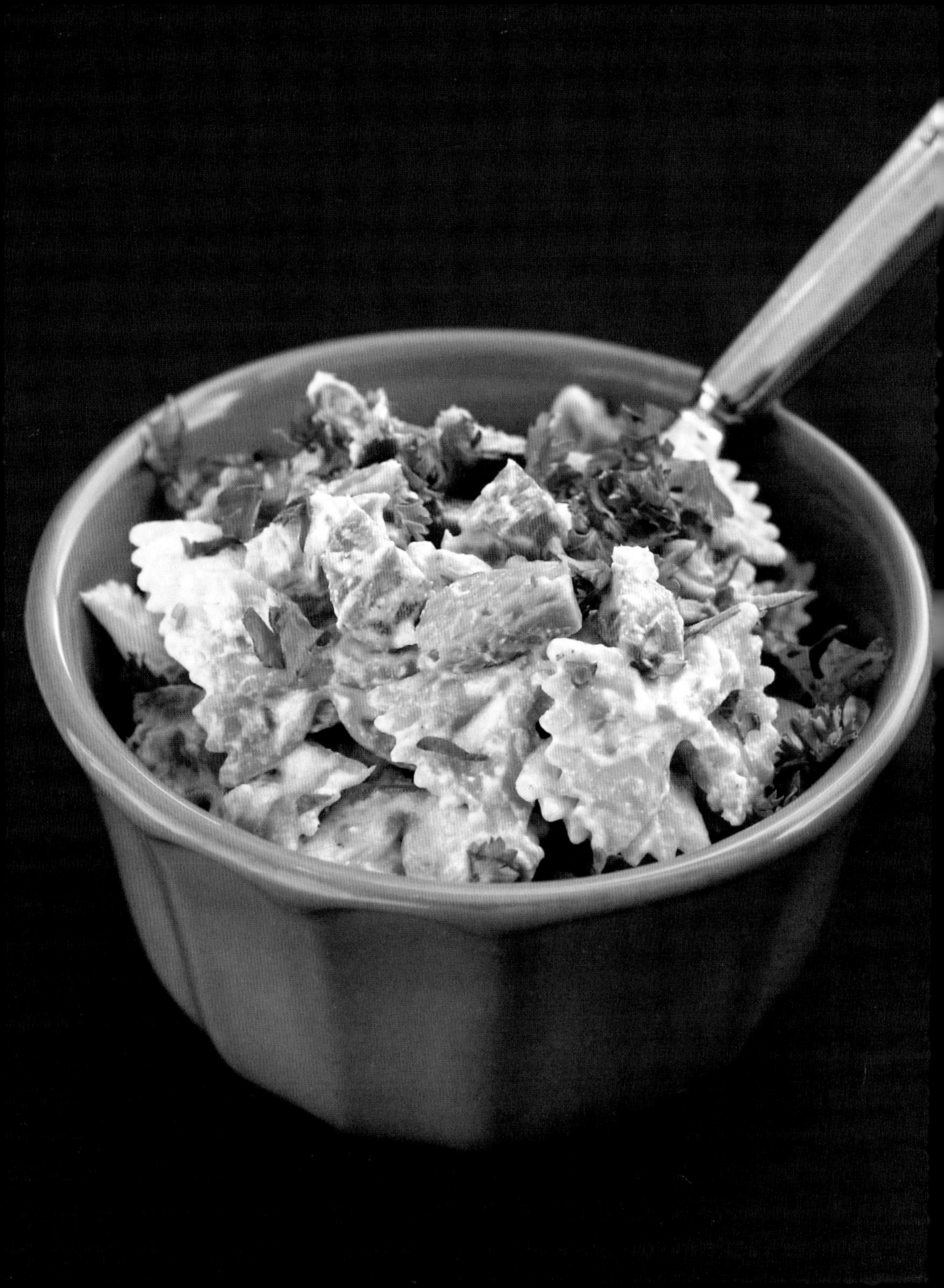

SERVINGS› 2
TIME› 20 minutes

Pasta with Smoked Salmon

This is a lighter take on a classic dish normally made with smoked salmon, cream, and butter. You can use cooked salmon or canned salmon instead of the smoked variety.

8 ounces farfalle (or other medium-size pasta)

3 ounces smoked salmon

1 cup yogurt (if using Greek yogurt add a splash of water)

½ cup low-sodium stock, water, or milk

1 small tomato, diced

½ cup carrots, diced

½ cup green peas (frozen peas and carrots are a fine substitute for fresh)

¼ cup chopped fresh parsley

OPTIONAL ADDITIONS

fresh tarragon, capers, and/or chopped green olives

1. Cook the pasta according to package directions to be al dente (10–11 minutes). Drain. Toss with a small amount of olive oil; set aside.
2. Remove any bones from the salmon and flake the meat with a fork.
3. In a large deep saucepan, whisk together the yogurt and stock. The consistency should be thick. Set over medium heat and bring to a gentle boil, stirring continually. Simmer.
4. Add tomato, carrots, peas, and parsley. Cook 5–6 minutes, or until carrots are tender. Add cooked pasta and salmon (and any optional ingredients), mix thoroughly, and remove from heat.

To finish the dish, add salt and pepper to taste, and offer grated parmesan and fresh lemon juice as condiments.

PER SERVING› **Energy** 584 cal • **Fat** 5 g • **Sodium** 1,032 mg • **Carbs** 106 g • **Fiber** 8 g • **Protein** 33 g

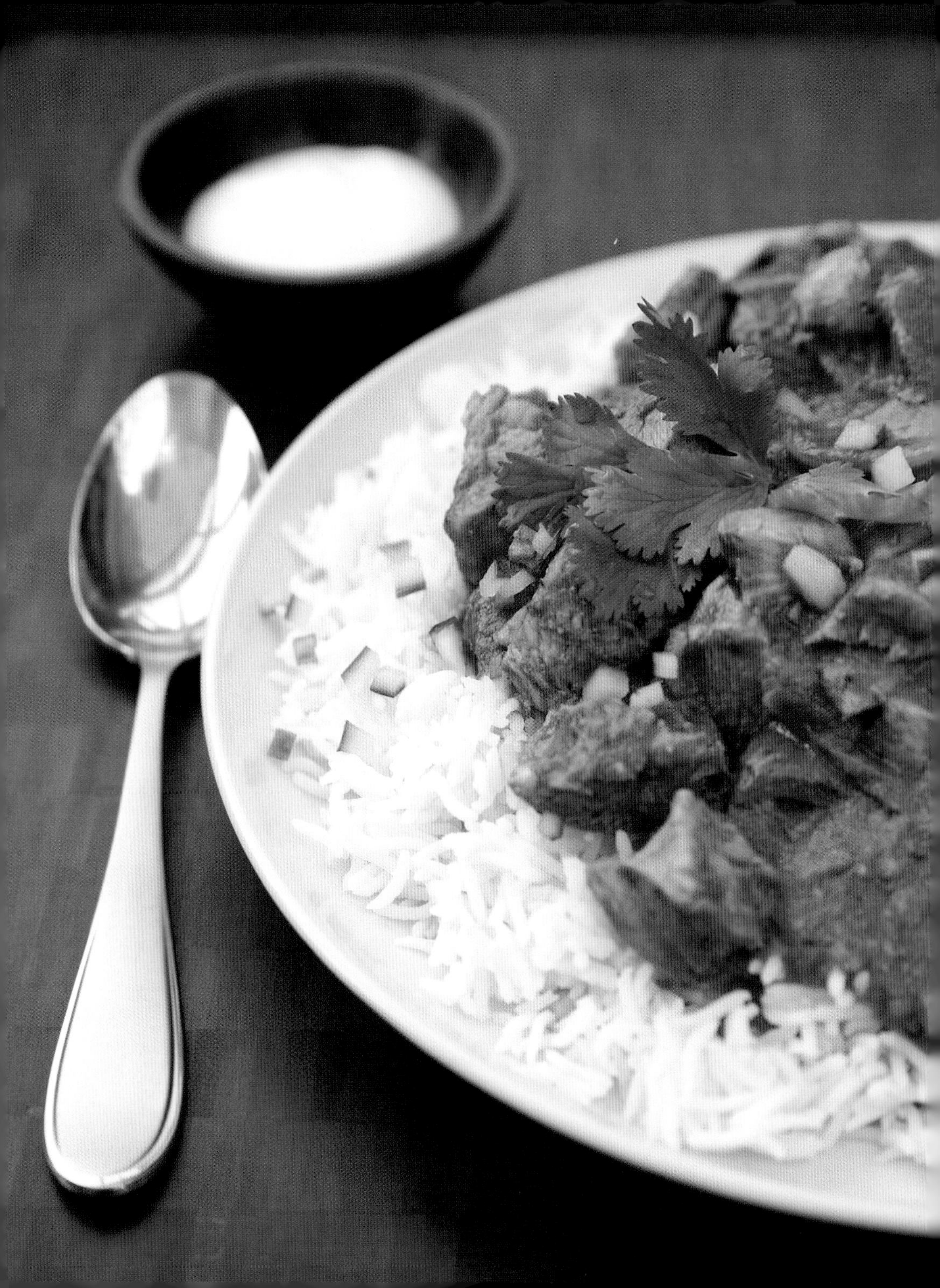

SERVINGS› 8
TIME› 1½ to 2 hours,
including time to marinate

Chicken Tikka Masala

Here's my version of the classic Indian dish reduced to the absolute basic ingredients. You should definitely experiment with adding more spices and heat as you're making this at home. Be sure to start marinating the chicken at least an hour before you plan to cook.

2 pounds chicken, cut into bite-size pieces

1 cup tomato sauce

1 cup plain yogurt

2 tablespoons curry powder

1 cup sliced onions

1 teaspoon salt

OPTIONAL ADDITIONS

minced fresh ginger

2–4 green chiles, cut into strips

1. Combine all ingredients (including optional additions, if desired) in a bowl. Let marinate for at least 1 hour in the fridge.
2. Heat oven to 375 degrees. Transfer chicken in marinade to a deep oven-proof dish; cover with foil. Bake until chicken is thoroughly cooked, about 1 hour. (Or prepare on stove top: Bring to a simmer and cook over medium heat for approximately 30 minutes.) Add salt and pepper to taste.

Garnish with chopped cilantro. Serve in bowl as a spicy stew or with steamed rice.

PER SERVING› **Energy** 399 cal • **Fat** 5 g • **Sodium** 574 mg • **Carbs** 8 g • **Fiber** 1 g • **Protein** 38 g
Nutrition for optional additions can be found in Appendix A.

SERVINGS› 4
TIME› 30 minutes

Grilled Chicken with Summer Orzo

This is a great way to combine good carbs with summer grilling while keeping the bad fats and mystery ingredients out. Coriander has a nice warm flavor that goes well with summer vegetables, but feel free to play around with other herbs and spices that sound good to you.

GRILLED CHICKEN

2 tablespoons olive oil

juice of ½ a lemon

1 teaspoon chopped garlic

1 teaspoon ground coriander or cumin

2 pounds boneless, skinless chicken breasts, cut into cubes

SUMMER ORZO

8 ounces orzo, toasted (see note)

2 large carrots, peeled and minced

¼ cup diced tomatoes

1 tablespoon minced parsley

1 teaspoon each of minced onion and minced garlic

2 tablespoons olive oil

1 tablespoon fresh orange juice

juice of ½ a lemon

2–3 tablespoons crumbled feta cheese

1. To make the grilled chicken: In a large bowl, mix together the oil, lemon juice, garlic, coriander or cumin, and a dash each of salt and pepper. Add the chicken and stir to coat all sides.
2. Either skewer and grill, or put in a hot sauté pan with a little oil until the chicken is golden on all sides and cooked through, about 12 minutes.
3. To make the orzo: Before adding the water, first toast the orzo in a dry pan over medium-high heat. Watch closely so that it doesn't burn. Then add water and cook orzo according to package directions. Drain.
4. Combine rest of ingredients with orzo in a medium bowl, adding salt and pepper to taste.

Spoon orzo onto a big plate. Set cooked skewers of chicken over pasta. Top with a dollop of yogurt, fresh chopped herbs, and a sprinkle of coarse salt.

NOTE› Toasting the orzo adds a nice nutty taste to the pasta.

PER SERVING› Energy 311 cal • Fat 14 g • Sodium 29 mg • Carbs 1 g • Fiber 0 g • Protein 53 g
ORZO (1 cup)› Energy 263 cal • Fat 9 g • Sodium 171 mg • Carbs 38 g • Fiber 1 g • Protein 7 g

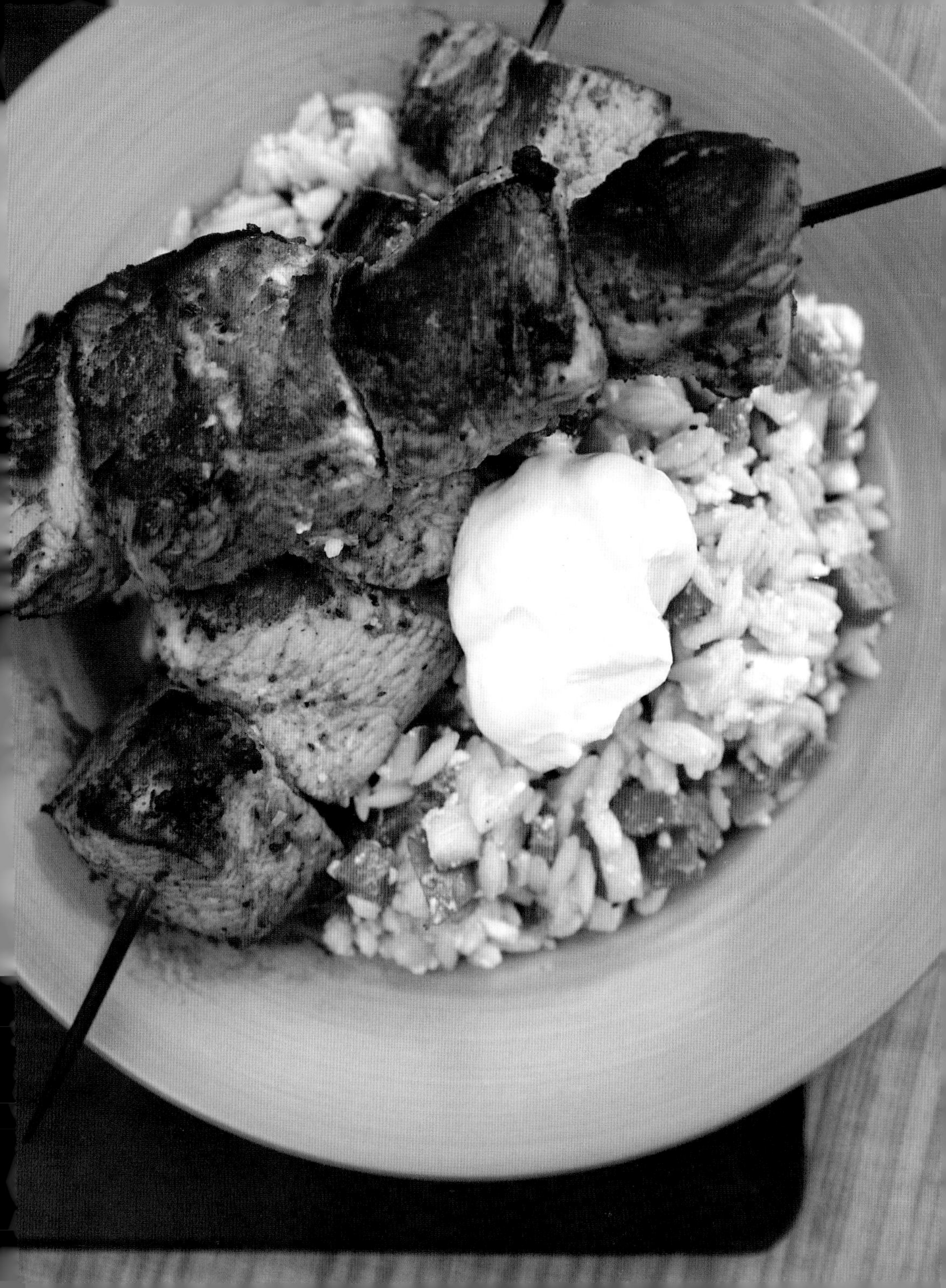

★ Millet Salad (page 278) is a great accompaniment to fish and full of protein.

SERVINGS› 2
TIME› 10 minutes

Lemon and Herb Salmon

This dish uses a very simple poaching technique to make a light and simply seasoned salmon. Salmon pairs well with simple carbs like rice or couscous, or you might try a millet salad like the one shown here. Millet has a nutty, crunchy flavor that is especially good with fish.

½ of a lemon, sliced

a few sprigs of fresh herbs: parsley, thyme, basil, cilantro

2 small salmon filets (3–4 ounces each)

1. In a wide pan bring to a gentle boil 1 inch of water. Add the lemon slices and herb sprigs.
2. Place salmon, skin side down, into the poaching liquid. It will begin to turn opaque in 3–4 minutes. Turn over; continue cooking until flesh is evenly pink. Remove the skin (it should pull off easily) and set filets on paper towels to drain.

Add salt, pepper, and lemon juice to taste, along with a touch of butter or olive oil.

PER SERVING› **Energy** 132 cal • **Fat** 4 g • **Sodium** 213 mg • **Carbs** 2 g • **Fiber** 1 g • **Protein** 23 g

SERVINGS› 6
TIME› 1½ hours

Meatballs in Red Wine Sauce

This is a one-pot dinner recipe to make you famous among your friends. Make sure your pot is large enough. It's really a three-step process: First make and brown the meatballs. Then, in the same pot, make the sauce. Last, return the meatballs to the sauce to stew while you revel in your kitchen skills.

MEATBALLS

1 pound ground beef
1 pound spicy Italian bulk sausage
2 eggs, lightly beaten
2 tablespoons grated parmesan
1 cup bread crumbs (see note)
dry basil leaves and red pepper flakes
¼ cup olive oil

RED WINE SAUCE

½ cup chopped onion
2 tablespoons minced garlic
½ cup diced bell peppers
½ cup diced fresh tomato
1 small can (4 ounces) tomato paste
1 cup water
1 cup crushed tomatoes
½ cup red wine
¼ cup balsamic vinegar
1 tablespoon brown sugar
chopped fresh parsley and basil

1. To make the meatballs: Place ingredients in a large bowl and blend together by hand, making sure that bread crumbs are worked evenly into mixture. Let rest in fridge for 30 minutes. Shape to be the size of golf balls.
2. Bring ¼ cup olive oil to medium-high heat in a large pot, then add a few meatballs and brown them on all sides. Remove them from the pot as they finish browning, adding more oil as needed. (The meatballs will finish cooking in the sauce.)
3. To make the sauce: Keeping the heat on medium, add the onions, garlic, peppers, and tomatoes to the pot and sauté until the onions are translucent.
4. Add the remaining ingredients in the order shown, thoroughly incorporating each item into the sauce before adding the next.
5. Keep scraping the bottom of the pan while the sauce cooks. Bring sauce to a low boil, then return the meatballs to the pot. Let simmer, covered, until cooked thoroughly, approximately 30–40 minutes. Adjust salt.

Makes 12 meatballs. Serve with your favorite pasta.

NOTE› To make bread crumbs, pulse stale or hard bread in a food processor.

PER SERVING (2 meatballs & sauce)› **Energy** 449 cal • **Fat** 27 g • **Sodium** 748 mg • **Carbs** 15 g • **Fiber** 2 g • **Protein** 33 g

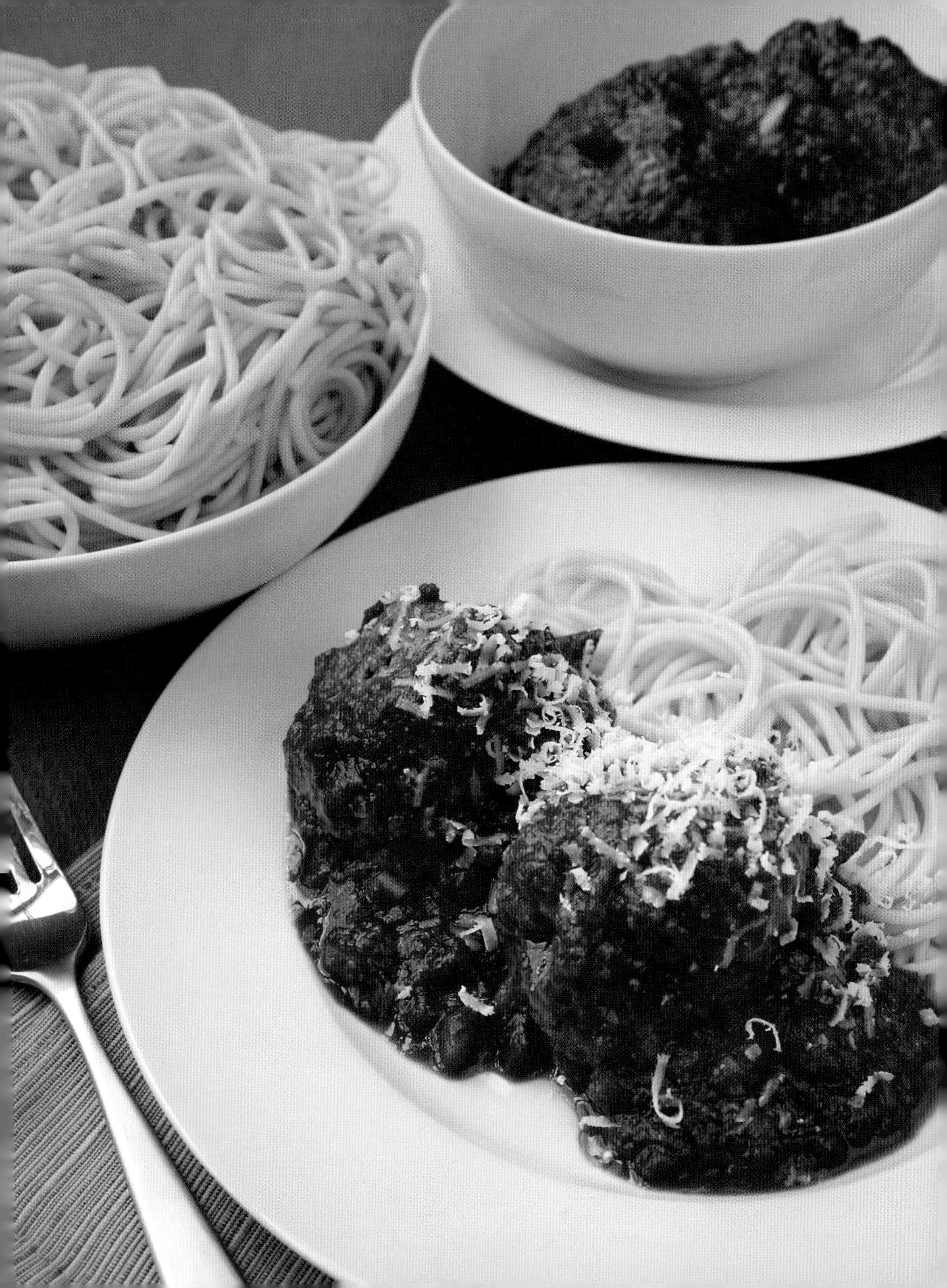

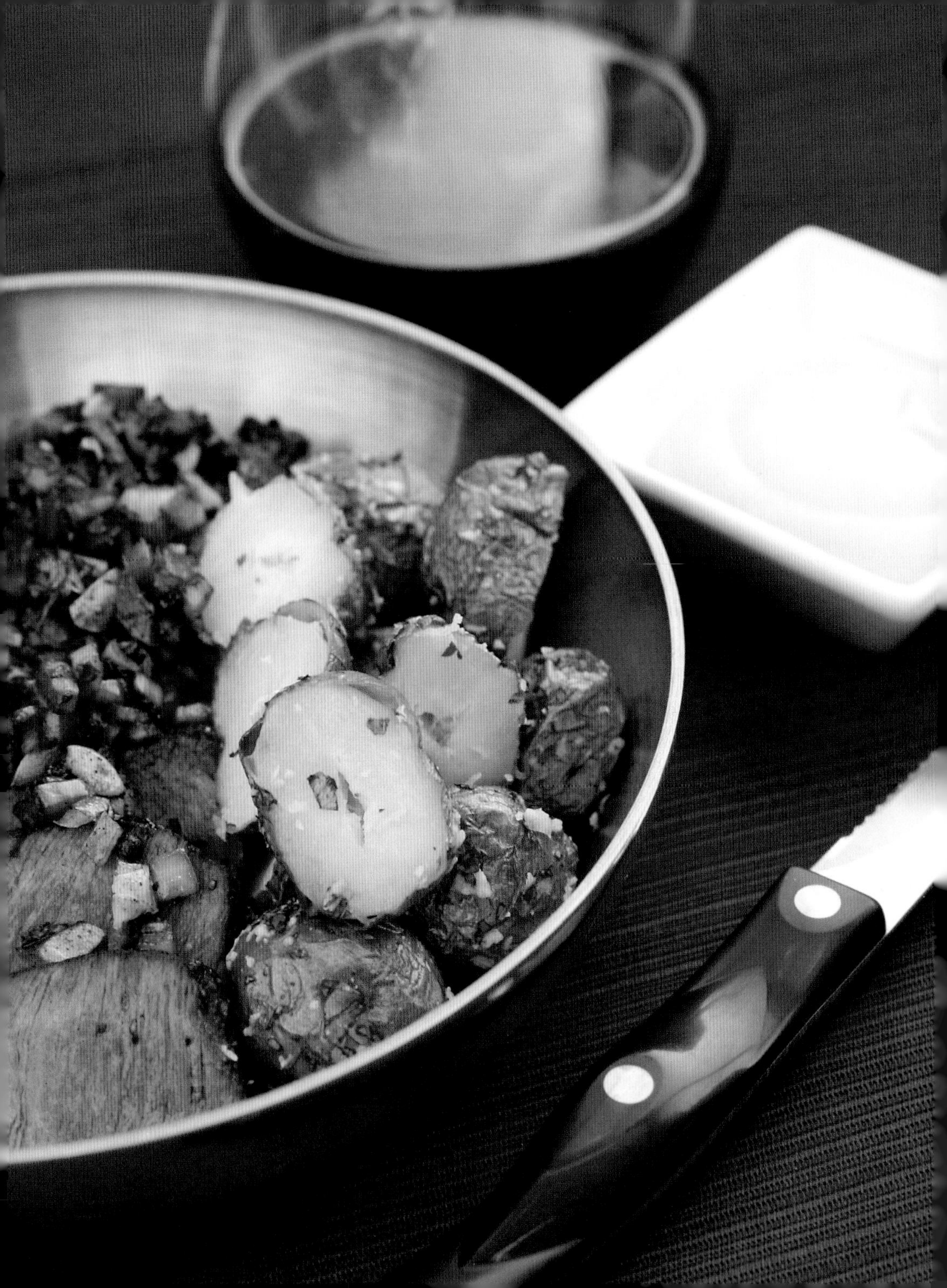

SERVINGS› 2–4
TIME› 25 minutes

Flatiron Steak with Mustard Sauce

I'm a fan of flatiron steak because I really like the texture, and it costs less than many other cuts. Skirt or flank steak also works well prepared this way.

1–2 pounds flatiron steaks, trimmed of excess fat

olive oil, salt, pepper, and sugar for rubbing the steak

1 tablespoon olive oil

1 teaspoon each minced garlic, onion, and parsley

1 teaspoon whole peppercorns (mixed color if you have them)

MUSTARD SAUCE

2 tablespoons Dijon or whole-grain mustard

¼ cup yogurt

1 tablespoon apple cider vinegar

1. Heat oven to 375 degrees. Rub steaks with a bit of oil, salt, pepper, and a sprinkle of sugar.
2. Place a large oven-safe sauté pan over high heat. When it is hot, add the steaks and sear each side. Add 1 tablespoon olive oil, the garlic, onion, and parsley, and the peppercorns to the side of the pan. Let cook for a few seconds, until the peppercorns get a nice shine and begin to plump.
3. Transfer sauté pan to the oven and let cook until steaks are done to your liking, about 8–10 minutes total. (I personally go with a medium to medium-rare.) Remove steaks from pan and let rest while you make the sauce.
4. To make the mustard sauce: Into the hot pan add mustard, yogurt, and vinegar (this may splatter, so keep a lid handy). Stir; add salt and pepper to taste.

Slice steaks against the grain. Arrange on plates, then spoon the mustard sauce over the steaks.

TIP This works best in a pan that is not nonstick.

PER SERVING (8 oz. steak)› **Energy** 448 cal • **Fat** 24 g • **Sodium** 160 mg • **Carbs** 11 g • **Fiber** 0 g • **Protein** 52 g
MUSTARD SAUCE (2 tbsp.)› **Energy** 21 cal • **Fat** 1 g • **Sodium** 239 mg • **Carbs** 1 g • **Fiber** 0 g • **Protein** 1 g

SERVINGS› 2
TIME› 50 minutes

Corn Cakes with Crisp Chicken

Corn cakes can feel like an indulgence after lots of pasta and rice. This is a beautiful dish, but it doesn't have to be difficult. If you are pressed for time, prepare the corn cake dough in advance and use rotisserie chicken.

CORN CAKES

1 cup masa harina (ground corn flour)

1 teaspoon salt

1 teaspoon brown sugar

¾ cup boiling water

1 tablespoon grapeseed or canola oil

CRISP CHICKEN

COOKED 2 cups cooked and shredded chicken

½ cup thinly sliced onions

1 tablespoon chopped garlic

1 jalapeno, sliced into thin strips

1 tablespoon ground cumin powder

¼ cup raisins

2 tablespoons chopped fresh cilantro

¼ cup queso fresca or soft goat cheese (optional)

1. To make the corn cakes: In a bowl, mix together all ingredients except oil until it forms a ball. Let rest for about 30 minutes. Separate into 8 smaller rounds. Press each into the palm of your hand to make a thick little cake about 3–4 inches in diameter.
2. Heat a dry nonstick sauté pan over medium-high heat. Toast the cakes on both sides and set aside. They are only partially cooked at this point. (You can wrap and store the cakes in the fridge at this stage and then finish right before you're ready to eat.)
3. Add 1 tablespoon of oil to the pan and heat to medium-high. Fry 2 or 3 cakes at a time, until each is crisp on both sides, about 3 minutes.
4. To make the crisp chicken: Place cooked chicken, onions, garlic, jalapeno, and cumin in a hot pan with a bit of oil; sauté. When chicken begins to crisp, add raisins and mix thoroughly. Turn off heat. Add cilantro and cheese, if using. Add salt and pepper to taste.

Onto each corn cake, pile cooked chicken mixture. Top with additional cilantro, crumbled cheese, a dash of salt, and lime juice.

CHICKEN› **Energy** 355 cal • **Fat** 7 g • **Sodium** 189 mg • **Carbs** 19 g • **Fiber** 2 g • **Protein** 55 g
CORN CAKES (3 cakes)› **Energy** 276 cal • **Fat** 9 g • **Sodium** 1,166 mg • **Carbs** 47 g • **Fiber** 8 g • **Protein** 4 g
Nutrition for optional addition can be found in Appendix A.

★ Top it off with Chocolate and Balsamic Vinegar (page 294).

SERVINGS› 1+
TIME› 20 minutes

Pan-Seared Steak

It's surprisingly easy to make a good steak. Coriander brings a hint of citrus and sage to the sugar, salt, and pepper rub used here. When you have the time to make some tomato jam, you'll find it enhances the flavor even more.

- 4–6 ounces ribeye or tenderloin steak per serving
- salt, pepper, sugar, and ground coriander to rub
- a few thick slices of rustic bread per serving
- Tomato Jam (page 289)
- 1 small bunch of radishes, sliced thin
- crumbled blue or goat cheese
- juice of ½ a lemon

1. Rub steaks with salt, pepper, a sprinkle of sugar, and a dash of ground coriander. Heat a lightly oiled sauté pan to medium-high.
2. Sear the steaks in the hot pan. After second side has seared, turn heat to medium and cook to desired degree of doneness, about 10–12 minutes total. Let rest for a few minutes while you grill the bread.
3. Brush both sides of bread with butter or oil. Grill in hot pan or under broiler until both sides are crisp.

Set steak (whole or sliced) atop grilled bread and spoon some tomato jam on top. Garnish with sliced radishes and crumbled cheese. Squeeze lemon over steak and add freshly ground black pepper to taste.

TIP It's important to let the steak rest before serving. A bit of extra time allows the delicious juices to be reabsorbed.

PER SERVING› **Energy** 629 cal • **Fat** 20 g • **Sodium** 1,085 mg • **Carbs** 66 g • **Fiber** 4 g • **Protein** 44 g

* Tomato Jam (page 289) tastes great with steak.

★ Peach Chutney (page 290) complements the salty pork flavors.

SERVINGS› 4
TIME› 30 minutes

Pork Loin with Chutney

This grilled pork is a delightful mix of salty and sweet. For an athlete in the midst of a challenging bout of training, this can be just what the body needs. Couscous with Currants (page 279) is one of my favorite carbs to serve with this dish because it shows off the spicy fruit flavors so well.

2 tablespoons Peach Chutney (page 290), plus additional for serving

2 tablespoons olive oil

1 pound pork loin

salt, pepper, and sugar to rub

1. In a small bowl, combine 2 tablespoons of chutney with an equal amount of olive oil to make a glaze for the pork.
2. Heat the grill. Rub the pork with a good sprinkle of salt, pepper, and sugar.
3. Grill pork to at least medium doneness, 12–15 minutes total. Just before pork is done, brush it generously with the glaze. Let rest for a few minutes before slicing.

Top sliced pork with chutney. Serve with couscous or grilled bread and your favorite sides.

TIP Pork chops are also great prepared this way.

PER SERVING› **Energy** 426 cal • **Fat** 17 g • **Sodium** 1,221 mg • **Carbs** 40 g • **Fiber** 3 g • **Protein** 30 g

SERVINGS› 4
TIME› 20 minutes prep,
1 hour to marinate

Bison with Spice Rub

Long popular in Europe, hanging tender (sometimes called hanger steak) is becoming more common in American restaurants and is available through local butchers. It's an intensely flavored, lean, slightly chewy and grainy cut that does well with strong marinades and sauces. If you can't find hanging tender, use another thin, low-fat cut of meat, such as skirt or flank steak. This cut is best served medium-rare or medium.

2 pounds bison or beef hanging tender

1 tablespoon brown sugar

1 teaspoon coarse salt

2 teaspoons curry powder

1 teaspoon ground cardamom

1 teaspoon coarse-ground black pepper

1. Trim meat of excess fat. Combine remaining ingredients in a small bowl and rub thoroughly over all sides of the meat. Let rest for at least 1 hour or overnight in fridge.
2. Bring a lightly oiled sauté pan to high heat. Sear meat on all sides; the sugar in the spice mixture will produce a nice crust.
3. Either finish cooking in the pan to desired doneness or place pan (check that it's ovenproof) in an oven heated to 400 degrees. Total cooking time will vary but shouldn't take more than 12–15 minutes.

Let steak rest for 3–5 minutes before being cut. Slice thinly against the grain. Serve with polenta, potatoes, rice, or salad.

TIP Once the meat is rubbed in the spice mixture, you can keep it refrigerated for up to 3 days.

PER SERVING› **Energy** 389 cal • **Fat** 11 g • **Sodium** 598 mg • **Carbs** 2 g • **Fiber** 0 g • **Protein** 67 g

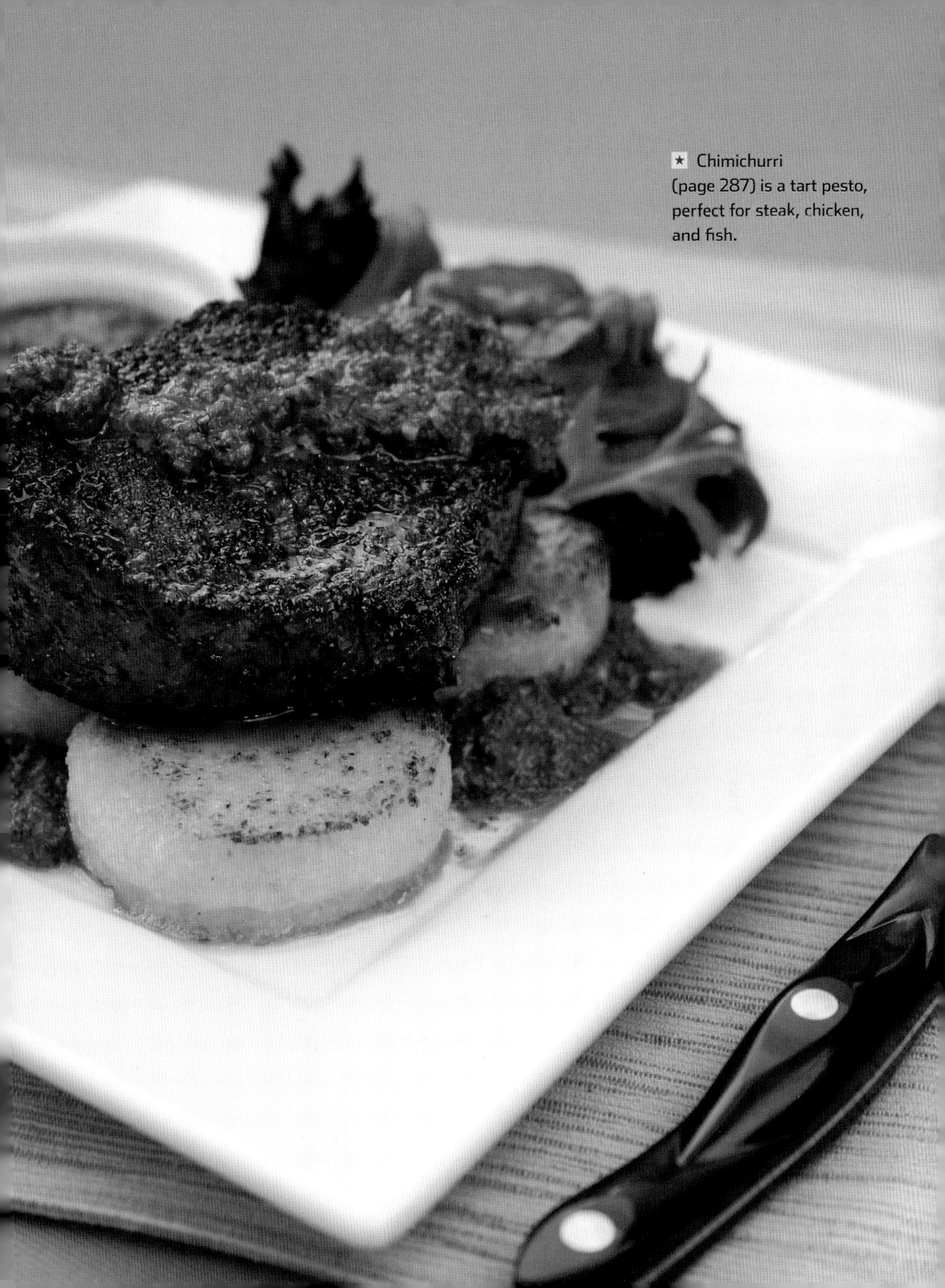

★ Chimichurri (page 287) is a tart pesto, perfect for steak, chicken, and fish.

SERVINGS› 4
TIME› 40 minutes

Ground Turkey Shepherd's Pie

This is a simple revision of a classic comfort food we all grew up eating. Ground turkey makes this dish a bit lighter, but you can still get your meat-and-potatoes fix.

2 pounds potatoes
1 tablespoon butter
¼ cup milk
dash each of ground nutmeg, salt, and pepper
1 pound ground turkey
½ onion, minced
2 cloves garlic, minced
1 tomato, diced
2 tablespoons molasses or brown sugar
¼ cup ketchup
splash of low-sodium soy sauce

OPTIONAL ADDITIONS
(1 teaspoon of any)

ground cinnamon, ground cumin, chili powder, celery salt, nutmeg

1. Boil potatoes on stove top or cook them in microwave on high heat until tender, approximately 8–10 minutes. Let cool and then peel skins and cut into large cubes.
2. In large bowl, combine cooked potatoes, butter, and milk. Mash thoroughly. Add a sprinkle of nutmeg, salt, and pepper to taste. Add more milk if mixture is too dry. Set aside.
3. In a large sauté pan, brown turkey on medium-high heat. Add remaining ingredients. Cover; let simmer for about 10 minutes, and then adjust seasonings to taste.
4. Heat oven to 375 degrees. Oil an 8-inch square or 9-inch round baking pan. Spread the cooked turkey in the bottom of the pan. Top with potato mixture. Bake 20 minutes or until peaks of potatoes turn golden.

Let cool a bit, garnish with fresh chopped herbs or freshly grated cheese, and serve.

PER SERVING› **Energy** 449 cal • **Fat** 4 g • **Sodium** 486 mg • **Carbs** 138 g • **Fiber** 26 g • **Protein** 65 g

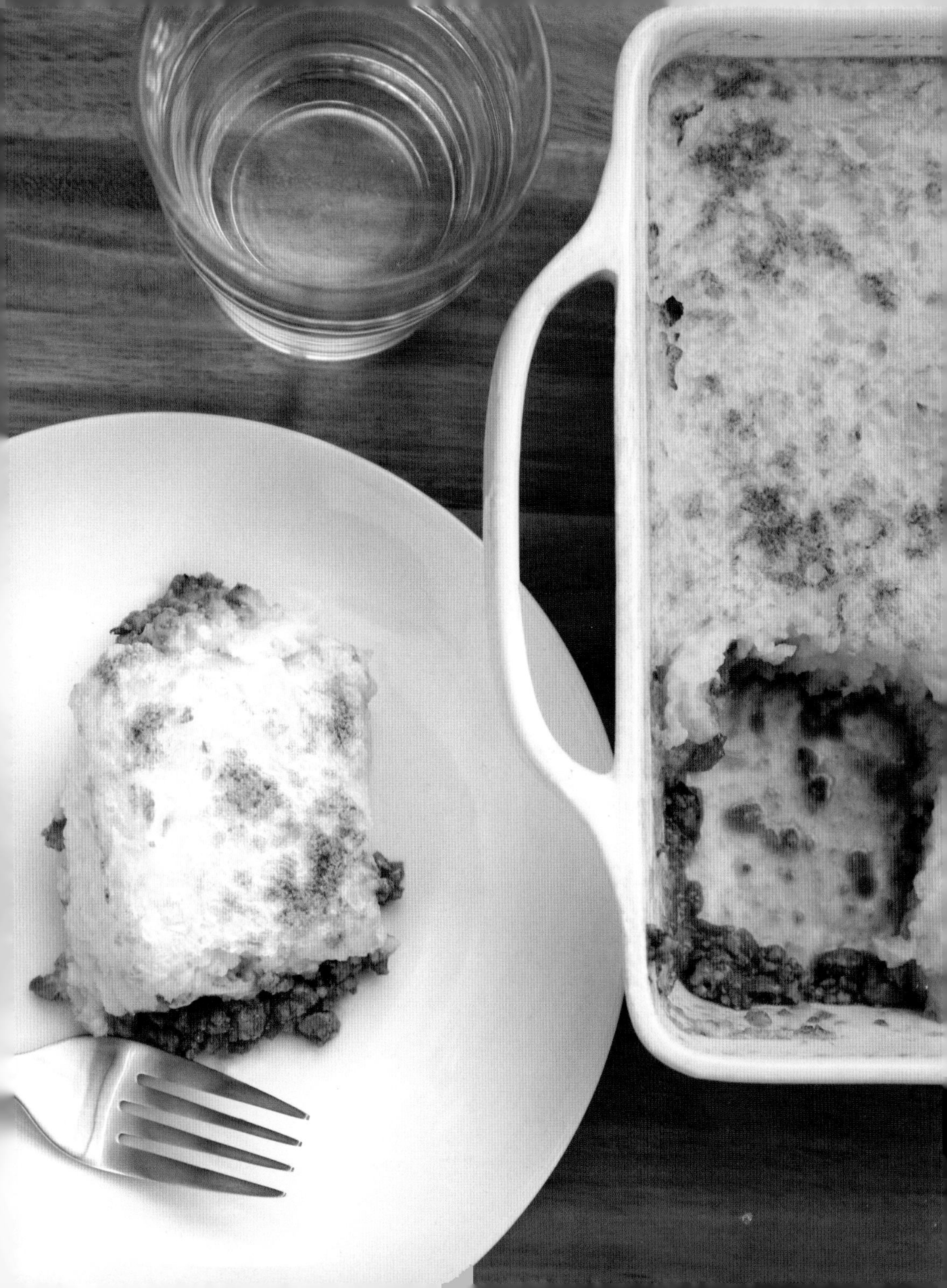

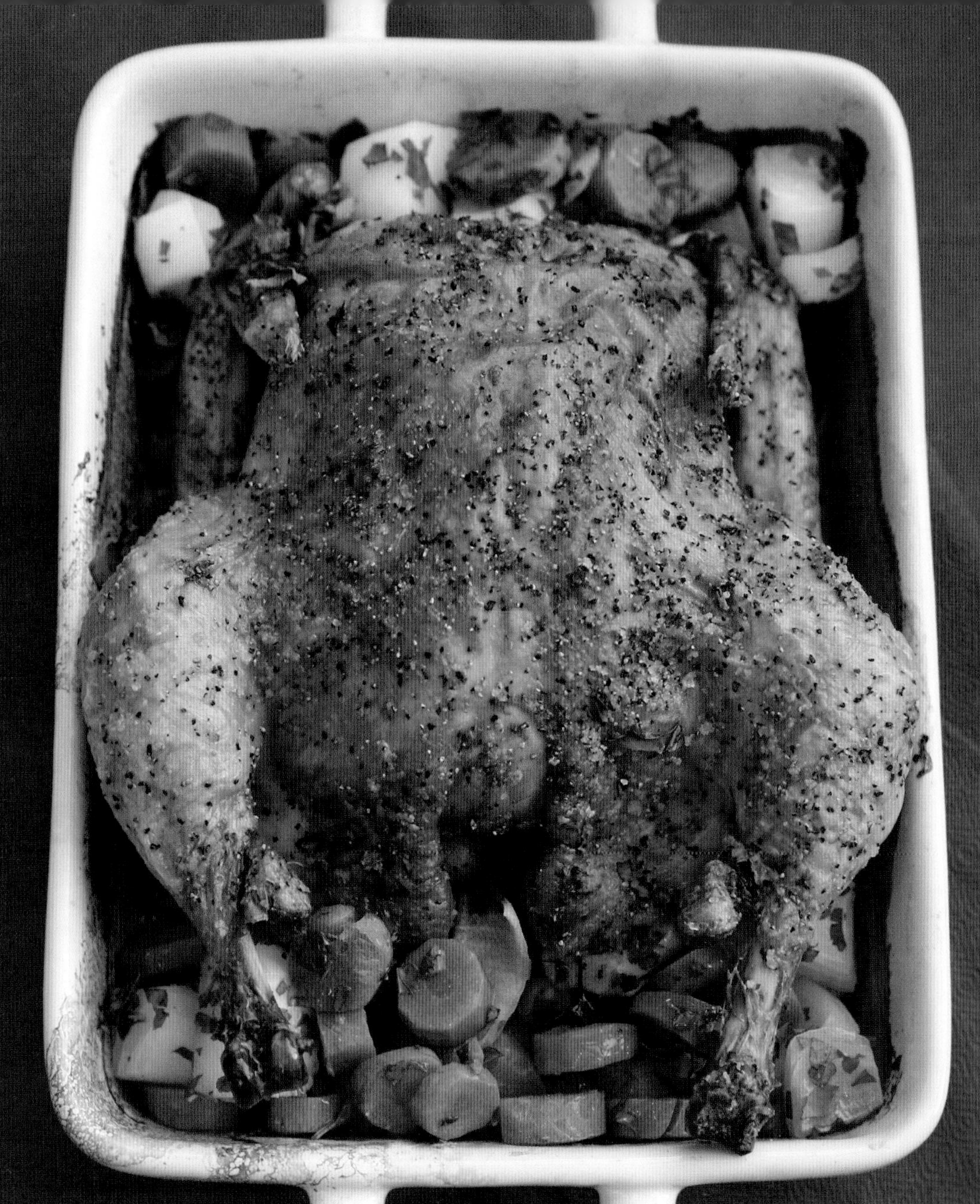

★ This goes great with Crushed Potatoes (page 283) or pasta with vegetables.

SERVINGS› 4
TIME› 15 minutes prep,
cook 90 minutes

Whole Roasted Chicken

Of course, you can easily and affordably purchase rotisserie chicken at your local market, but there's something special about roasting your own. And the leftovers are great when used in other recipes.

- **1 whole roasting chicken (about 6 pounds)**
- **¼ cup olive oil, divided use**
- **1 cup coarsely chopped carrots**
- **1 onion, cut into large chunks**
- **4–6 garlic cloves, peeled and crushed**
- **½ cup chopped fresh parsley**

OPTIONAL ADDITIONS

large chunks of potatoes, beets, parsnips, and/or turnips

1. Heat oven to 350 degrees and move racks if needed to accommodate a large roasting pan.
2. Brush chicken with some of the olive oil, then coat thoroughly with coarse salt and pepper. Place chicken, breast up, in a deep roasting pan.
3. In a bowl, combine carrots, onions, garlic, and parsley (and any optional ingredients). Add remaining olive oil to coat all surfaces, along with coarse salt and pepper to taste. Transfer vegetables to the pan alongside the chicken. Wrap in foil and let cook 1 hour.
4. Remove foil and stir vegetables. Baste (spoon the rendered fat from the bottom of the pan over the chicken). Replace foil and let cook 20 minutes.
5. Remove foil; baste. Continue to roast, uncovered, in oven until chicken has cooked thoroughly, about 90 minutes in total. Juices will run clear, outside skin will be nicely crisp, and the chicken will be tender to the touch.

Let chicken cool before cutting or taking apart.

PER SERVING› **Energy** 324 cal • **Fat** 19 g • **Sodium** 179 mg • **Carbs** 8 g • **Fiber** 2 g • **Protein** 31 g
Nutrition for optional additions can be found in Appendix A.

★★★

Every once in a while it is great to indulge. Because of this we've included some tasty desserts to satisfy your sweet tooth, finish off a great meal, or provide you with some fast and dense calories after a hard day of training.

While we normally think of desserts as a bad thing, all the reasons that make them bad—their high glycemic index, sugar and fat, and their ability to make us eat way too much—**may actually make them pretty good immediately after exercise.** Knowing this, and knowing that some people might actually sneak some dessert immediately after a ride, we use a lot of fresh fruit. For the times when you need a real morale booster, try Biju's chocolate bread pudding or flourless chocolate cake.

That all said, if you're really conscious about what you're eating, as many of the athletes we work with are, you may want to **stick with the dish that most of them eat after a race: a bowl of fresh fruit, berries, and yogurt, topped with honey and a sprinkle of Biju's ever popular toasted nut mix.**

DESSERTS

DRINKS

DESSERTS

V **VEGETARIAN**
G **GLUTEN-FREE**

MENU

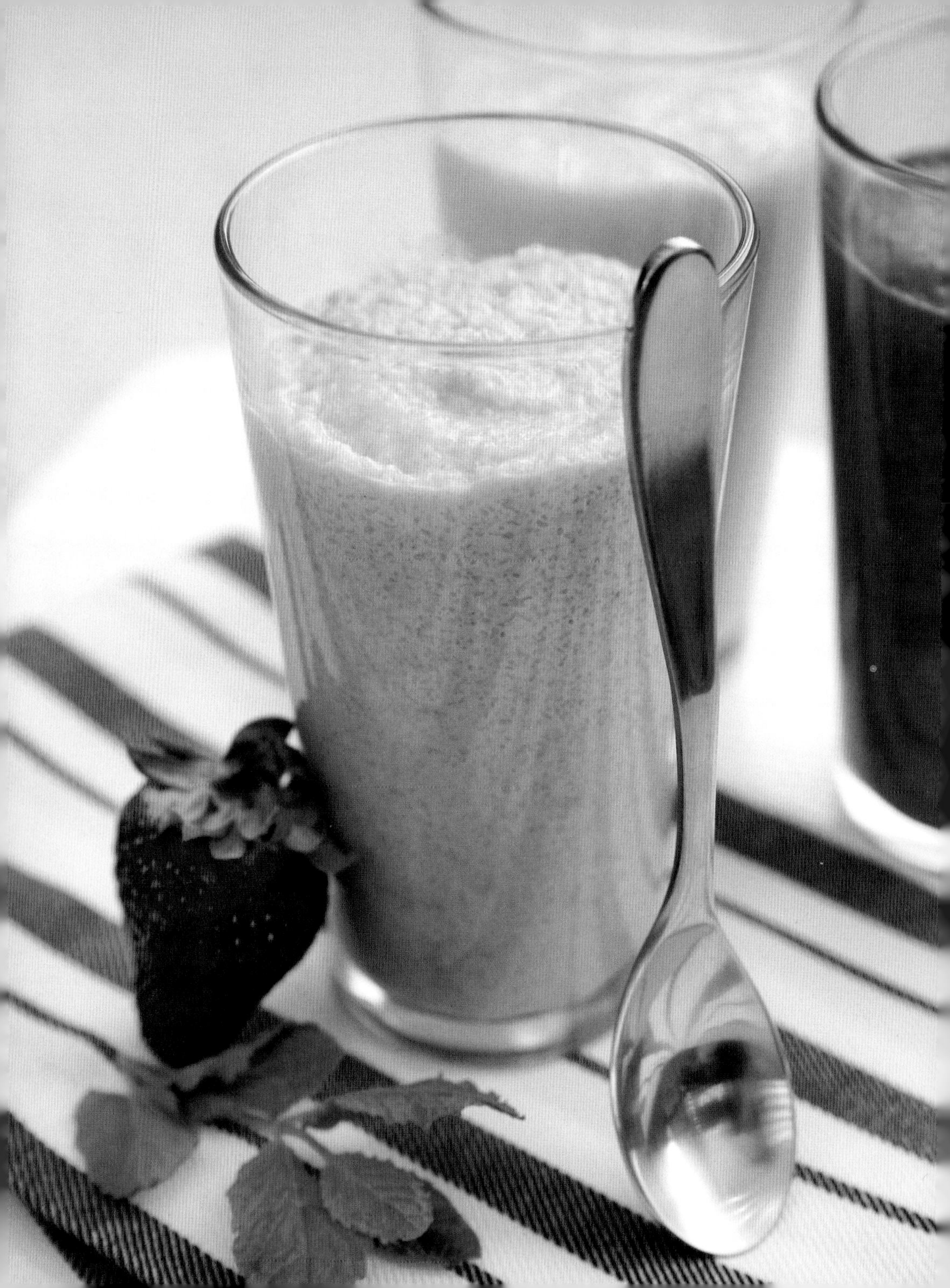

SERVINGS› 2
TIME› 5 minutes

Rice Smoothies

This smoothie works best immediately after a ride. Add ice to give it a bit more thickness, or keep a pile of ripe bananas in the freezer at all times and just add those to the blender with the other ingredients.

COOKED **1¼ cup cooked rice**
¼ cup yogurt
½ cup milk

1 ripe banana
OR
2 tablespoons Nutella
OR
½ cup strawberries

OPTIONAL ADDITIONS
protein powder
more milk to adjust thickness

1. Place all ingredients in blender and mix thoroughly, adding milk or ice to achieve desired consistency.

BANANA› **Energy** 221 cal • **Fat** 1 g • **Sodium** 60 mg • **Carbs** 49 g • **Fiber** 2 g • **Protein** 6 g
NUTELLA› **Energy** 277 cal • **Fat** 6 g • **Sodium** 69 mg • **Carbs** 47 g • **Fiber** 2 g • **Protein** 7 g
STRAWBERRY› **Energy** 179 cal • **Fat** 1 g • **Sodium** 60 mg • **Carbs** 38 g • **Fiber** 2 g • **Protein** 6 g

SERVINGS> 4
TIME> 10 minutes

Fruit and Ginger Cream

Fresh fruit and berries is a pleasant everyday dessert, but a dollop of ginger cream takes it to a whole new level. St. Germain is an elderflower liqueur with a bright flavor of berries and ginger.

1 cup mixed fresh berries and other fruit (bananas, mangos, kiwi), washed

1 cup heavy whipping cream

1 tablespoon St. Germain elderflower liqueur (see note)

1 teaspoon finely minced or grated fresh ginger

1. Slice the fruit if necessary. Set aside.
2. Using an electric mixer, whip the cream until it forms thick peaks. Fold in the St. Germain and ginger. Taste; if you want it sweeter, add more St. Germain or a bit of sugar.

Spoon whipped cream over fruits and berries. Serve with biscotti or cookies.

NOTE> If you don't have St. Germain liqueur, substitute 1 tablespoon honey.

PER SERVING (½ cup)> **Energy** 224 cal • **Fat** 23 g • **Sodium** 24 mg • **Carbs** 4 g • **Fiber** 0 g • **Protein** 0 g
Nutrition includes only ginger cream; fruit options can be found in Appendix A.

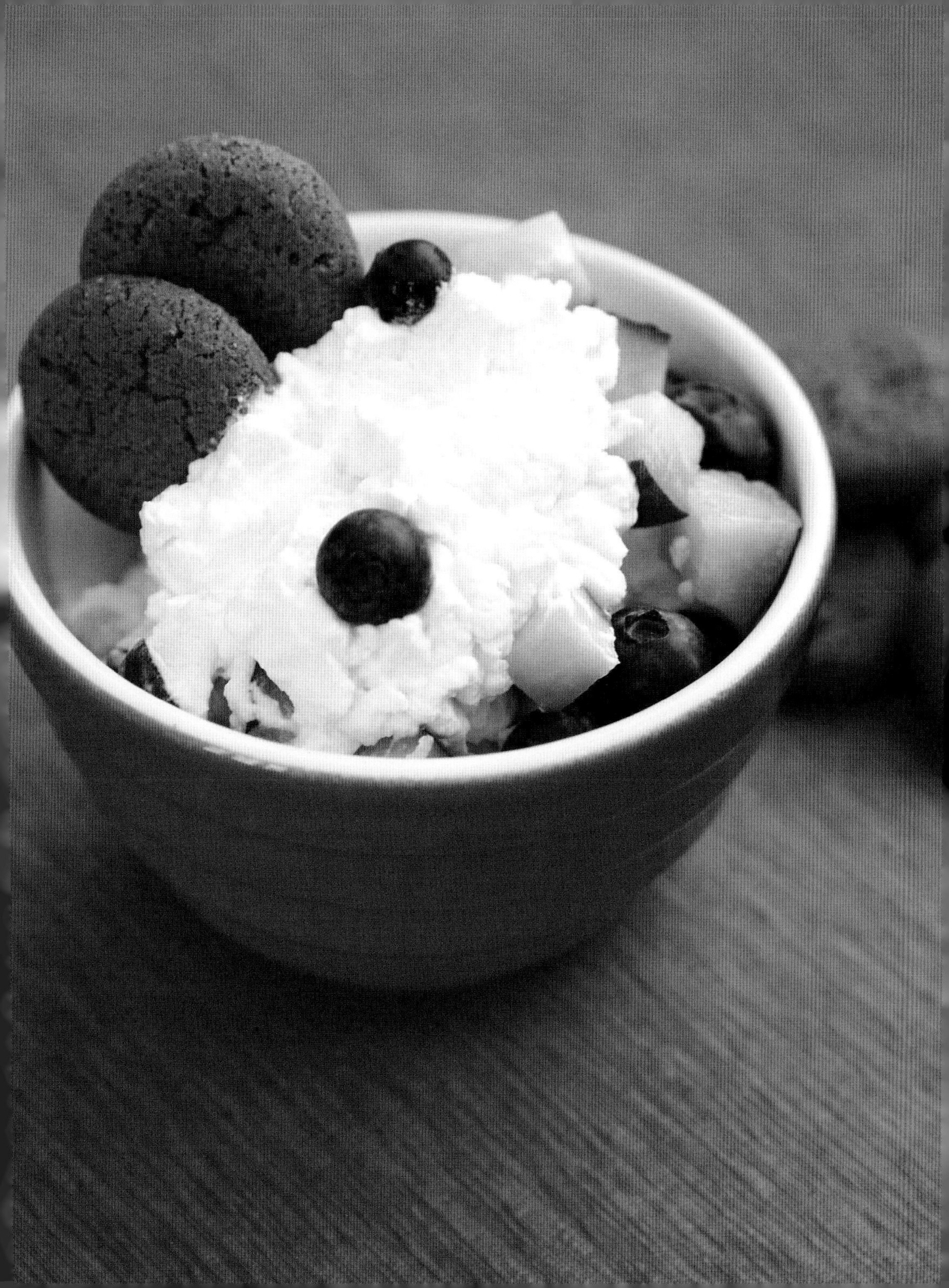

SERVINGS› 6
TIME› 40 minutes

Peach Crisp

Though this recipe features fresh peaches, you can substitute apples or other seasonally available fruits. Adjust for sweetness depending on how ripe your available fruit happens to be.

2 cups fresh peaches, peeled and sliced

½ cup flour (all-purpose or gluten-free bread mix)

½ cup "old-fashioned" rolled oats

¼ cup brown sugar

½ cup butter

OPTIONAL ADDITIONS

¼ cup chopped nuts and/or dried fruit

1 teaspoon cinnamon

1. Heat oven to 375 degrees. Lightly butter a 2-quart oven-safe dish. Arrange peach slices in bottom of dish.
2. In a bowl, mix together the flour, oats, brown sugar, and butter (a fork works well for cutting the butter into the dry ingredients). Add optional ingredients, if using.
3. Spread the mixture evenly over the peaches. Bake until top is golden brown and peaches are tender, approximately 25–35 minutes.

Serve warm, topped with ice cream or a drizzle of molasses.

PER SERVING› **Energy** 271 cal • **Fat** 16 g • **Sodium** 156 mg • **Carbs** 31 g • **Fiber** 3 g • **Protein** 3 g

Nutrition for optional additions can be found in Appendix A.

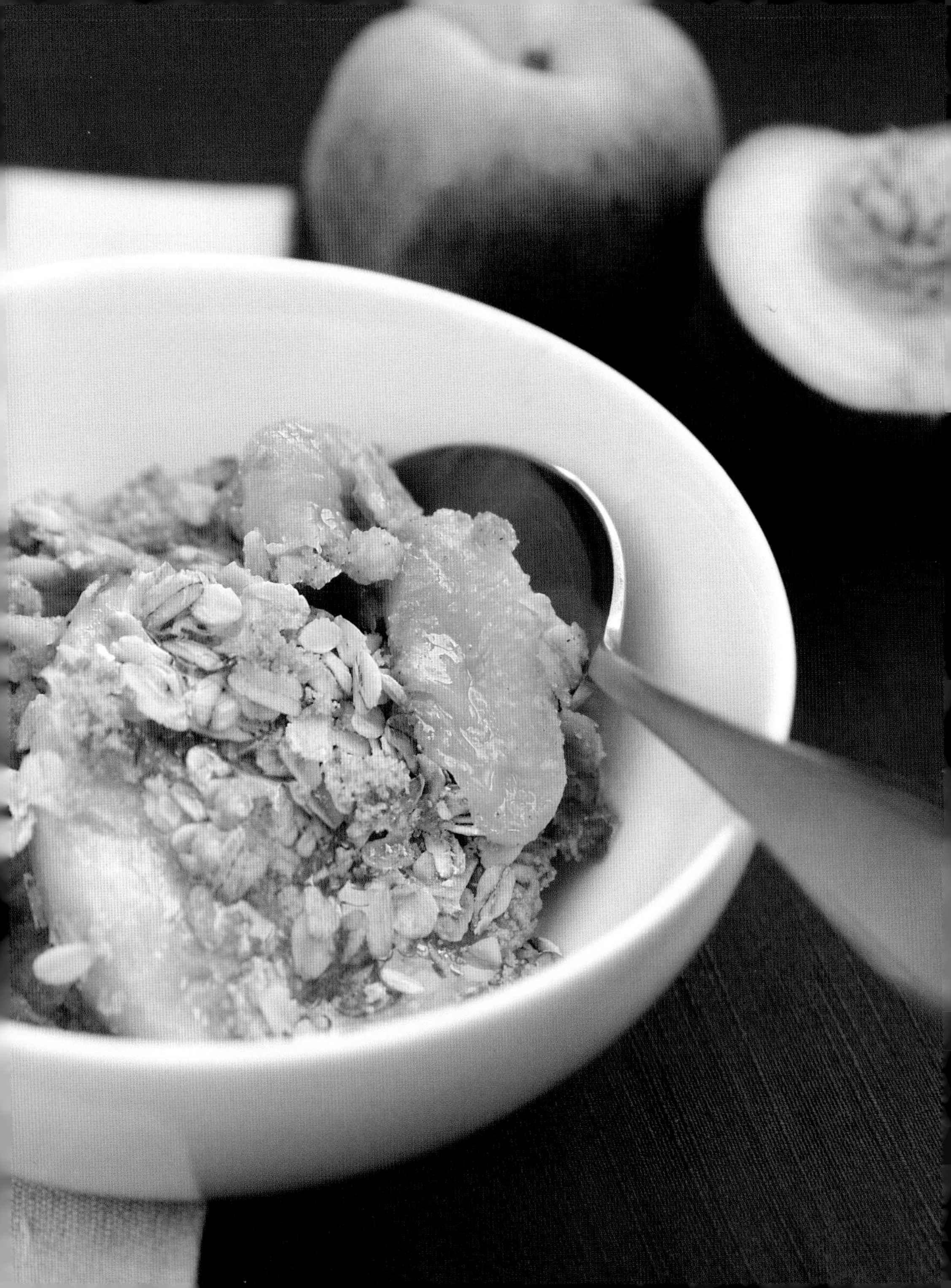

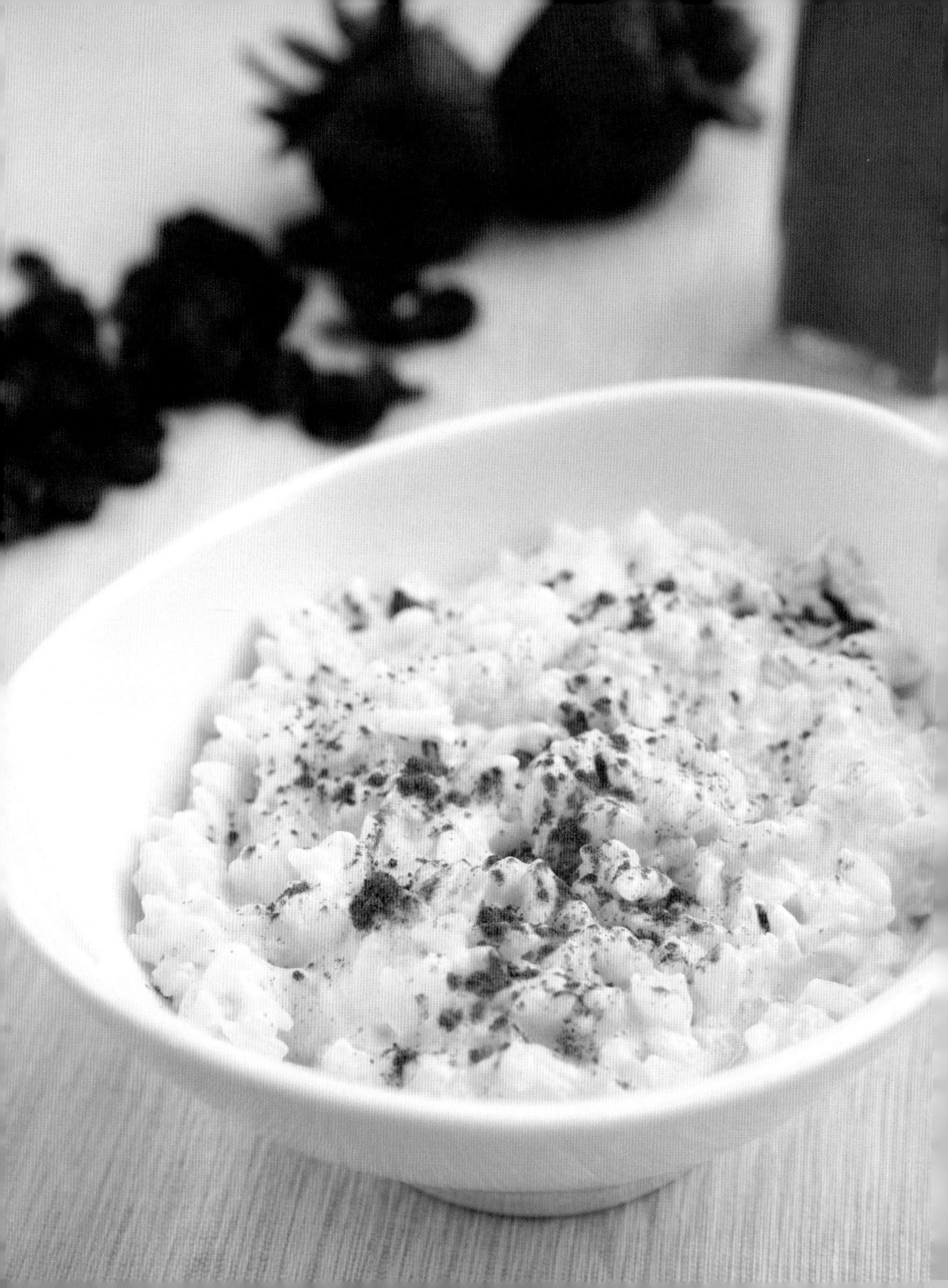

SERVINGS> 4
TIME> 5–15 minutes

Leftover Rice Pudding

This is a practical dessert that can be quickly prepared. For the best flavor, wait a few hours before eating the pudding, or make enough to have some leftover for tomorrow.

2 cups milk (any kind)

3 egg yolks

COOKED 2 cups cooked rice (see note)

2 tablespoons brown sugar

¼ teaspoon vanilla extract

OPTIONAL ADDITIONS

2 tablespoons each of your favorite dried fruits or nuts

ground cinnamon, nutmeg, or allspice

¼ cup ground pumpkin or sweet potatoes, yogurt, applesauce, or fruit jam

TO PREPARE ON THE STOVE

1. Combine the milk and egg yolks in a medium saucepan and bring to a gentle boil. Simmer.
2. Add rice, brown sugar, and vanilla. Stir, then add a dash of salt and any optional additions (see list). Simmer for a few minutes or until the mixture thickens; remove from heat and let cool.

TO PREPARE IN THE MICROWAVE

1. Combine milk, egg yolks, rice, brown sugar, and vanilla in a large bowl. Cover and heat on high for 1½ minutes.
2. Stir thoroughly, then add a dash of salt and any optional additions. Cook for 1–2 more minutes and let cool.

NOTE> If you don't have rice cooked and ready, let it cool before using.

PER SERVING> **Energy** 208 cal • **Fat** 5 g • **Sodium** 125 mg • **Carbs** 30 g • **Fiber** 2 g • **Protein** 12 g
Nutrition for optional additions can be found in Appendix A.

SERVINGS› 8
TIME› 45–60 minutes

Chocolate Bread Pudding

This is a fantastic last-minute dessert that requires no real precision. Slightly stale or older bread works best. If the bread is too soft the pudding may become soggy.

2 cups cubed bread
4 eggs, beaten
¼ cup sugar
½ cup almond milk
½ cup chocolate chips, melted
1 tablespoon vanilla extract
sprinkle of cinnamon
½ cup chopped bananas

1. Heat oven to 350 degrees. Butter a 9-inch round baking dish.
2. Combine all ingredients except bread in a large mixing bowl. Add bread cubes and let soak until cubes are thoroughly coated, about 10 minutes. Add a bit more milk if all liquid has been absorbed.
3. Pour into prepared pan and bake in oven for 30–45 minutes, or until a toothpick inserted in the middle comes out clean.

Scoop bread pudding into a small bowl and garnish with fresh fruit.

TIP The simplest way to make bread pudding is to prepare your favorite French toast batter, add cut bread, soak, add fruit, and then bake until firm.

PER SERVING› **Energy** 215 cal • **Fat** 11 g • **Sodium** 94 mg • **Carbs** 23 g • **Fiber** 1 g • **Protein** 4 g

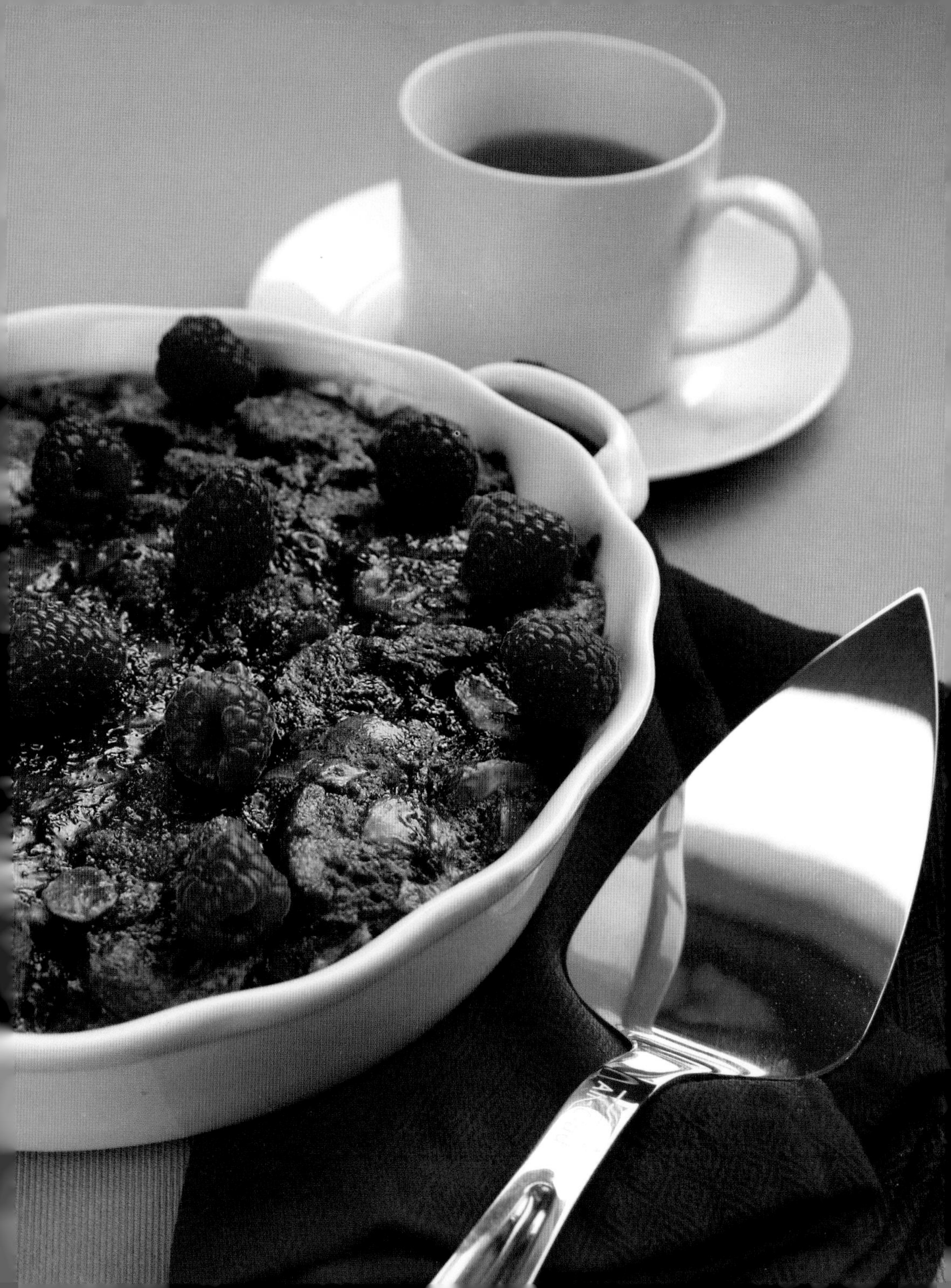

SERVINGS› 4
TIME› 10 minutes prep, freeze overnight

Simple Granita

Most sorbets are made using an ice cream maker, an expensive piece of equipment that most of us won't use except a few times a year. This version requires only a blender or a small food processor.

¼ cup Simple Syrup (see below)

1½ cups fresh fruit

1 teaspoon lemon juice

SIMPLE SYRUP

¼ cup sweetener of your choice (honey, agave nectar, maple syrup, or jam)

¾ cup warm water

SUGGESTED COMBINATIONS

banana and strawberry

cantaloupe and ginger

cucumber and fresh basil

mango and raspberry

peach and mint leaves

1. To make the syrup: Stir together sweetener and water. Taste; add more sweetener if needed.
2. Put all ingredients in a blender or small processor and process until very smooth. Pour into a plastic container with a lid and freeze several hours or overnight.

PER SERVING› Energy 90 cal • Fat 0 g • Sodium 2 mg • Carbs 23 g • Fiber 2 g • Protein 1 g

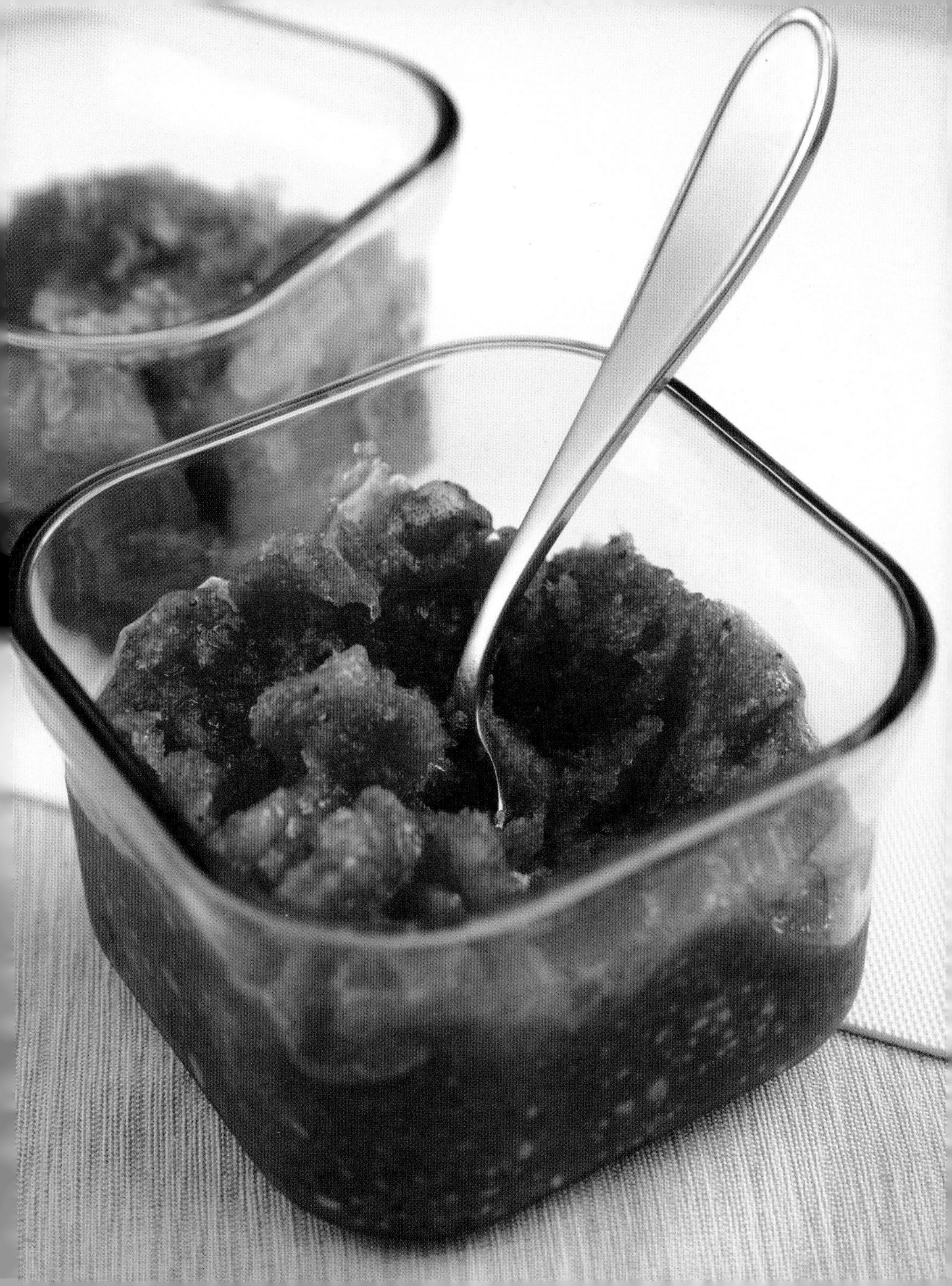

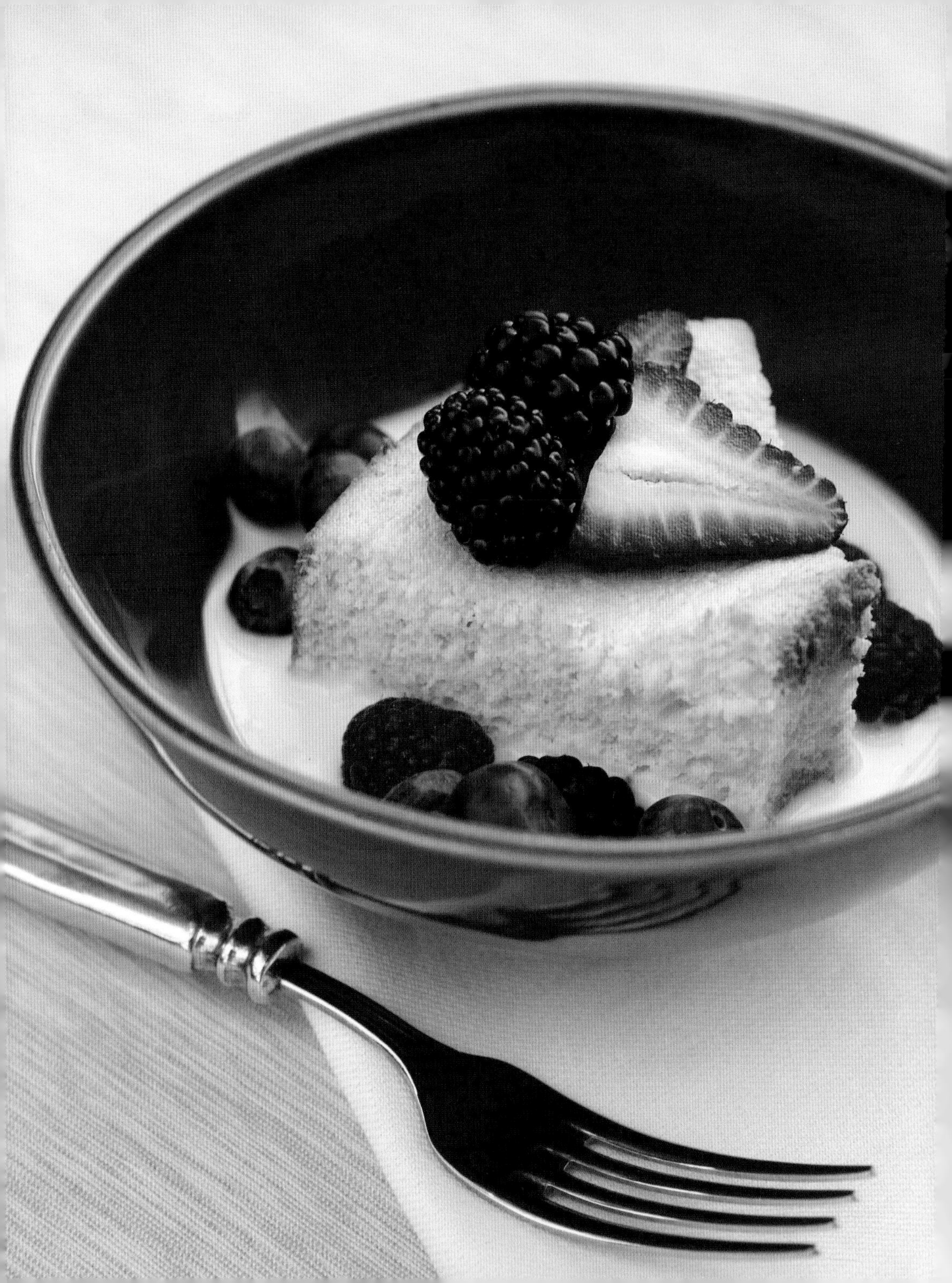

SERVINGS› 8
TIME› 20 minutes prep,
bake 35 minutes

Angel Food Cake

Low in fat and versatile enough to make everyone happy, this is a beautiful dessert. A purchased angel food cake can be used, but it's easy to make the cake from scratch—just three basic steps to follow.

1 cup flour

1 tablespoon cornstarch

¾ cup powdered sugar

12 egg whites, at room temperature

¾ teaspoon salt

1½ teaspoons cream of tartar

1 teaspoon vanilla or almond extract

in-season berries or fruit, cut into bite-size pieces

milk

1. Heat oven to 350 degrees. Sift together flour, cornstarch, and ½ cup of the sugar. Set aside.
2. Using an electric mixer, beat egg whites and salt until foamy, then add cream of tartar and continue to beat until soft peaks form. Add the remaining ¼ cup of sugar and beat until stiff. The mixture should have a nice shine but should not be dry. Fold in the vanilla extract.
3. Gradually add the flour mixture into the egg mixture and fold in together. Spoon batter into an ungreased tube pan and bake for 30–35 minutes. Cool upside-down with a bottle in the middle of the pan.

Makes 8 slices. In a bowl, top sliced cake with fresh fruit or berries. Pour milk over the cake and drizzle with honey, if desired.

PER SERVING› **Energy** 144 cal • **Fat** 0 g • **Sodium** 297 mg • **Carbs** 28 g • **Fiber** 1 g • **Protein** 7 g
Nutrition includes 1 cup of blueberries for fruit.

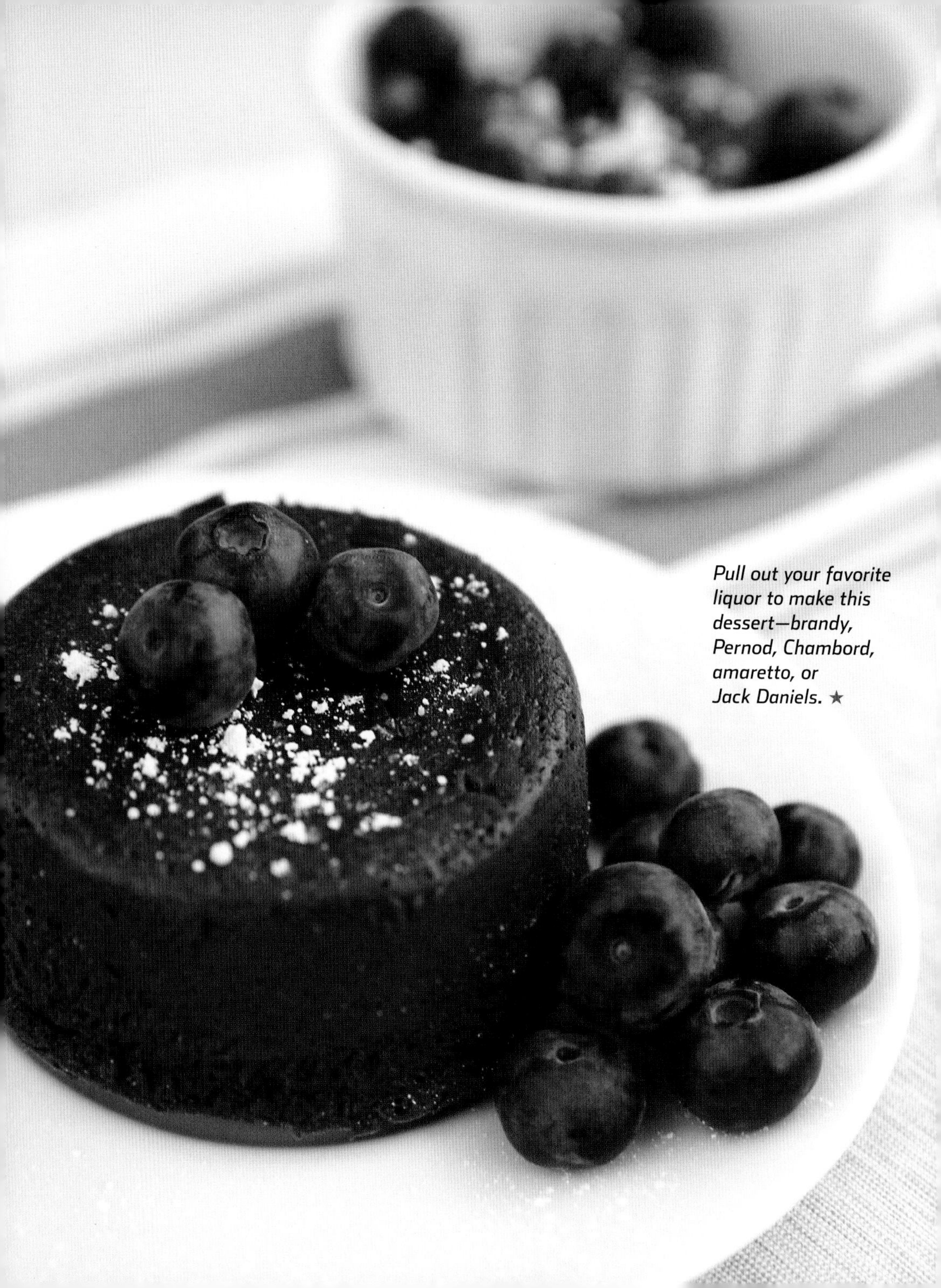

Pull out your favorite liquor to make this dessert—brandy, Pernod, Chambord, amaretto, or Jack Daniels. ★

SERVINGS> 12
TIME> 30 minutes

Flourless Chocolate Cake

Many a cyclist has indulged in this dessert, which is a favorite of Lance Armstrong and his friend "College." These cakes are blissfully laden with chocolate and a hint of your favorite liquor.

2 cups semi-sweet chocolate chips
1 cup (2 sticks) unsalted butter
¼ cup liquor
10 large eggs
¼ cup sugar
1 teaspoon vanilla extract
½ teaspoon salt
sprinkle of cayenne pepper

1. Heat oven to 325 degrees. Grease a 12-cup muffin tin or use foil cupcake liners in the tin.
2. Put water in bottom half of a double boiler, or fill a small saucepan halfway with water. Bring to a gentle boil.
3. Into top of double boiler or metal bowl in sauce pan (see note), add chocolate chips, butter, and liquor. When the chocolate and butter begin to melt, blend thoroughly. It should have an even, shiny finish. Remove from heat.
4. While the chocolate is melting, whip eggs in a separate bowl until frothy. Add sugar, vanilla, salt, and cayenne.
5. Ladle a bit of the egg mixture to the warm chocolate mixture and whisk quickly so that the eggs don't cook. Continue adding egg mixture and whisking until about one-third of it is incorporated into the chocolate mixture. Then pour the chocolate mixture back into the larger bowl containing the remaining eggs, and stir to combine.
6. Pour batter into muffin tin, filling each tin halfway. Bake 15–20 minutes. Cakes should be light and dry on the outside (with cracks on top) and dense and moist on the inside.

Let cakes cool to touch or chill in the fridge before serving. Add powdered sugar and fresh berries, if desired.

NOTE> If you don't have a double boiler, a metal bowl that is big enough to rest on top of your saucepan will do just fine.

PER SERVING> **Energy** 439 cal • **Fat** 30 g • **Sodium** 152 mg • **Carbs** 32 g • **Fiber** 0 g • **Protein** 5 g

★★★

Here you will find instruction and recipes for the items we consider to be staples. You're likely to find yourself using many of these recipes repeatedly—basil marinara, pizza crust, crushed potatoes. **It's here that you can begin exploring different flavors, inventing your own recipes, or adding a new twist to many of our own.**

This section opens with some basic techniques and instruction on how to have your favorite carbs and other common ingredients cooked and ready, which saves you valuable time. You'll find a variety of recipes: beans, various forms of carbohydrates, and dough. When paired with the right flavors, these foods are the athlete's base for every meal.

Our recipes in other menus will at times refer back to the recipes and instructions here. **Take some time to explore this section because cooking and storing a lot of these basics can make life simpler, more delicious, and extremely nutritious.** Learning to prepare the basics will give you a huge advantage and will help to solve the age-old question of what to eat in a practical and creative way.

BASICS

SIMPLE TECHNIQUES

COOKED AND READY

CARBS

SIDES

FLAVORS ON THE SIDE

V VEGETARIAN
G GLUTEN-FREE

Simple Techniques

HOW TO TOAST NUTS

Heat a cast-iron or other metal pan (not nonstick) over medium-high heat. Add the nuts and stir constantly until nuts begin to turn dark brown, about 3–5 minutes. **See also Toasted Nut Mix, page 276.** ★

★★★

HOW TO BLANCH VEGETABLES

Boil a pot of salted water on the stove. Add the vegetables to the boiling water and keep in the pot until they are just cooked through but still tender and brightly colored. Then immediately immerse vegetables into a bowl of ice-cold water. Keep them in cold water until the vegetables lose all their warmth. This process will destroy the enzymes and will keep them fresher longer.

★★★

HOW TO PEEL TOMATOES AND FRUITS

Boil a pot of salted water on the stove. Use a knife to lightly mark an "x" on the bottom of each fruit. Use a slotted spoon to place each piece in the boiling water for about 30 seconds, or just long enough for the skin to begin to loosen. Immediately transfer the fruit to a bowl of ice water while you finish up. Once the fruit has cooled, gently peel away the skin.

HOW TO COOK EGGS

Scramble› Warm a lightly oiled sauté pan over medium heat. Crack as many eggs as you like over the pan, and stir until the eggs clump together and are no longer runny. Add salt and pepper to taste.

Poach› Bring a pan of water with a splash of vinegar to a gentle boil. Crack the egg into a small cup or ladle, and gently transfer the egg to the pan. Don't touch the egg until it turns white and you can see the yolk. Cook approximately 4–5 minutes. Use a slotted spoon or spatula to remove the poached egg.

Boil› Place eggs in the bottom of a pot full of water. Bring the water to a boil. Cook 3 minutes for soft-boiled eggs; 10 minutes for hard-boiled eggs. Either store the eggs in the fridge for later use or run them under cold water, peel the shells, and put them in a container to cool.

★ Toasted Nut Mix goes great with Biju's Oatmeal (page 34) or Sweet Rice and Fruit (page 114). See recipe on page 276.

Cooked and Ready

HOW TO COOK POTATOES

Oven› Wash and wrap the potatoes in foil and place them in the oven to bake for 1 hour at 350 degrees. Pierce with a knife, and when it comes out clean the potatoes are done.

Microwave› Wash the potatoes and use a fork to poke holes throughout. Place the potatoes in the microwave and cook on high for 8–10 minutes (5–8 minutes for a single potato, depending on the size). Let stand for 5 minutes. Once the potatoes have cooled, peel and coarsely chop, storing in 2-cup increments.

Sweet potatoes tend to cook quicker in the oven, but they typically require the same time in the microwave. It all depends on the size of the potato.

★★★

HOW TO COOK BEETS

Oven› The dry heat of the oven gives beets a slight sweetness and more consistent texture. Wash and wrap the beets in foil and place in an oven-safe dish with a splash of water. Bake for 1 hour or until tender at 350 degrees. Let cool and then peel the skins by hand.

Microwave› Wash the beets, poke some holes using a fork, and put in the microwave for 8 minutes. Turn, and microwave 3–4 more minutes or until tender. Let cool and then peel the skins by hand.

HOW TO COOK PASTA

Boil› For most all pasta (Italian cut) or noodles (Asian cut), add a pinch of salt to a pot of water and bring to a boil. Cooking times will vary according to the type of pasta. Drain water and toss pasta or noodles with a bit of oil to keep from sticking.

Cooked and Ready Pasta› *Al dente* means "to the tooth." The pasta will be a little raw in the middle and have a bite to it. Cook the pasta to three-quarters of the time specified on the package, or the lower end of the range. When you reheat the pasta later it will be cooked to perfection.

★★★

HOW TO COOK CHICKEN

Boil› Cover chicken (boneless, skinless, etc.) with salted water in a large pot. Bring the water to a boil, let it simmer for 10 minutes, then cover and let it sit for 45 minutes. Pull out the chicken, let it cool, and then shred or cut it for desired purposes.

Fry/Grill› For a quicker method, you can pan-sear the chicken until cooked through (20 minutes), or grill it (12–15 minutes).

Roast› Toss chicken in olive oil and add salt and pepper. Put the chicken in the oven for 20–25 minutes at 400 degrees. **See also Whole Roasted Chicken, page 249.** ★

SERVINGS› 2
TIME› 20 minutes

Basmati Rice

1 cup basmati rice

1½ cups of water

1 teaspoon salt

1 tablespoon white vinegar

1. Rinse the rice in warm water twice (put rice and water in bowl, slowly tip water out, repeat).
2. Put rice and remaining ingredients in a medium pot over medium-high heat. Bring to a boil; stir, turn heat to low, and cover with a tight-fitting lid. Simmer until all the moisture is cooked out, about 15 minutes. Turn heat off and let sit a few minutes with lid on.

Serve with any meats, fish, or stew. Makes 2 cups.

Basmati rice is lighter than the medium-grain rice used in many of our recipes. ★

PER SERVING (1 cup)› **Energy** 320 cal • **Fat** 0 g • **Sodium** 1,163 mg • **Carbs** 70 g • **Fiber** 2 g • **Protein** 8 g

SERVINGS› 4–5
TIME› Soak overnight, cook 1½–2 hours

Dry Beans

1 pound (about 2 cups) dry beans, such as adzuki or red beans

salt

1. Rinse the dried beans in cold water, then cover with water and set in fridge overnight or for at least 2 hours.
2. Pour off soaking water and transfer the beans to a large pot. Cover with double the water as beans and bring to a rolling boil. Turn heat down to a simmer and cook covered until tender—in most cases 1½–2 hours. Rinse thoroughly before using.

Makes 4–5 cups.

Whenever possible, use dry beans in your recipes. Not only can you control the amount of sodium, but the flavor and texture are better. ★

PER SERVING (1 cup)› **Energy** 226 cal • **Fat** 1 g • **Sodium** 280 mg • **Carbs** 40 g • **Fiber** 13 g • **Protein** 16 g

SERVINGS› 4
TIME› 20 minutes

Quinoa

1 cup quinoa

2 cups water or low-sodium stock

½ tablespoon apple cider vinegar

1. Rinse the quinoa in water. Put it in a medium saucepan along with the water or stock and vinegar. Bring to a boil, reduce heat to a simmer, cover with a lid, and let cook until most of the liquid has been absorbed, about 10 minutes.
2. Turn off heat and let rest, covered, 5 minutes. Quinoa should be tender and light, not overly chewy, when properly cooked.

Finish with salt and a touch of olive oil or butter to taste. Makes 4 cups.

Quinoa (pronounced keen-wa) is a grain that is high in fiber and has all eight amino acids. ★

PER SERVING (1 cup)› Energy 185 cal • Fat 5 g • Sodium 146 mg • Carbs 30 g • Fiber 3 g • Protein 7 g

SERVINGS› 4
TIME› 15–40 minutes

Polenta

4 cups water (see note)

½ teaspoon salt

1 cup instant polenta or finely ground cornmeal

2 tablespoons olive oil or butter

2 tablespoons julienned fresh basil

2 tablespoons minced fresh parsley

1. In a heavy-bottomed pot, bring the water and salt to a rolling boil. Slowly pour in the polenta, stirring constantly with a wooden spoon. Let cook until thick (about 15 minutes for instant, 30–40 minutes for cornmeal); it will begin to pull away from the sides of the pot.
2. Add remaining ingredients, stir, and turn off heat.

NOTE› Alternatively, you can use 2 cups water, 2 cups low-sodium chicken or vegetable stock.

Instant polenta cooks in less than half the time of regular cornmeal. Look for it at your local grocery store. ★ *You can serve the polenta soft or pour it into a deep dish and set it in the fridge overnight to harden. Cut polenta into bars to be wrapped and taken on rides.*

PER SERVING (1 cup)› Energy 170 cal • Fat 8 g • Sodium 302 mg • Carbs 24 g • Fiber 3 g • Protein 3 g

SERVINGS› 8
TIME› 15 minutes prep,
1 hour to rise,
cook 12–15 minutes

Pizza Dough

This is my favorite pizza crust recipe. It is super-fast, easy, and always produces a very thin crust—which puts the focus on the flavors of whatever seasonal ingredients you have *(see recipes, pages 207–210)**. Once you've mastered the basic recipe, try using other flours such as whole wheat, garbanzo, or almond flour.*

1 cup warm tap water

1 package (1 scant tablespoon) active dry yeast

½ teaspoon sugar

3 cups all-purpose flour, plus more for dusting surfaces

2 tablespoons olive oil

1 teaspoon coarse salt

a pinch of cornmeal to dust pan or stone (optional)

1. In a large bowl combine water, yeast, and sugar, and gently mix. Set aside for about 5 minutes or until the mixture is foamy.
2. Stir in 2½ cups of the flour, 1 tablespoon of the olive oil, and the salt. The dough will be sticky.
3. Transfer dough to a floured surface and knead while adding remaining ½ cup of flour in small amounts until you get a consistent, nonsticky, elastic ball.
4. Coat another large bowl with the remaining olive oil. Place dough in bowl, turning to coat evenly with oil. Cover with a damp cloth and let rise in a warm place until dough has doubled in size, about 1 hour. (If you can't wait for dough to rise, roll out the dough right away. It will make a very thin "cracker" crust, but this is also very good.)
5. Divide the dough into 2 balls. Roll out each ball on a floured board with a rolling pin or a wine bottle. Dust with flour as needed, flip it once or twice, and continue stretching the dough from the center outward.
6. Transfer dough to a pizza pan or stone dusted with cornmeal, top with favorite ingredients, and bake at 400 degrees until crust is a light golden brown underneath, 12–15 minutes.

Makes 2 thin 10-inch crusts.

TIP Freeze leftover dough and thaw it at room temperature when you are ready to use it.

PER SERVING (¼ crust)› **Energy** 200 cal • **Fat** 4 g • **Sodium** 292 mg • **Carbs** 36 g • **Fiber** 1 g • **Protein** 2 g

SERVINGS› 8
TIME› 15 minutes

★ See photos, pages 196 and 199.

Pie Crust

3 cups flour

½ teaspoon salt

½ teaspoon ground cinnamon (optional)

⅔ cup cold butter, cut into ½-inch cubes

½ cup cold water

1. In a small food processor pulse together flour, salt, and cinnamon. Add butter and blend until the butter pieces are no longer visible.
2. Transfer the mixture to a large bowl and add cold water a little bit at a time, using a spatula to turn the dough and mix in dry ingredients. Once they are worked in, add more water or a bit more flour if needed to obtain a firm pie dough.

Makes 6–8 empanadas.

Chill in the fridge until you are ready to use the dough. ★

PER SERVING (⅛ crust)› Energy 305 cal • Fat 16 g • Sodium 149 mg • Carbs 36 g • Fiber 5 g • Protein 5 g

SERVINGS› 24
TIME› 10 minutes

Toasted Nut Mix

1 cup slivered almonds

1 cup pine nuts

1 cup unsweetened shredded coconut

½ cup currants or raisins

1. Heat a cast-iron or other metal pan (not nonstick) over medium-high heat. Add the almonds and pine nuts and stir constantly until nuts begin to turn dark brown, about 3–5 minutes.
2. Turn heat off, add coconut and currants, stir, and remove pan from heat.

Makes about 3 cups. Store in an airtight container in the fridge or pantry.

TIP Vary ingredients based on what you have. Use unsalted and unsweetened items whenever you can.

PER SERVING (2 tbsp.)› Energy 137 cal • Fat 11 g • Sodium 3 mg • Carbs 9 g • Fiber 2 g • Protein 5 g

SERVINGS› 2
TIME› 10 minutes

Rice Salad

3 cups cooked rice COOKED

¼ cup olive oil

¼ cup chopped carrots

¼ cup chopped fresh parsley

¼ cup grated parmesan

OPTIONAL ADDITIONS

(about ¼ cup of each or all)

fresh sweet corn kernels

chopped peppers

chopped cucumbers

raisins

1. In a large bowl, mix together all ingredients. Add a squeeze of lemon juice and salt and pepper to taste.

Serve with fish or lighter meats.

PER SERVING› **Energy** 578 cal • **Fat** 31 g • **Sodium** 222 mg • **Carbs** 67 g • **Fiber** 2 g • **Protein** 9 g › Nutrition for optional additions can be found in Appendix A.

SERVINGS› 2
TIME› 10 minutes

Mediterranean Rice Salad

3 cups cooked rice COOKED

¼ cup olive oil

¼ cup chopped carrots

¼ cup chopped fresh basil

¼ cup crumbled feta cheese

½ cup cherry tomatoes

¼ cup chopped red onion

OPTIONAL ADDITIONS

½ cup cooked or canned tuna

½ cup cooked or canned white beans, rinsed

1. In a large bowl, mix together all ingredients. Add a squeeze of lemon juice and salt and pepper to taste.

Serve cold with grilled meats and fish.

PER SERVING› **Energy** 583 cal • **Fat** 31 g • **Sodium** 198 mg • **Carbs** 70 g • **Fiber** 3 g • **Protein** 8 g › Nutrition for optional additions can be found in Appendix A.

SERVINGS› 2
TIME› 45 minutes ★ See photo, page 232.

Millet Salad

Millet is another in a line of ancient "super" grains that provide all sorts of nutritional value while offering something different from the norm. It has a nutty flavor and crunchy texture that complements meat, chicken, and fish nicely.

1 cup millet

3 cups water

½ cup plain yogurt

juice of 1 lemon

1 cup chopped tomatoes

½ cup each chopped carrots and cucumbers

¼ cup each chopped fresh chives and parsley

¼ cup chopped green olives

1. Toast and cook the millet: Bring a large, deep pot with a lid to medium-high heat. Add the dry millet, stirring constantly with a wooden spoon until millet turns golden brown.
2. Carefully pour in 3 cups water. Stir once, reduce heat to low, and cover with the lid. Let cook for approximately 30 minutes, stirring occasionally to keep from clumping. When all the water has been absorbed, remove from heat and set aside with lid on. Let cool.
3. Combine cooked millet with remaining ingredients, adding olive oil, salt, and pepper to taste.

TIP To save time, chop the vegetables while the millet is cooking or cooling.

PER SERVING› **Energy** 450 cal • **Fat** 13 g • **Sodium** 722 mg • **Carbs** 79 g • **Fiber** 7 g • **Protein** 13 g

SERVINGS› 2
TIME› 15 minutes

Quinoa Salad

3 cups cooked quinoa, chilled COOKED

1 cup cooked or canned black beans

1 cup chopped sweet peppers

1 tablespoon minced hot peppers

½ cup chopped parsley

¼ cup olive oil

2 teaspoons Southwestern or Mexican seasoning

juice of 1 lemon

1. In a large bowl, mix together all ingredients, adding salt and pepper to taste. Chill to allow flavors to blend. Top with chopped cilantro.

Serve with chicken or fish.

PER SERVING› **Energy** 535 cal • **Fat** 31 g • **Sodium** 610 mg • **Carbs** 53 g • **Fiber** 12 g • **Protein** 15 g

SERVINGS› 2
TIME› 10 minutes

Couscous with Currants

1½ cups couscous

dash of salt

1 tablespoon olive oil

2 tablespoons currants, raisins, or other dried fruit

2 tablespoons chopped fresh parsley

1 small garlic clove, minced

2 tablespoons pine nuts or other nuts, chopped

1. Bring 2 cups of water to a boil. Put couscous and salt in a heat-proof bowl. Pour boiling water over couscous. Stir thoroughly, then cover and set aside for about 5 minutes.

2. While couscous is resting, heat olive oil in a large sauté pan. Add currants, parsley, garlic, and nuts. Stir and cook over medium-high heat for 2–3 minutes. Add couscous and gently mix all ingredients. Add salt and pepper to taste.

Makes 4–5 cups.

Couscous is a very fast and easy pasta to keep around. Serve it with pork, poultry, fish, or eggs. ★

PER SERVING› **Energy** 500 cal • **Fat** 15 g • **Sodium** 468 mg • **Carbs** 75 g • **Fiber** 6 g • **Protein** 16 g

SERVINGS› 2
TIME› 15 minutes

Quick Pasta with Parsley Pesto

Because fresh parsley is less expensive than fresh basil and is stocked at most groceries, I often make this easy pesto. It's great with both chunky and long types of pasta.

1 cup fresh parsley, roughly chopped

1 garlic clove, chopped

2 tablespoons olive oil, plus extra if needed to thin

2 tablespoons grated parmesan

juice of ½ a lemon

⅛ teaspoon salt

COOKED **2 cups cooked pasta, warm or at room temperature**

OPTIONAL ADDITIONS

1 teaspoon red pepper flakes

1 tablespoon white wine vinegar

1. Put all ingredients except pasta in a food processor or blender. Pulse to a coarse mixture, adding a bit more oil if pesto is too thick. Taste, and adjust seasonings.
2. Combine cooked pasta with pesto in a large serving bowl.

Serve it with chicken or steak. Makes about ½ cup pesto.

TIP Flat-leaf Italian parsley has a more pronounced flavor, but you can also use curly parsley—which is especially easy to find in stores.

PER SERVING› **Energy** 302 cal • **Fat** 16 g • **Sodium** 268 mg • **Carbs** 32 g • **Fiber** 6 g • **Protein** 8 g

SERVINGS› 4
TIME› 25–30 minutes

Basil Marinara

In my opinion, the best marinara sauces are a bright and chunky mix of the freshest vegetables you can find. I personally use this sauce as an excuse to eat as much seasonal produce as possible. This recipe works great as a pasta sauce or a soup.

2 tablespoons olive oil

2 tablespoons chopped garlic

2 onions, chopped

2 tablespoons dried Italian herb mixture: basil, oregano, parsley

½ cup tomato paste

¼ cup balsamic vinegar

½ cup red wine

4 ripe tomatoes, chopped

¼ cup fresh basil

COOKED **4 cups cooked pasta**

OPTIONAL ADDITIONS
(chopped or minced)

carrots

sweet bell peppers

fresh parsley

1. In a deep, heavy non-aluminum pot, warm olive oil over medium heat.
2. Add the garlic and stir. Add the onions and stir. Add the dried herbs, tomato paste, vinegar, and wine, and stir. Finally, add the tomatoes. Stir, bring to a gentle boil, then reduce the heat so that the sauce barely simmers and begins to thicken.
3. Add basil and any of the optional ingredients, if desired; stir again. Adjust flavor with salt, pepper, and a bit of molasses or brown sugar.
4. Combine cooked pasta with marinara in a large serving bowl.

Makes about 4 cups marinara.

TIP Adjust thickness with wine, stock, or water. For a great soup, thin sauce and serve with crusty bread.

CARBS

PER SERVING› **Energy** 383 cal • **Fat** 9g • **Sodium** 114 mg • **Carbs** 61 g • **Fiber** 7 g • **Protein** 11 g

Nutrition for optional additions can be found in Appendix A.

SERVINGS› 4
TIME› 30 minutes prep, chill 1 hour

Potato Cakes

Dipped in bread crumbs, these pan-fried potato cakes have a crunchy golden-brown crust and a warm, rich center. They are just a bit different from the Sweet Potato Cakes stuffed with Swiss (page 51), but no less tasty. Wrap one up for lunch on the go or for your next ride.

- COOKED **2 cups peeled potatoes, mashed and cooled**
- **2 egg yolks**
- **1 tablespoon chopped fresh parsley**
- **2 tablespoons grated parmesan**
- **⅛ teaspoon each of salt and pepper**
- **2 tablespoons crumbled goat cheese**
- **egg wash: 1 whole egg blended with a splash of cold water**
- **¾ cup bread crumbs or panko**
- **1 tablespoon grapeseed or canola oil**

1. Thoroughly combine mashed potatoes, egg yolks, parsley, parmesan, salt, and pepper in a medium bowl. Let chill for about an hour in the fridge.
2. Shape into small rounds or ovals about 3 or 4 inches wide and ½-inch thick. Stuff a small amount of goat cheese into the center of each cake.
3. Dip cakes in egg wash, then roll in bread crumbs.
4. Pour oil into a sauté pan and turn heat to medium-high. Fry cakes, two or three at a time or as room allows, turning after first side is golden brown, about 6–8 minutes. Cook on second side until golden, then remove to a plate lined with paper towels. Cover cakes to keep them warm while you fry the remaining cakes.

Serve with cool yogurt sauce or your favorite jam. Makes about 4 cakes.

PER SERVING› **Energy** 268 cal • **Fat** 10 g • **Sodium** 264 mg • **Carbs** 36 g • **Fiber** 3 g • **Protein** 9 g

SERVINGS› 2
TIME› 20 minutes

Crushed Potatoes

- 1 pound potatoes
- small handful of fresh chopped herbs (parsley, basil, thyme, chives, etc.)
- 1 cup total chopped fresh vegetables (carrots, bell peppers, celery, garlic, etc.)
- 2–4 tablespoons olive oil, depending on how dry the potatoes are after cooking

1. Place potatoes in a microwave-safe bowl and microwave for 8–10 minutes, until fork tender. Let cool then peel (if desired) and cut into cubes.

2. Add remaining ingredients and crush together using your hands. Add salt and pepper to taste.

Serve with any grilled or roasted meat. Makes about 3 cups.

Fresh vegetables and herbs give these potatoes great texture and brightness. ★

TIP Leave the skins on the potatoes if you are eating this dish after training.

PER SERVING› **Energy** 480 cal • **Fat** 21 g • **Sodium** 192 mg • **Carbs** 70 g • **Fiber** 10 g • **Protein** 9 g

SERVINGS› 6
TIME› 45–60 minutes

Savory Bread Pudding

- 1 cup mixed vegetables, chopped (mushrooms, celery, and leeks or onions)
- 2 cups cubed bread
- ½ cup milk
- 4 eggs, beaten
- 1 teaspoon ground nutmeg
- ¼ cup shredded Swiss cheese
- sprinkle of sea salt and freshly ground black pepper

1. Heat oven to 375 degrees. Sauté the vegetables in a bit of butter; set aside to cool slightly.
2. Combine all ingredients in a bowl. Let the bread soak up the liquid, about 10 minutes.
3. Pour mixture into a lightly oiled 8-inch square pan. Bake for 30–45 minutes or until a toothpick comes out clean.

Serve with roast chicken and turkey or beside a salad.

PER SERVING› **Energy** 174 cal • **Fat** 12 g • **Sodium** 149 mg • **Carbs** 9 g • **Fiber** 2 g • **Protein** 7 g

SERVINGS› 2
TIME› 10 minutes

★ See photo, page 200.

Spiced Black Beans

2 tablespoons olive oil

½ onion, chopped

2 tablespoons taco spice

1 teaspoon each of whichever you have: ground cumin, cinnamon, black pepper, chili powder

1 can (16 ounces) black beans, drained and rinsed

chopped fresh parsley

lime juice

1. Pour oil in a medium sauté pan and turn heat to medium-high. Add onions and cook, stirring, until they start to brown, 3–5 minutes.
2. Add dry spices and stir for a few seconds. Turn down the heat and fold in the beans and parsley. Squeeze in fresh lime juice just before serving.

TIP When you have the time, prepare this with cooked Dry Beans (page 273).

PER SERVING› Energy 329 cal • Fat 15 g • Sodium 903 mg • Carbs 75 g • Fiber 14 g • Protein 15 g

SERVINGS› 4
TIME› 20 minutes

★ See photo, page 131.

Spicy Cabbage Slaw

1 tablespoon lime juice

¼ cup apple cider vinegar

½ tablespoon brown sugar

1 teaspoon kosher salt

¼ head red cabbage, thinly shredded

¼ head green cabbage, thinly shredded

½ jalapeno, minced

small handful of cilantro leaves

1. In a small bowl, whisk together lime juice, vinegar, brown sugar, and salt.
2. Combine the shredded cabbages, jalapeno, and cilantro in a large bowl. Pour dressing over and toss well.

Serve with tacos, burgers, and wraps.

PER SERVING› Energy 10 cal • Fat 0 g • Sodium 583 mg • Carbs 3 g • Fiber 1 g • Protein 1 g

SERVINGS› 4
TIME› 5 minutes

★ See photo, page 200.

Bitter Greens

2 cups washed loosely packed bitter greens, cut up as you'd like

juice of 1 lemon

1 teaspoon coarse salt

½ tablespoon apple cider vinegar (more if needed)

½ teaspoon brown sugar

1. Mix together all ingredients. Allow flavors to meld a couple of minutes. Taste; add a splash of olive oil if the flavors are too harsh.

Serve with fish or chicken dishes, stuff into burritos and wraps, or give brightness to an otherwise heavy dish.

My favorite greens are kale, chard, dandelion, mustard, and collard. The heartier greens will need to marinate just a bit longer than the more tender ones. ★

PER SERVING› Energy 9 cal • Fat 0 g • Sodium 646 mg • Carbs 2 g • Fiber 1 g • Protein 1 g

SERVINGS› 2
TIME› 5 minutes

★ See photo, page 220.

Mixed Greens

3 cups loosely packed mixed greens

2 ripe bananas, sliced

sprinkle of black sesame seeds (optional)

HONEY DRESSING

2 tablespoons honey

2 tablespoons olive oil

1 tablespoon apple cider vinegar

1 teaspoon minced green chiles

1. Make the dressing by whisking together the ingredients in a bowl. Add salt to taste.
2. In a salad bowl, combine greens and bananas. Add dressing and toss gently. Sprinkle with sesame seeds, if desired.

Serve with steamed rice and grilled chicken, or in a wrap.

Bananas are super-versatile and easy to cook with, making a great addition to everything from fresh salads to cooked meats and seafood items. ★

PER SERVING› Energy 306 cal • Fat 14 g • Sodium 198 mg • Carbs 48 g • Fiber 2 g • Protein 3 g

SERVINGS› 4
TIME› 10–20 minutes

Salsa

I make two versions of this salsa. One is fresh, and the other includes roasted or grilled vegetables. Both are easy to make and far superior to most purchased salsas. If you're at the height of the cycling season you may want to peel the tomatoes to make them easier to digest. (See "How to Peel Tomatoes and Fruits," page 270.)

- **3–4 ripe tomatoes**
- **2–3 jalapenos or other medium-heat chiles**
- **1 small onion**
- **juice of 1 lime or 1 tablespoon apple cider vinegar**
- **small handful of cilantro, chopped**
- **salt**
- **2 tablespoons olive oil (if roasting)**
- **1 teaspoon brown sugar or honey (optional)**

SALSA FRESCA ★ See photo, page 134.

1. In a blender or by hand, chop the tomatoes, chiles, and onion. Add lime juice, cilantro, and salt to taste.

ROASTED SALSA ★ See photo, page 131.

1. Coat the whole tomatoes, chiles, and onion in olive oil. Roast them over high heat until the skin blackens. This can be done on a hot grill, in a pan on the stove, or under the broiler in an oven. Remove from heat and let cool, then pulse in a blender or chopper—or just chop by hand, keeping the juices. Add lime juice, cilantro, and salt to taste.

FRESCA› **Energy** 47 cal • **Fat** 1 g • **Sodium** 159 mg • **Carbs** 12 g • **Fiber** 2 g • **Protein** 2 g
ROASTED› **Energy** 106 cal • **Fat** 7 g • **Sodium** 159 mg • **Carbs** 12 g • **Fiber** 2 g • **Protein** 2 g
Nutrition for optional additions can be found in Appendix A.

SERVINGS› 2
TIME› 5 minutes

★ See photo, page 132.

Pico de Gallo

1 large tomato, diced

1 jalapeno (cut off stem but use the seeds), diced

½ onion, diced

small handful of cilantro, chopped

lime juice

1. In a food processor or chopper, combine all ingredients, adding lime juice and salt to taste.

Serve with tacos, burritos, and eggs. Makes about 1 cup.

PER SERVING (½ cup)› Energy 37 cal • Fat 0 g • Sodium 302 mg • Carbs 10 g • Fiber 4 g • Protein 2 g

SERVINGS› 8
TIME› 10 minutes

★ See photo, page 245.

Chimichurri

½ cup olive oil

1 bunch parsley, rinsed and shaken or pat dry

½ ripe tomato

½ jalapeno (or 1 tablespoon red pepper flakes)

1 clove garlic

½ cup apple cider or white vinegar

1 teaspoon brown sugar or honey

juice of 1 lemon or lime

1. Put all ingredients into a blender or food processor. Process until it is a nice, even consistency—it should be a bit thinner than regular pesto. Add more vinegar or lemon/lime juice if it is too thick. Add salt and pepper to taste.

Serve with chicken, fish, or steak. Makes about 1 cup. Keeps in the fridge for 3–4 days.

Chimichurri is a tart and oily pesto of dried or fresh herbs commonly used in Caribbean and South American cooking. My version is a simple parsley vinaigrette. ★

PER SERVING (2 tbsp.)› Energy 124 cal • Fat 14 g • Sodium 73 mg • Carbs 2 g • Fiber 0 g • Protein 0 g

FLAVORS

SERVINGS› 12
TIME› 20 minutes

★ See photo, page 66.

Romesco

This is my take on a classic coastal Spanish dish that is packed with all sorts of goodness from the toasted almonds to the rustic hint of anchovy. You can make a decent romesco using just toasted bread, almonds, anchovies, olive oil, and salt. My recipe has a few more items, but include whatever sounds good to you.

- 2 cups coarsely chopped rustic bread
- ½ cup whole almonds
- 3 tomatoes, cut in half
- 1 red bell pepper, coarsely chopped
- 1 onion, peeled and cut into quarters
- 1 jalapeno, coarsely chopped
- 2 garlic cloves
- ¼ cup olive oil
- ½ cup red wine vinegar
- 1 tablespoon chopped anchovies (optional)
- 1 tablespoon brown sugar
- ½ tablespoon coarse salt
- lemon juice

1. Bring a dry sauté pan to medium-high heat. Add bread, almonds, tomatoes, bell pepper, onion, jalapeno, and garlic. Toast the ingredients, stirring often, about 5–10 minutes. Remove from heat.
2. In a small bowl, combine oil, vinegar, anchovies (if using), brown sugar, and salt. Pour over the toasted items in the pan; stir well. Let everything sit for a few minutes so the bread soaks up the liquid. Add more vinegar or oil if it's dry.
3. Transfer pan contents to a food processor or blender. Process briefly; the sauce should remain chunky. Add lemon juice, salt, and pepper to taste.

This goes great with any number of hearty egg and meat dishes, or just some bread and wine! Makes about 4 cups.

PER SERVING (¼ cup)› Energy 99 cal • Fat 6 g • Sodium 91 mg • Carbs 9 g • Fiber 1 g • Protein 3 g

FLAVORS

SERVINGS› 8
TIME› 1–1½ hours

★ See photo, page 199.

Tomato Jam

2 pounds tomatoes, chopped (about 8–10 medium tomatoes)

1 cup sugar

2 tablespoons minced jalapeno

2 tablespoons molasses

1. Put everything in a heavy pot and add a splash of water. Turn heat to medium. Let cook, covered, until the mixture becomes dark and thickens, approximately 1–1½ hours, stirring occasionally. Remove from heat.
2. Transfer jam to a blender or food processor and quickly blend to achieve an even texture.

Makes 1–1½ cups. Store in covered container in fridge for up to 10 days.

Tomato Jam has a slightly sweet and earthy flavor. Serve with grilled chicken and steak. ★

PER SERVING (2 tbsp.)› **Energy** 136 cal • **Fat** 0 g • **Sodium** 15 mg • **Carbs** 34 g • **Fiber** 2 g • **Protein** 1 g

SERVINGS› 6
TIME› 5 minutes

Orange Jalapeno Jam

½ cup orange marmalade

2 tablespoons light olive oil

1 tablespoon chopped jalapeno

1 tablespoon chopped fresh parsley

1. Combine all ingredients in a small bowl, adding salt to taste.

Makes about ¾ cup. Keeps in the fridge 3–4 days.

Last-minute sauce or marinade, especially good on chicken. ★

PER SERVING (2 tbsp.)› **Energy** 106 cal • **Fat** 5 g • **Sodium** 97 mg • **Carbs** 17 g • **Fiber** 0 g • **Protein** 0 g

SERVINGS› 6
TIME› 30 minutes

★ See photo, page 242.

Peach Chutney

- 4–6 medium peaches, coarsely chopped (no need to remove skin)
- ½ cup brown sugar
- ½ cup white or apple cider vinegar
- juice of ½ a lemon
- 1 jalapeno, chopped
- 1 teaspoon chopped fresh ginger
- ½ medium onion, chopped
- 2 teaspoons salt

1. Place all ingredients in a large heavy pot. Cook over medium-high heat, stirring occasionally, until peaches have softened and the syrup has turned a caramel color, about 20 minutes. Let cool.
2. Run in food processor or blender for a few seconds to achieve an even, chunky consistency.

Serve with most grilled meats and roasted chicken. Makes about 1½ cups. Keeps in the fridge 3–4 days.

PER SERVING (¼ cup)› Energy 106 cal • Fat 0 g • Sodium 776 mg • Carbs 27 g • Fiber 2 g • Protein 1 g

SERVINGS› 4
TIME› 10 minutes

Cilantro Chutney

- 2 cups washed and drained spinach leaves
- 1 cup chopped cilantro
- 2 tablespoons apple cider vinegar (see note)
- 2 tablespoons light olive oil
- 1 teaspoon chopped jalapeno
- 1 teaspoon chopped red onion
- 1 teaspoon brown sugar
- juice of ½ a lime

1. Put the spinach in a food processor and process a few seconds to chop it. Add the remaining ingredients and process until smooth. Add salt to taste.

Serve on salads, grilled meats, or fish. Makes about 1 cup. Keeps in the fridge 3–4 days.

NOTE› Depending on the amount of moisture in your spinach, you may have to add a bit more vinegar.

PER SERVING (¼ cup)› Energy 70 cal • Fat 7 g • Sodium 160 mg • Carbs 8 g • Fiber 1 g • Protein 1 g

SERVINGS› 4
TIME› 5 minutes

★ See photo, page 68.

Cilantro-Mint Yogurt

⅔ cup plain Greek-style yogurt

⅓ fresh jalapeno, stemmed, seeded, and minced

3 tablespoons fresh mint leaves

3 tablespoons cilantro leaves

1½ tablespoons honey

⅓ teaspoon ground cumin

1. Combine all ingredients in a blender or food processor and process until smooth. Add salt to taste.

Serve with tacos, wraps, and pitas. Makes about 1 cup.

PER SERVING (¼ cup)› Energy 57 cal • Fat 2 g • Sodium 19 mg • Carbs 8 g • Fiber 0 g • Protein 3 g

SERVINGS› 12
TIME› 10 minutes

Raisin-Mango Relish

¾ cup prepared mango chutney

½ cup golden raisins

⅓ cup diced ripe mango

1½ tablespoons freshly squeezed lime juice

3 tablespoons chopped cilantro

¾ teaspoon red pepper flakes

1. Combine the chutney, raisins, mango, and lime juice in a heavy 1-quart saucepan and heat over low heat, stirring often, until raisins are plumped, about 5 minutes. Remove from heat; cool. Stir in cilantro and red pepper flakes.

Serve as you would a classic relish, on burgers and sandwiches. Makes about 1½ cups. Keeps in the fridge 3–4 days.

PER SERVING (2 tbsp.)› Energy 82 cal • Fat 0 g • Sodium 171 mg • Carbs 20 g • Fiber 0 g • Protein 0 g

SERVINGS› 4
TIME› 5 minutes

Dijon Sauce with Yogurt

- 1 tablespoon olive oil
- 1 teaspoon each minced garlic, onion, and parsley
- 1 teaspoon whole peppercorns (mixed color if you have them)
- 2 tablespoons Dijon or whole-grain mustard
- ¼ cup plain yogurt
- 1 tablespoon apple cider vinegar

1. In a small saucepan over medium heat, sauté olive oil, garlic, onion, parsley, and peppercorns until the peppercorns begin to plump (this takes only a few seconds). Turn heat off, then add the mustard, yogurt, and vinegar (this may splatter, so keep a lid handy). Stir well. Add salt and pepper to taste.

Depending on the dish you're making, either leave the sauce chunky (rustic), or run in a blender and make smooth. Serve with steaks and other grilled meats. Makes about ½ cup.

PER SERVING (2 tbsp.)› **Energy** 51 cal • **Fat** 4 g • **Sodium** 186 mg • **Carbs** 2 g • **Fiber** 0 g • **Protein** 1 g

SERVINGS› 8
TIME› 10 minutes

★ See photo, page 43.

Red Pepper Mayonnaise

- 2 fresh egg yolks
- 2 tablespoons apple cider vinegar
- 2 tablespoons oil
- ½ teaspoon ground mustard
- juice of ½ a lemon
- 1 roasted red pepper (seeded and skinned or from a jar)

1. Combine all ingredients in a blender or food processor, adding salt to taste. Refrigerate any leftover mayonnaise.

Serve with sandwiches and burgers. Makes about ½ cup.

TIP For an easy shortcut, combine the roasted red pepper, lemon juice, and salt in a blender with ½ cup purchased mayonnaise.

PER SERVING (1 tbsp.)› **Energy** 49 cal • **Fat** 5 g • **Sodium** 36 mg • **Carbs** 1 g • **Fiber** 0 g • **Protein** 1 g

SERVINGS› 8
TIME› 15 minutes

Bacon Dressing

4 ounces bacon, chopped

½ cup thinly sliced red onion

¼ cup balsamic vinegar

1 teaspoon brown sugar

2 tablespoons walnuts

¼ cup olive oil

juice of ½ a lemon

1. In a sauté pan over medium-high heat, fry the bacon until it begins to crisp. Drain excess fat; add sliced onions and cook until onions are softened, about 3–5 minutes.
2. Add vinegar and sugar. Cook for a few more minutes, until the sauce thickens a bit. Turn off heat.
3. Add nuts and oil. Adjust flavor with lemon juice, salt, and pepper.

Serve warm over grilled vegetables, salads, or seared chicken. Makes about 1 cup. Keeps about 4 days in the fridge.

PER SERVING (2 tbsp.)› Energy 92 cal • Fat 9 g • Sodium 80 mg • Carbs 1 g • Fiber 0 g • Protein 1 g

SERVINGS› 4
TIME› 5 minutes

Lemon and Honey Dressing

1 teaspoon minced jalapeno

2 tablespoons olive oil

2 tablespoons honey

juice of ½ a lemon

OPTIONAL ADDITIONS

1 tablespoon chopped herbs (parsley, chives, tarragon)

juice of ½ an orange

1. Whisk together all ingredients in a small bowl. Add salt to taste.

Makes about ½ cup.

This is my everyday dressing. The sweet citrus flavor will taste familiar because it's used in a lot of our dishes. ★

PER SERVING (2 tbsp.)› Energy 92 cal • Fat 7 g • Sodium 70 mg • Carbs 9 g • Fiber 0 g • Protein 0 g

FLAVORS

SERVINGS› 6
TIME› 5 minutes

Orange Maple Vinaigrette

¼ cup olive oil

1 tablespoon chopped fresh tarragon or parsely

1 small clove garlic

¼ cup white or apple cider vinegar

¼ cup maple syrup

1 tablespoon orange marmalade

1 teaspoon vanilla extract

1. Combine oil, tarragon, and garlic in a blender or food processor. While motor is running at low speed, drizzle in the vinegar. Add maple syrup, marmalade, and vanilla extract; blend. Add salt and pepper to taste.

Serve with fish or chicken. Makes about ¾ cup.

PER SERVING (2 tbsp.)› Energy 122 cal • Fat 9 g • Sodium 98 mg • Carbs 65 g • Fiber 0 g • Protein 0 g

SERVINGS› 8
TIME› 5 minutes

★ See photo, page 239.

Chocolate and Balsamic Vinegar

1 cup balsamic vinegar

¼ cup sugar

2 tablespoons Mexican hot chocolate mix, such as Abuela brand

1 teaspoon ground cayenne pepper

1. Bring vinegar and sugar to a gentle boil in a small pot. Stir in chocolate mix and cayenne; remove from heat. Adjust flavor with salt, sugar, or more chocolate depending on the strength of your balsamic vinegar.

Serve warm or chilled with chicken or pork. Makes about 1 cup.

PER SERVING (2 tbsp.)› Energy 33 cal • Fat 1 g • Sodium 1 mg • Carbs 7 g • Fiber 0 g • Protein 0 g

SERVINGS› 48
TIME› 5 minutes

Taco Spice

1 cup chili powder

3 tablespoons coarsely ground black pepper

3 tablespoons coarse salt

2 tablespoons ground cumin

OPTIONAL ADDITIONS

1 tablespoon garlic powder

2 tablespoons onion powder

1 tablespoon brown sugar

2 tablespoons mild paprika

2 tablespoons dried oregano

1. Combine all ingredients (including any optional additions) and store in a tightly sealed container.

Makes about 1½–2 cups.

Use this spice mix wherever taco seasoning is called for in this book. Adjust the heat to your liking. ★

PER SERVING (½ tbsp.)› Energy 0 cal • Fat 0 g • Sodium 436 mg • Carbs 0 g • Fiber 0 g • Protein 0 g

SERVINGS› 56
TIME› 5 minutes

Spice Rub

1 cup brown sugar

½ cup kosher salt

1 tablespoon celery salt

2 tablespoons coarsely ground black pepper

OPTIONAL ADDITIONS

dried ground sage, rosemary, and/or thyme

ground cardamom, cinnamon, and/or nutmeg

ground cayenne pepper

ground mustard

peppercorns

red pepper flakes

1. Thoroughly combine all ingredients. Keep in ziplock bag or airtight container. Use generously as a dry rub on meat prior to cooking.

Makes about 1¾–2 cups.

Our photographer friend Lucas Gilman perfected this spice rub after years of experimenting. Our simplified version will work with most any meat. Adjust flavors as you like. ★

PER SERVING (½ tbsp.)› Energy 0 cal • Fat 0 g • Sodium 25 mg • Carbs 3 g • Fiber 0 g • Protein 0 g

APPENDIXES

APPENDIX A>

Nutrition for Additions and Alternatives

CARBS	ENERGY (cal)	FAT (g)	SODIUM (mg)	CARBS (g)	FIBER (g)	PROTEIN (g)
BREADS & GRAINS						
Bread, gluten-free> *1 slice*	110	2	230	22	0	1
Bread, rustic> *1 slice*	150	2	332	28	2	5
Bread, whole wheat> *1 slice*	69	1	132	12	2	4
Couscous> *1 cup cooked*	176	0	8	36	2	6
Millet> *1 cup cooked*	207	2	3	41	2	6
Pita> *1 whole*	165	1	322	33	1	5
Polenta> *1 cup cooked*	170	8	302	24	3	3
Quinoa> *1 cup cooked*	185	5	146	30	3	7
Tortilla, corn> *1 whole*	40	1	0	9	1	1
Tortilla, whole wheat> *1 whole*	110	3	320	18	3	5
PASTA> *1 cup cooked*						
Angel hair	221	1	1	42	3	8
Egg noodles	213	2	11	40	2	8
Elbow pasta	221	1	1	43	3	8
Gluten-free	205	1	4	46	4	4
Orzo	200	1	0	42	2	7
Whole wheat	174	1	4	37	6	7
RICE> *1 cup cooked*						
Brown	218	2	2	46	4	5
White	242	0	0	53	0	5

FRUITS	ENERGY (cal)	FAT (g)	SODIUM (mg)	CARBS (g)	FIBER (g)	PROTEIN (g)
BERRIES> *½ cup*						
Blackberries	31	1	1	7	6	1
Blueberries	42	0	1	11	2	1
Raspberries	32	1	1	8	4	1
Strawberries	25	0	1	6	2	1
DRIED FRUIT> *½ cup*						
Cranberries	185	2	2	50	3	0
Currants	204	0	6	54	5	3

FRUITS *(continued)*	ENERGY *(cal)*	FAT *(g)*	SODIUM *(mg)*	CARBS *(g)*	FIBER *(g)*	PROTEIN *(g)*
Dates	20	0	0	5	1	0
Figs	220	0	0	52	10	2
Goji berries	197	0	242	41	2	6
Raisins	247	1	9	66	3	3
WHOLE FRUIT> *1 piece*						
Apple	29	0	1	8	2	0
Banana	67	0	1	17	2	1
Kiwi	56	0	3	13	3	1
Lemon	22	0	3	12	5	1
Lime	20	0	1	7	2	0
Mango	135	1	4	35	4	1
Orange	62	0	0	15	3	1
Peach	51	0	0	12	2	1
Pineapple> *½ cup*	37	0	1	10	0	1

VEGETABLES	ENERGY *(cal)*	FAT *(g)*	SODIUM *(mg)*	CARBS *(g)*	FIBER *(g)*	PROTEIN *(g)*
Asparagus> *½ cup*	13	0	1	3	1	1
Beets> *½ cup*	37	0	176	9	2	1
Bell pepper> *½ cup*	15	0	2	4	2	1
Broccoli> *½ cup*	16	0	15	3	1	2
Butternut squash> *½ cup*	47	0	3	12	0	2
Cabbage> *½ cup*	9	0	7	2	1	1
Carrot> *1 piece*	25	0	42	6	2	1
Celery> *½ cup*	8	0	41	2	1	1
Cucumber> *½ cup*	8	0	1	2	1	1
Green chile> *1 piece*	15	0	856	4	1	1
Jalapeno> *½ cup*	14	1	1	3	2	1
Kale> *½ cup*	17	0	15	4	1	1
Mushrooms> *½ cup*	11	0	3	2	1	1
Onion> *½ cup*	32	0	3	8	2	1
Parsnips> *½ cup*	50	0	7	12	4	1
Peas> *½ cup*	59	0	4	10	4	4
Potato> *1 piece*	149	0	13	34	4	4
Radish> *½ cup*	10	0	23	2	1	1
Spinach> *½ cup*	4	0	12	1	1	1
Sun-dried tomatoes> *½ cup*	70	1	566	15	4	4
Sweet corn> *½ cup*	66	1	12	15	2	2
Sweet potatoes> *½ cup*	57	0	37	14	2	1
Tomatoes> *½ cup*	22	0	13	5	1	1
Turnips> *½ cup*	26	0	19	6	3	1

PROTEIN

PROTEIN	ENERGY (cal)	FAT (g)	SODIUM (mg)	CARBS (g)	FIBER (g)	PROTEIN (g)
BEANS> *1 cup cooked*						
Adzuki	294	0	18	57	17	17
Garbanzo beans	269	4	11	45	13	15
Red kidney	225	1	4	40	13	15
White	249	1	11	45	11	17
EGGS> *1 egg*						
Fried	90	7	94	0	0	6
Hard-boiled	78	5	62	1	0	6
Poached	71	5	147	0	0	6
Scrambled	102	7	171	1	0	7
MEATS						
Bacon, cooked> *2 oz.*	84	6	384	0	0	6
Chicken, roasted> *1 cup*	214	6	71	0	0	38
Ham, shaved> *2 oz.*	100	6	744	2	0	10
Salmon, canned> *3 oz.*	118	5	64	0	0	17
Sausage> *2 oz.*	155	13	410	2	1	8
Tuna, canned> *3 oz.*	99	1	287	0	0	22
NUT BUTTERS> *2 tbsp.*						
Almond butter	202	18	144	6	2	4
Nutella	200	10	20	23	2	3
Peanut butter	188	16	147	6	2	8
NUTS & SEEDS						
Almonds, raw> *10 pieces*	69	6	0	3	2	3
Cashews> *1 oz.*	157	12	3	9	1	5
Pecans> *½ cup*	377	39	0	8	6	5
Pine nuts> *½ cup*	455	46	2	9	3	9
Sesame seeds> *½ cup*	413	36	8	17	9	13
Walnuts> *½ cup*	386	37	1	6	5	15

DAIRY

DAIRY	ENERGY (cal)	FAT (g)	SODIUM (mg)	CARBS (g)	FIBER (g)	PROTEIN (g)
CHEESE> *1 oz.*						
Cheddar	113	9	174	0	0	7
Feta	75	6	316	1	0	4
Fontina	109	9	224	0	0	7
Goat	103	8	146	1	0	6
Monterey jack	104	8	150	0	0	7
Mozzarella	72	5	175	1	0	7
Parmesan	111	7	454	1	0	10
Swiss	106	8	54	2	0	8

DAIRY *(continued)*	ENERGY *(cal)*	FAT *(g)*	SODIUM *(mg)*	CARBS *(g)*	FIBER *(g)*	PROTEIN *(g)*
CREAM CHEESE & YOGURT						
Cream cheese, low-fat> *1 tbsp.*	30	2	70	1	0	1
Yogurt, Greek, nonfat> *8 fl. oz.*	133	0	87	9	0	24
Yogurt, plain, low-fat> *8 fl. oz.*	154	4	172	17	0	13
MILK> *½ cup*						
1%	51	1	54	6	0	4
2%	61	3	50	6	0	4
Almond	20	2	90	1	0	1
Rice	40	2	85	6	0	1
Skim	43	0	64	6	0	4
Soy	50	1	45	9	1	2
Whole	73	4	49	6	0	4

FLAVORS	ENERGY *(cal)*	FAT *(g)*	SODIUM *(mg)*	CARBS *(g)*	FIBER *(g)*	PROTEIN *(g)*
OILS & VINEGARS> *1 tbsp.*						
Balsamic vinegar	20	0	0	5	0	0
Butter	102	12	82	0	0	0
Oils: canola, grapeseed, olive, truffle	120	14	0	0	0	0
Vinegars: apple cider, red wine	0	0	0	0	0	0
SALTY> *2 tbsp.*						
Capers	4	0	510	0	0	0
Liquid amino acids	0	0	1,800	0	0	0
Olives	80	8	480	2	0	0
Soy sauce, low-sodium	16	0	1,066	2	0	2
SPICY> *2 tbsp.*						
Hot sauce/Sriracha sauce	0	0	180	0	0	0
Salsa, prepared	9	0	192	2	1	0
SUGARY> *2 tbsp.*						
Agave nectar	120	0	0	32	0	0
Applesauce	42	0	2	11	1	0
Brown sugar	209	0	16	54	0	0
Chocolate chips, semi-sweet	56	3	0	8	0	0
Honey	128	0	2	34	0	0
Jam	112	0	12	28	0	0
Maple syrup	104	0	4	26	0	0
Molasses	116	0	14	30	0	0

APPENDIX B>

Conversions

COOKED AND READY INGREDIENTS

If your recipe calls for cooked ingredients and you don't have them on hand, use the charts below to determine the uncooked quantities so you can prepare the ingredients for the recipe. Conversions are approximate and can vary depending on different varieties or brands.

These conversions are meant to be helpful, but try not to overthink specific measurements. Most cooked and ready ingredients are carbohydrates, so measurements can be adjusted according to the demands of your training, or more simply, how hungry you are.

INGREDIENT	UNCOOKED	COOKED
BEANS		
Beans	1 cup	2–2½ cups
GRAINS		
Couscous	1 cup	2 cups
Millett	1 cup	3½ cups
Oats	1 cup	2½ cups
Polenta	1 cup	4 cups
Quinoa	1 cup	4 cups
MEAT		
Bacon	8 oz.	¾–1 cup
Chicken	8 oz.	1 cup
PASTA		
Angel hair	8 oz.	4½ cups
Egg noodles	8 oz.	5 cups
Elbow	8 oz.	4 cups
Farfalle	8 oz.	5 cups
Fettuccine	8 oz.	3 cups
Fusilli	8 oz.	3 cups
Orzo	8 oz.	3 cups
Penne	8 oz.	3½ cups

INGREDIENT	UNCOOKED	COOKED
RICE		
Brown	1 cup	3 cups
Long grain> *basmati*	1 cup	3 cups
Medium grain> *jasmine*	1 cup	2½–3 cups
Short-grain> *calrose/sushi*	1 cup	2 cups
VEGETABLES		
Beets	8 oz.	1½ cups
Potatoes> *cubed, diced, or mashed*	8 oz.	1 cup
Potatoes> *sliced*	8 oz.	1¼ cups
Sweet potatoes	8 oz.	1 cup

VOLUME

U.S. STANDARD		
3 tsp.	↔	1 tbsp.
4 tbsp.	↔	¼ cup
8 tbsp.	↔	½ cup
16 tbsp.	↔	1 cup

IMPERIAL		
1 tbsp.	↔	½ fl. oz.
1 cup	↔	8 fl. oz.
1 cup	↔	½ pint
2 cups	↔	1 pint
4 cups	↔	1 quart
2 pints	↔	1 quart
4 quarts	↔	1 gallon

METRIC		
1 tsp.	↔	5 ml
1 tbsp.	↔	15 ml
¼ cup	↔	60 ml
½ cup	↔	125 ml
¾ cup	↔	175 ml
1 cup	↔	250 ml
1 pint	↔	480 ml
1 quart	↔	1 liter

WEIGHTS

METRIC		
1 oz.	↔	30 grams
2 oz.	↔	60 grams
4 oz.	↔	115 grams
8 oz.	↔	225 grams
1 pound	↔	450 grams
2 pounds	↔	900 grams

NOTE› Conversions have been rounded to make measuring easier.

APPENDIX C>

Shopping List

FRUITS

- ○ Apples
- ○ Bananas
- ○ Berries
- ○ Dried fruit
- ○ Lemons/Limes
- ○ Peaches
- ○ ____________
- ○ ____________
- ○ ____________

VEGETABLES

- ○ Beets
- ○ Broccoli
- ○ Carrots
- ○ Garlic
- ○ Greens, bitter
- ○ Greens, salad mix
- ○ Onions
- ○ Peppers
- ○ Potatoes/ Sweet potatoes
- ○ Spinach
- ○ Squash
- ○ Tomatoes
- ○ ____________
- ○ ____________
- ○ ____________

FRESH HERBS

- ○ Basil
- ○ Cilantro
- ○ Mint
- ○ Parsley
- ○ Thyme
- ○ ____________
- ○ ____________
- ○ ____________

PASTA, RICE & GRAINS

- ○ Couscous
- ○ Oatmeal
- ○ Pasta/Gluten-free
- ○ Quinoa
- ○ Rice
- ○ ____________
- ○ ____________
- ○ ____________

MEAT & FISH

- ○ Bacon
- ○ Beef/Bison/Steak
- ○ Chicken
- ○ Fish
- ○ Sausage
- ○ Turkey
- ○ ____________
- ○ ____________
- ○ ____________

BREADS

- ○ Gluten-free
- ○ Pitas
- ○ Rustic
- ○ Tortillas
- ○ Whole wheat
- ○ ____________
- ○ ____________
- ○ ____________

DAIRY

- ○ Butter
- ○ Cheese
- ○ Eggs
- ○ Milk
- ○ Yogurt
- ○ ____________
- ○ ____________
- ○ ____________

CANNED GOODS

- Beans
- Stock
- Tomato sauce
- Tuna/Salmon
- ______________
- ______________
- ______________

BAKING

- Baking powder
- Chocolate chips
- Flour
- Sugar
- ______________
- ______________
- ______________

SPICES

- Chile powder
- Cinnamon
- Curry powder
- Nutmeg
- Pepper
- Sea salt
- ______________
- ______________
- ______________

CONDIMENTS

- Honey
- Hot sauce
- Jam
- Maple syrup
- Nut butter
- Salsa
- ______________
- ______________
- ______________

SAUCES & OILS

- Olive oil
- Soy sauce/ Liquid aminos
- Vinegar
- ______________
- ______________
- ______________

FOOD STORAGE

- Aluminum foil
- Freezer bags
- Paper foil
- Plastic wrap
- ______________
- ______________
- ______________

FROZEN FOODS

- Vegetables
- Waffles
- ______________
- ______________
- ______________

Index

NOTE› Page numbers in italics refer to illustrations.

Acknowledgments

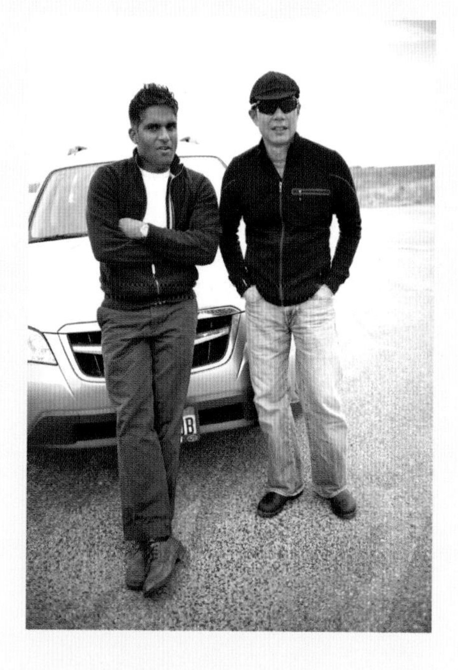

FIRST AND FOREMOST, I'd like to thank Allen Lim for bringing me along on this ride; Renee Jardine, Kara Mannix, and Ted Costantino at VeloPress for their saintly patience and support through the process; and Caroline Treadway, Megan Forbes, Vicki Hopewell, and Jeanine Thurston for their vision and many long hours.

Research help came from Courtney Thompson, Gus Flottman, and Lucas Euser. Production help—cooking, tasting, fine-tuning recipes, washing loads of dishes—came from Chef James Mazzio, Meagan McCorkle, and Kirsten Wedde.

Special thanks to Michelle and Corrina at Prana Apartments for letting us take over the building during our long photo shoot days. I'd also like to thank Mike Kaeske and Rusty and Deborah Perry for their kitchens and a special thanks to Gloria Borglum and Alex E'Aton for all of the years and countless meals.

Finally, a great big thanks to Robin at MapMyRide, Levi Leipheimer and Team RadioShack, and the athletes, friends, and family who have endured many strange meals and ideas, a small portion of which is here.

BIJU THOMAS

IF IT WERE NOT FOR the unconditional support and amazing food fed to me by my parents, the seeds for this book would not have been planted. Culture is more than what your mom fed you. It's the culmination of any meal or any recipe shared with others and it is the joy that we experienced cooking and eating with those closest to us. With that in mind, I'd like to thank those whom I have shared most of my meals with: my parents, George and Margarita, my brother Almerick, all of my cousins, aunts, uncles, friends, and athletes who took the time to cook me a meal or took a chance eating one of mine.

This book, however, would never have actually been written if it were not for the incredible work of Renee Jardine and her talented crew at VeloPress that included Kara Mannix and Ted Costantino. Because Renee's head did not literally explode while coaxing us to meet deadlines and while forcing us to actually sit down somewhere in this world and write, this book exists.

A huge thanks to Megan Forbes for all of her work on the nutritionals and for always being an invaluable sounding board when I needed someone to help me solve the most complex nutritional dilemmas.

I'd also like to give a special thanks to Dr. William Byrnes, my mentor at the University of Colorado at Boulder. Whenever I would come up with a crazy theory, Dr. Byrnes was the first to shake his head at me and challenge me with one line, "Young man, you don't know that." It was his critical eye and extraordinary care that provided me with the foundation for my career in professional cycling and it's been that single line that has checked me as a simple voice of reason ever since graduating.

Of course my untold thanks and immense respect to Chef Biju Thomas for never saying no to hitting the road to cook with me in the worst possible conditions with the least possible sleep for nothing more than our sheer love for food and cycling.

ALLEN LIM

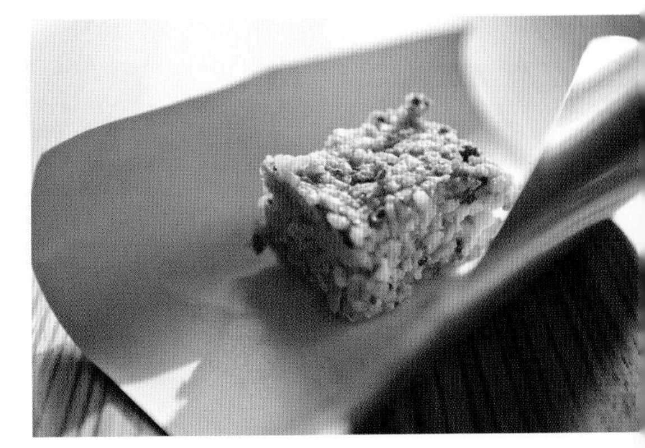

About the Authors

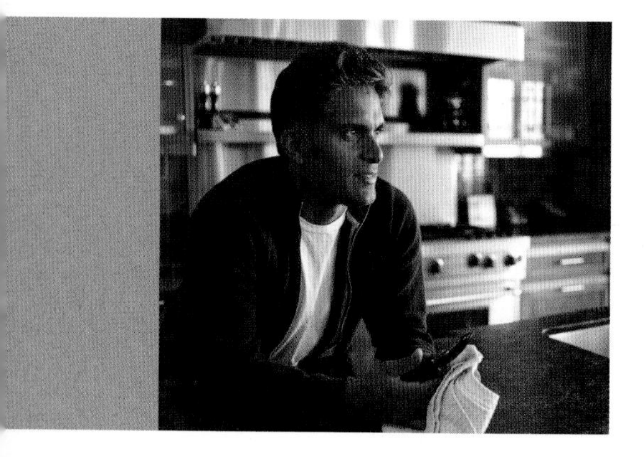

BORN IN SOUTH INDIA, BIJU THOMAS first came to the United States at the age of three. Part of a large extended family, including five siblings and several cousins, he learned to love food by watching his mother and grandmother cook for and feed large groups with ease. The entire family found joy and comaraderie in cooking, constantly upstaging one another in the kitchen.

A self-taught chef, Biju soon discovered he had a deep passion for cooking. He began working in restaurants at age 15, moving quickly to the top of his field as an in-demand chef in Colorado, and then finally as an instructor and consultant to the industry, writing menus and helping to start restaurants around the country.

However, he had another great passion—cycling. Growing up in Colorado in the 1980s meant that he was surrounded by many of the greats of American cycling, including the 7-Eleven team and a generation of young cyclists who went on to define the sport.

In an attempt to marry his two greatest passions, Biju began to work with various cycling- and sports-related fund-raisers and events. This led him to Andy Hampsten, then to Jonathan Vaughters and an early Garmin pro cycling team, where he befriended Allen Lim.

Through those relationships, Biju has cooked and shared his love of food with many top cyclists, including Lance Armstrong; Levi Leipheimer; Tommy Danielson; Christian Vande Velde; and a new generation of riders, including Ben King and Matt Busche.

Biju contributes to MapMyRide and to other online media and various magazines while doing TV spots and heading up workshops and classes—all the while doing his best to remain a skinny chef on the roads around Boulder, Colorado.

"I WISH BIJU HAD COOKED FOR ME ALL THOSE YEARS I RACED BECAUSE IT WOULD HAVE MADE ME FASTER."

—Axel Merckx, former pro cyclist, Olympic medalist, and Belgian national champion

BORN IN THE PHILIPPINES, DR. ALLEN LIM began watching and helping his parents (who are originally from China) cook in the kitchen at the age of four—the same age that he taught himself to ride a bicycle. By age eight, Lim's affinity for food and cycling was in full bloom. He began spending hours on his dirt bike roaming the streets just outside of Los Angeles and teaching his parents classic Western recipes, like the Denver omelet, picked up at sleepover parties with his American friends.

This merging of cultures eventually led Lim to search for ways to turn his love for cycling and food into a legitimate career—a search that culminated with Lim earning his doctorate in 2004 in the Department of Integrative Physiology at CU Boulder. Having worked almost exclusively with pro cycling teams since 2004, Dr. Lim was the director of sport science for the RadioShack pro cycling team for the 2010 and 2011 seasons and formerly held the same title for the Garmin pro cycling team. He has the unique distinction of being the only American scientist to have worked and cooked at the Tour de France, guiding countless riders, including Floyd Landis and Lance Armstrong—controversial and inspiring winners of cycling's most prestigious race.

Through these experiences, Lim has come to know firsthand the complexity of sport—an arena where ambition, emotion, and culture can both fuel and oppose the practice of science, innovation, and fair play. These dichotomies have led Lim to look for ways to redefine his love for cycling and food as a legitimate tool for social change—a conversation he is eager to discuss on a ride or at the dinner table.

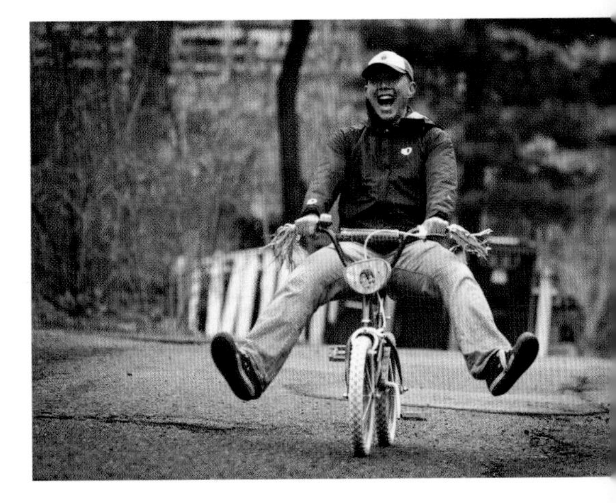

"SOME OF LIM'S FOODS ARE SCIENTIFIC AND OTHERS JUST FEEL GOOD, BUT ONE INGREDIENT WAS ALWAYS PRESENT: PASSION FROM THE ASIAN EQUATION."

—Christian Vande Velde, Team Garmin-Cervélo

★

Cover design by **Katie Jennings**

Cover, recipe photos, and photos on pages vi (left), vii (right), 17, and 23 by **Jeanine Thurston, Fototails Photography**

Photo shoot location> **Prana Apartments**, Lafayette, CO

Art direction, design, and composition by **Vicki Hopewell**

Photos on pages v, vi–vii (spread), ix, 1–2, 4–6, 9, 11, 19, 22, 24, 27, 84–85, and 312–314 by **Caroline Treadway**

Photo on page xi by **Casey B. Gibson**

Photo on page 15 by **Graham Watson**

Photo on page 315 by **Jamie Kripke**

Nutrition facts by **Megan Forbes, RD, Forbes Nutritional Consulting**